Topics in Integrative Neuroscience

Neuroscience is progressing so rapidly that even expressions such as "by leaps and bounds" fail to capture the pace of its growth. Questions that once were thought to be unanswerable – perhaps even unaskable – have now been both asked and answered, and new questions, once unthinkable, are routine. *Topics in Integrative Neuroscience* has singled out four of the most important problems in neuroscience: higher order perception; language; memory systems; and sensory processes. The volume presents original contributions by many of the leading researchers in those fields, and with an initial chapter covering neuroethics. It is impossible to capture fully the sweep of discoveries that emerged from the "Decade of the Brain" within the covers of a single volume. It is possible, however, to provide a sample, both in recognition of what has been accomplished and as a harbinger of what is surely to come.

JAMES R. POMERANTZ is Professor of Psychology at Rice University and Adjunct Professor of Neuroscience at Baylor College of Medicine. He is currently President of the Foundation for the Advancement of Behavioral and Brain Sciences in Washington DC.

Topics in Integrative Neuroscience

From Cells to Cognition

Edited by
JAMES R. POMERANTZ
Rice University

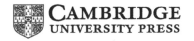

CAMBRIDGE
UNIVERSITY PRESS

CAMBRIDGE UNIVERSITY PRESS
Cambridge, New York, Melbourne, Madrid, Cape Town, Singapore,
São Paulo, Delhi, Dubai, Tokyo, Mexico City

Cambridge University Press
The Edinburgh Building, Cambridge CB2 8RU, UK

Published in the United States of America by Cambridge University Press, New York

www.cambridge.org
Information on this title: www.cambridge.org/9780521143400

First published 2008
First paperback printing 2010

A catalogue record for this publication is available from the British Library

Library of Congress Cataloguing in Publication data
Topics in integrative neuroscience: from cells to cognition / James R. Pomerantz, editor.
   p. ; cm.
Includes bibliographical references and index.
ISBN-13: 978-0-521-86913-3 (hardback : alk. paper)
1. Higher nervous activity.   2. Perception.   3. Language and languages.
4. Memory.   I. Pomerantz, James R.
[DNLM: 1. Higher Nervous Activity – physiology.   2. Auditory Perception – Physiology.
3. Language.   4. Memory – physiology.   WL 102 T674 2007]
QP395. T67   2008
612.8–dc22   2007016477

ISBN 978-0-521-86913-3 Hardback
ISBN 978-0-521-14340-0 Paperback

Additional resources for this publication at www.cambridge.org/9780521143400

Contents

List of contributors

Hong Bao
Section of Neurobiology, College of Natural Sciences
The University of Texas at Austin
Austin, TX 78712

Elizabeth P. Bauer
W. M. Keck Foundation Laboratory of Neurobiology
Center for Neural Science
6 Washington Place, Room 276
New York University
New York, NY 10003

Hugh T. Blair
Department of Psycology
University of California
1285 Franz Hall
Box 951563
Los Angeles, CA 90095-1563

Charlotte A. Boettiger
Department of Psychology
University of California
3210 Tolman Hall #1650
Berkeley, CA 94720-1650

Patricia S. Churchland
Professor, Department of Philosophy
University of California, San Diego
La Jolia, CA 92093-0119

Peter De Weerd
Laboratory of Perception & Actions
Department of Psychology (Room 518)
University of Arizona
1503 E. University Blvd.
PO Box 210068
Tucson, AZ 85721

Allison J. Doupe
University of California
UCSF, 513 Parnassus (HSE-818)
Box 0444
San Francisco, CA 94143-0444

Ruth Anne Eatock
Eaton-Peabody Laboratory
Department of Otology and Laryngology
Harvard Medical School
Boston, MA 02114

Howard B. Eichenbaum
Director, Cognitive Neurobiology Laboratory
Director, Center for Memory and Brain
University Professor and Chairman, Department of Psychology
Boston University
Center for Memory and Brain
2 Cummington Street
Boston, MA 02215

Jin Fan
Department of Psychiatry
Icahn Medical Institute
1425 Madison Avenue, Room 20-82
Mount Sinai School of Medicine
One Gustave L. Levy
Place, Box 1228
New York, NY 10029

Charles Gilbert
Professor, Neurobiology
Laboratory of Neurobiology
The Rockefeller University
1230 York Avenue
New York, NY 10021

Naida L. Graham
MRC Cognition & Brain Science Unit
15 Chaucer Road
Cambridge CB2 2EF, UK

Martin Hackl
Department of Linguistics and Cognitive Science
Pomona College
Mason Hall 211B
550 Harvard Ave – 110B Mason Hall
Claremont, CA 91711

Neal A. Hessler
Keck Center for Integrative Neuroscience
Department of Physiology
Box 0444
University of California
San Francisco, CA 94143-0444

John R. Hodges
MRC Cognition & Brain Sciences Unit
University of Cambridge
15 Chaucer Road
Cambridge
CB2 2EF
UK

Karen M. Hurley
Department of Clinical Studies at New Bolton Center
School of Veterinary Medicine
382 West Street Road
Kennett Square, PA 19348

Sabine Kastner
Department of Psychology
Center for the Study of Brain, Mind & Behavior
Princeton University
Green Hall (3-N-1E)
Princeton, NJ 08544-1010

Matthew A. Lambon Ralph
The University of Manchester
Oxford Road
Manchester
M13 9PL
UK

Joseph E. LeDoux
University Professor
Professor of Neural Science and Psychology
Center for Neural Science
New York University
4 Washington Place, Room 809
New York, NY 10003

Jacques Mehler
Director, Language, Cognition and Development Lab
International School of Advanced Studies
SISSA/ISAS CNS (ORO, rm 13)
Via Beirut 4
34014 Trieste
Italy

Karim Nader
Department of Psychology
McGill University, Canada
Stewart Biological Sciences Building
Room N8/8, 398-3511
1205 Dr Penfield Avenue
Montreal, Quebec, H3A 1B1

Kazu Nakazawa
National Institute of Mental Health
Genetics of Cognition and Behavior Unit, NIMH
Porter Neuroscience Research Center
Building 34, Room IC-915
35 Convent Drive, MSC 3710
Bethesda, MD 20892-3710

Marina Nespor
University of Milan Bicocca
Psychology Department
Edificio U6 Piazza dell' Ateneo Nuovo,
1-20126 Milano

Helen J. Neville
Director, Brain Development Lab
Professor, Psychology and Neuroscience
University of Oregon
Eugene, Oregon 97403-1227

Karalyn Patterson
Senior Scientist, MRC Cognition and Brain Science Unit
University of Cambridge
15 Chaucer Road,
Cambridge CB2 2EF, UK

Marcela Peña
Cognitive Neuroscience Sector
SISSA/ISAS
Via Beirut 4
34014 Trieste
Italy

David Poeppel
Professor, Department of Linguistics
Cognitive and Neuroscience Language Lab
University of Maryland
1401 Marie Mount Hall
College Park, MD 20742

James R. Pomerantz
Professor/Director of Neuroscience
Psychology Department (MS-25)
Rice University
6100 Main Street
PO Box 1892
Houston, TX 77005-1892
Office: 429 A Sewall Hall

Michael I. Posner
Professor Emeritus
Psychology Department
University of Oregon
Eugene, Oregon 97403 1227

Seth J. Ramus
Department of Psychology and Program in Neuroscience
Bowdoin College
Brunswick, ME 04011

Sarina M. Rodrigues
W. M. Keck Foundation Laboratory of Neurobiology
Center for Neural Science
New York University
New York, New York 10003

Lisa D. Sanders
Department of Psychology
University of Massachusetts at Amherst
Tobin Hall, 135 Hicks Way
Amherst, MA 01003

Glenn E. Schafe
Department of Psychology and Interdisciplinary Neuroscience Program
Yale University
2 Hillhouse Avenue
New Haven, Connecticut 06511-6814

Michele M. Solis
5733 26th Ave NE
Seattle, WA 98105

Larry R. Squire
Professor of Psychiatry, Neurosciences, and Psychology
University of California
3350 La Jolla Village Drive
San Diego, CA 92161

Craig E. L. Stark
Assistant Professor
Department of Psychological and Brain Sciences
The Johns Hopkins University
204 Ames Hall
3400 N. Charles Street
Baltimore, MD 21218

Susumu Tonegawa
Director, Picower Center for Learning and Memory
Massachusetts Institute of Technology
77 Massachusetts Avenue
Building E17, Room 353
Cambridge, MA 01239-4307

Leslie G. Ungerleider
Chief, Laboratory of Brain and Cognition
National Institute of Mental Health
Building 10, Room 4C104
10 Center Drive, MSC 1148
Bethesda, MD 20892-1366

Christine M. Weber-Fox
Speech, Language, and Hearing Sciences
Purdue University
West Lafayette, IN 47907

Matthew A. Wilson
Center for Learning and Memory
RIKEN-MIT Neuroscience Research Center
Department of Brain & Cognitive Science and Biology
Massachusetts Institute of Technology (46-5233)
77 Massachusetts Avenue
Cambridge, MA 02139-4307

Julian R. A. Wooltorton
Department of Clinical Studies at New Bolton Center
School of Veterinary Medicine
382 West Street Road
Kennett Square, PA 19348

Preface

The field of neuroscience is progressing so rapidly that even expressions such as "by leaps and bounds" fail to capture the pace of its growth. Questions that at one time were thought to be unanswerable – perhaps even unaskable – have now been asked and in some cases answered, and new questions once unthinkable are now asked matter-of-factly. Much of this acceleration is due to the maturing of the field – advances in techniques as well as in theory – fueled by an infusion of research support during the 1990s "Decade of the Brain" effort.

It is impossible to capture fully the sweep of discoveries and advances that emerged from that decade within the covers of a single volume. It is possible, however, to provide a sample of the best of that work, both as recognition of what has been accomplished during that period of time and since, and as a harbinger of what is surely to come as the pace of neuroscience shows no hint of slowing down.

Our goal in the present volume is to provide that sample through carefully chosen topics and even more carefully chosen researchers in those fields. Singling out the four most important problems in neuroscience is probably an unwise goal and is a surefire way to start an argument. That said, however, few would argue that the four featured here are anything less than powerful candidates for that inner circle: higher order perception; language; memory systems; and sensory processes.

Within these four categories, even fewer would contest the preeminence of the research programs carried out by the authors of this volume's chapters. In Higher Order Perception, we have Michael Posner leading a group including both Charles Gilbert and Leslie Ungerleider and her colleagues. In Language we see Helen Neville leading a distinguished international team of scholars including David Poeppel, Karalyn Patterson, Jacques Mehler, and their co-workers.

Our part on Memory Systems is led by Larry Squire and includes Howard Eichenbaum, Joseph E. LeDoux, Susumu Tonegawa, and their co-authors. Finally, a part on Sensory Processes includes chapters by Allison J. Doupe, Ruth Anne Eatock, and their colleagues.

As a special treat, we have an additional chapter, not part of these four parts, dealing with the intersection of neuroscience and philosophy. This chapter is written by Patricia Churchland and deals with changing conceptions of choice and responsibility as we better understand the neural processes underlying human behavior.

No effort of this magnitude takes place without a great deal of effort, stemming first and most importantly from those neuroscientists and other scholars who have conducted the work described here and who have written about it for this volume. We are grateful to them, their co-authors, and for the many students and other collaborators who helped them along the way.

Our second round of thanks goes out to C. M. and Demaris Hudspeth of Houston Texas, whose generosity and support made this volume possible. The inspiration and impetus for this book lies with a De Lange Conference held in March 2001 on the campus of Rice University, entitled "The Neurobiology of Perception and Communication: From Synapse to Society." This book is based to a considerable extent on updated, written versions of presentations first given on that occasion. The De Lange Conference series is made possible by an endowment established at Rice University by the Hudspeths in memory of the parents of Demaris, Albert, and Demaris De Lange. These conferences are held every few years and have the flexibility to range broadly in subject matter and discipline. All are intended to bring to the Rice University campus top experts and major figures to focus on a topic of great concern to society. Rice University owes a great debt to Hank and Demaris Hudspeth, two alumni whose contributions to this institution have been so great and who are a source of both pride and admiration for all who are fortunate enough to know them and work with them.

Our third round of thanks goes to the two institutions that provided additional support, both financial and human, that this effort possible: Rice University and its neighbor across Main St., Baylor College of Medicine. Our partnership in this and other ventures is a source of great satisfaction to both institutions and multiplies the contributions we can make both locally and globally. The steering committee behind this effort included, on the Baylor side, Michael C. Crair, Kathryn J. Kotrla, James W. Patrick, and J. David Sweatt. The Rice side included Don Johnson, Randi Martin, and James Pomerantz. Additional valuable support was provided by Rice University's outstanding Glasscock School of Continuing Studies and their fine group of staff.

On the Rice side in particular, our largest rounds of applause are reserved first for Kathleen Minadeo Johnson, who served as the De Lange Conference Coordinator, handling the myriad duties that go along with a major, multi-institutional event. Kathleen handled all her assignments with a combination of efficiency, grace, and good cheer and kept the morale high even during times when by all rights it should have been low. Great thanks and gratitude go as well to Ellen Butler, who since has taken over as the permanent Executive Assistant for the De Lange Conferences and who has done much of the organizational work needed to convert the set of manuscripts from which we began into a complete draft volume to present to the Cambridge University Press. Picking up on a complex task that another person has begun is rarely easy, and it is a testament to the skill and patience of both of these individuals that the final result is as good as it is. I give my great personal thanks to both, not only for their hard work but also for their friendship.

Finally, we thank the editors and staff at Cambridge University Press for their efforts in publishing this volume and their patience in dealing with setbacks experienced along the way. We especially thank Martin Griffiths (Commissioning Editor) and Jeanette Alfoldi (Production Editor), at Cambridge for their careful work and attention.

As progress in neuroscience continues at its blistering pace, it will not be long before another decade of the brain is in order. Perhaps when that time arises, we will produce another De Lange Conference and published volume summarizing where we have come. In the meantime, please read and enjoy the chapters that follow and appreciate the advances that these pioneers in the field have worked so hard to achieve.

Overview of neuroscience, choice and responsibility

JAMES R. POMERANTZ

Neuroethics overview

The reach of neuroscience is unusually broad. As the title of this book indicates, our present interest in neuroscience extends all the way from cells to cognition – from how neurons operate at the microscopic level to how people think, speak, perceive, and remember at the macroscopic level. Given that the brain is the most complex structure in the known universe, this breathtaking breadth may come as no surprise and makes it understandable why neuroscience is of compelling interest to engineers, physicians, computer scientists, and even to musicians.

The reach of our concerns is so great that it engages even philosophers, including those grappling with the most difficult – perhaps intractable – questions of them all, those touching on the question of human choice and free will. In this special chapter with which we lead off this book, the noted philosopher Patricia Churchland takes on the challenge of reconciling the seemingly deterministic neurological system underlying human choice behavior, the common belief in free will, and the question of who, if anyone, is responsible for the behavior of human beings. When people commit crimes or other ethical breeches, may they rightfully claim that "their neurons made them do it"? Or, is there lurking within their nervous systems an accountable agent that must take responsibility for decisions made?

Topics in Integrative Neuroscience: From Cells to Cognition, ed. James R. Pomerantz. Published by Cambridge University Press. © Cambridge University Press 2008.

Neuroscience, choice and responsibility

PATRICIA S. CHURCHLAND

1.1   Introduction

Much of human social life depends on the notion that agents have control over their actions and are responsible for their choices. In daily life it is commonly assumed that it is fair to punish and reward behavior so long as the person is in control and makes choices knowingly and intentionally. Without the assumptions of agent control and responsibility, human social commerce is hardly conceivable. As members of a social species, we recognize co-operation, loyalty, honesty, and helping as prominent features of the social environment. We react with hostility when group members disappoint certain socially significant expectations. Inflicting disutilities (e.g., shunning, pinching) on the socially erring and rewarding civic virtue help restore the standards.

In other social species too, social unreliability, such as a failure to reciprocate grooming or food-sharing, provokes a reaction likely to cost the erring agent, sooner or later. In social mammals at least, mechanisms for learning and keeping the social order seem to be part of what evolution has bequeathed to our brain circuitry. Given that the stability of the social-expectation baseline is sufficiently important for survival, individuals are prepared to incur some cost in enforcing those expectations. Just as anubis baboons learn that tasty scorpions are to be found under rocks but cannot just be picked up, so they learn that failure to reciprocate grooming when it is duly expected may incur a slap.

In social species, parents invest heavily not only in the production, feeding, and protection of the young, but also in their socialization. The young of the social species must learn how to navigate the physical world, but their survival and flourishing also depends on their acquiring appropriate habits to navigate the social world. In both cases, the reward system plays a crucial role, enabling the brain to improve its predictions about what will satisfy, and what will bring pain.

Topics in Integrative Neuroscience: From Cells to Cognition, ed. James R. Pomerantz. Published by Cambridge University Press. © Cambridge University Press 2008.

If the reward and punishment system is to be effectively engaged in shaping social behavior, the actions for which the agent is rewarded or punished must be under the agent's control; that is, reward and punishment should make some difference to the agent's future predictions of an action's consequences and hence of his behavior. What does it mean, for us to have control over our behavior? Are we ever *really* responsible for our choices and decisions? Will neuroscientific understanding of the neuronal mechanisms for decision-making change how we think about these fundamental features of social commerce? These are the places where issues about free will bump up against practical reality of negotiating of what is fair, what is reasonable, and what is effective.

1.2   Are we in control if our choices and actions are *caused*?

One tradition bases the conditions for free will and control on a contrast between being *caused* to do something and *not* being so caused. For example, if someone falls on me and I hit you, then my hitting you was caused by the falling body; I did not choose to hit you. I am not, therefore, responsible for hitting you. Were you to punish me for hitting you, it would not help me avoid such events in the future. Examples emanating from this prototype have been extended to the broader idea that in order for *any* choice to be free, it must be absolutely *uncaused*; that is, it is suggested that a free choice is made when, without any prior cause and constraints, a decision comes into being and an action results. An example allegedly illustrating this idea is Eisenhower's decision to send troops into Little Rock to enforce school desegregation. Or my decision to go to the coffee shop for a cappuccino. This *contracausal* construal of free choice is known as "libertarianism."[1] Is it plausible? That is, are the paradigm cases of free choices actually *uncaused* choices?

As Hume proposed in 1739,[2] the answer is *no*. Hume argued that our choices and decisions are in fact caused by other events in the mind – desires, beliefs, preferences, feelings, and so forth. Thus Eisenhower's decision was the outcome of his beliefs about the situation, and his desire to ensure that the federal school integration law was not flaunted. His decision did not suddenly and without preceding beliefs, thoughts, hopes, and worries spring uncaused into existence. I went to get a cappuccino because I usually have one about this time in the afternoon, I wanted to have one, and I knew I had enough money to pay for it, and so on. Save for these causal antecedents, albeit *cognitive* causal antecedents, I would not have gone for coffee. By contrast, suppose that without any antecedent causes, I suddenly enter a saloon, ask for a glass of vodka, and swig it back. I had no antecedent desire for vodka, no habit of going to a saloon anytime, let alone in the afternoon, and the behavior would be considered utterly at odds with my cognitive state and temperament. Is *this* the paradigm of free choice? Is *this* prototypically responsible behavior?

Reflecting on these sorts of possibilities, Hume made the deeper and more penetrating observation that an agent's choices are not considered freely made *unless* they are caused by his desires, intentions, and so forth. Randomness, pure chance, and utter unpredictability are not preconditions for attribution of responsible choice. Hume puts the issue with memorable compactness: "Where [actions] proceed not from some cause in the characters and disposition of the person, who perform'd them, they infix not themselves upon him, and can neither redound to his honor if good, nor infamy, if evil."[3]

Logic reveals, Hume argued, that responsible choice is actually *inconsistent* with libertarianism (uncaused choice). Someone may choose to climb onto his roof because he does not want the rain to come into his house, he wants to fix the loose shingles that allowed the rain in, and he believes that he needs to get up on the roof to do that. His desires, intentions, and beliefs are part of the causal antecedents resulting in his choice, though he may not be introspectively aware of them *as* causes. If, without any determining desires and beliefs, he simply went up onto the roof – as it were, *for no reason* – his sanity and hence his control is seriously in doubt.

More generally, a choice undetermined by anything the agent believes, intends, or desires is the kind of thing we consider *out* of the agent's control, and is not the sort of thing for which we hold someone responsible. Furthermore, desires or beliefs that are uncaused (assuming that is physically possible) rather than caused by other stable features of the person's character and temperament are likewise useless in producing the conditions for responsible choice. If a powerful desire with no antecedent connection to my other desires or my general character were to spring into my mind – say, the serious desire to become a seamstress – I would suspect that someone must be "messing with my mind." The brain presumably has no mechanism for introspectively recognizing a desire to fix the roof *as* a cause, just as it has no way of detecting through introspection that growth hormone has been released or that blood pressure is at 110/85. A cause, nevertheless, a desire most certainly is.

Neither Hume's argument that choices are internally caused nor his argument showing that libertarianism is absurd have ever been convincingly refuted. Notice, moreover, that his arguments hold regardless of whether the mind is a separate *Cartesian substance*, or a pattern of activity of the physical brain. And they hold regardless of whether the etiologically relevant states are conscious or unconscious.

In fact, the brain does indeed appear to be a causal machine. So far, there is no evidence at all that events at the neuronal or network or systems levels happen without any cause. True enough, neuroscience is still in its early stages, and we cannot absolutely rule out the possibility that evidence will be forthcoming at some later stage. Given the data, however, the odds are against it. Importantly, even were uncaused neuronal events to be discovered, it is a *further* and substantial matter to show that precisely *those* neural events constitute free choice. They might, for all we can tell now, have to do with features of growth hormone release or variations in the sleep–wake cycle.

Nonetheless, the idea that randomness in the physical world is somehow the key to what makes free choice *free* remains appealing to those inclined to believe that free choice must be uncaused choice. With the advent of quantum mechanics and the respectability of the idea of quantum indeterminacy (i.e. the physical description of a state is necessarily incomplete), the suggestion that somehow or other quantum-level indeterminacy is the basis for a "solution" to the problem of free will remains attractive to some libertarians.[4] Stripped to essentials, the hypothesis claims that although an agent may have the relevant desires, beliefs, etc., he still can make a choice that is truly independent of all antecedent causal conditions. On this view, the agent, not the agent's brain or his desires or his emotions, freely chooses between cappuccino and latte, for example. It is at the moment of deciding that the indeterminacy or the non-causality or the break in the causal nexus – whatever one wants to call it – occurs. The subsequent choice is therefore absolutely free.

This is meant to be an empirical hypothesis and, as such, it needs to confront neurobiologically informed questions. For example, what exactly, in neural terms, is the *agent who chooses*? How does that fit with what we understand about self and self-representational capacities in the brain? Under exactly what conditions do the supposed noncaused events occur? Does noncausal choice exist only when I am dithering or agonizing between two equally good – or perhaps equally bad – alternatives? What about when, in full conversation, I use the word "very" rather than the word "extremely"? Does it exist with respect to the *generation* of desires? Why not? There are also questions from quantum physics such as these: What is the mechanism of amplification of the non-deterministic events? Were quantum effects of the envisioned kind to exist in the brain, how could they fail to be swamped by thermal indeterminacy?

These are just the first snowballs in an avalanche of empirically informed questions. Part of their effect is to unmask the flagrantly ad hoc character of the hypothesis; that is, it is based more on a desire to prop up a wobbling ideology than on factual matters. Rather than fully discussing its merits and flaws now, however, we shall defer a closer analysis of the hypothesis of a quantum-level origin for uncaused choice until further details of the neurobiology of decision-making are on the table. That will allow us to see what bearing the neurobiological data have on the question of causality and choice in the brain, and hence provide a richer context for evaluating the hypothesis of noncausal choice. Therefore, we return to this hypothesis and its critics in Section 1.6 to see how it fares.

Provisionally, therefore, let us adopt the competing hypothesis, namely that Hume is essentially right, and all choices and all behavior *are* caused, one way or another. The absolutely critical point, however, is that not all causes are equal before the tribunal of responsibility: some are such as to excuse us from culpability; others precisely render us culpable. The important question concerns the relevant differences among causes of behavior such that some kinds play a role in free choice and others play a role in forced choice; that is: Are there systematic *brain-based* differences between voluntary and involuntary actions that will support the notion of agent responsibility? This is the crucial question, because we do hold people responsible for what we take to be *their* actions. When those actions are intentionally harmful to others, punishment, varying from social disapproval to execution, may be visited upon the agent. When, if ever, is it fair to hold an agent responsible? When, if ever, is punishment justified?

Many possibilities have been explored to explain how the notions of control and responsibility can make sense in the context of causation. These fall under the general rubric, "Compatibilism," meaning that our work-a-day notion of responsibility is, at bottom, *compatible* with the probable truth that the mind-brain is a causal machine. First we shall consider some obvious but unsuccessful attempts, and then we shall raise the possibility that increased understanding of the brain will aid in piecing together a plausible account.[5]

1.3   Caused choice and free choice: some traditional hypotheses

1.3.1   *Voluntary causes are* internal *causes*

Can we rely on this rule: you are responsible if the causes are internal, otherwise not? No, for several reasons. A patient with Huntington's disease makes nonpurposeful, jerky movements as a result of internal causes. But we do not hold the Huntington's patient responsible for his movements, since they are the outcome of a disease that causes destruction in the striatum. He has no control over his movements, and they are not consistent with his actual desires and intentions, which he cannot execute. A sleepwalker may unplug the phone or kick the dog. Here too the causes are internal, but the sleepwalker is not straightforwardly responsible. In a rather attenuated sense, the sleepwalker may *intend* his movements, though he is apparently unaware of his intentions.

1.3.2   *Voluntary causes are* internal, *they involve the agent's intentions,*
      and *the agent must be aware of the intention*

This strategy also fails. A patient with obsessive-compulsive disorder (OCD) may have an overwhelming urge to wash her hands. She wants and intends to wash her hands, and she is fully aware of her desire and her intention. She knows that the desire is her desire; she knows that it is she who is washing her hands. Nevertheless, in patients with OCD, obsessive behavior such as hand-washing or footstep-counting is considered to be out of the agent's control. They often indicate that they wish to be rid of hand-washing or footstep-counting behavior, but cannot stop. Pharmacological interventions, such as Prozac, may enable the subject to have what we would all regard as normal choice about whether or not to wash her hands.

1.3.3   *Voluntary causes* feel *different from the inside*

Another strategy is to base the distinction on *felt* differences in inner experience between those actions we choose to do and those over which we feel we have no control. Thus it allegedly feels different when we evince a cry as a startle response to a mouse leaping out of the compost heap, and when we cry out to get someone's attention and help. Is introspection a reliable guide to responsibility? Can introspection – attentive, careful, knowledgeable introspection – distinguish those internal causes for which we are responsible from those for which we are not? (See also Crick 1994.)

Probably not. There are undoubtedly many cases where introspection is no guide at all. Phobic patients, the OCD patients just mentioned, and those with Tourette's syndrome are obvious examples that muddy the waters. In a patient with claustrophobia, the desire not to go into a cave feels as much *his* as his desire not to go rafting without a life jacket. He can even give reasons for both – it could be unsafe, avoidable injuries could happen, etc. His desire not to go into a cave may be very very strong, but so may be his desire to eat when hungry or sleep with his wife. So mere *strength* of desire will not suffice to distinguish actions for which the agent has undiminished responsibility and those for which he is not fully responsible.

The various kinds of addictions present a further range of difficulties. A smoker feels that the desire for a cigarette is indeed *his*. His reaching for a cigarette may feel every bit as free as reaching to turn on the television or scratching his nose. He might wish it were not his, but so far as the *feeling* itself is concerned, it is as much his as his desire to quit smoking. The increase in intensity of sexual interest and desire at puberty is surely the result of hormonal changes on the brain, not something over which one has much control. Yet all of that interest, inclination, and alteration of behavior *feels* – from the inside at any rate – entirely free.

More problematic, perhaps, are the many examples from everyday life where one may suppose the decision was entirely one's own, only to discover that subtle manipulation of desires by others had in fact been the decisive factor.

According to the fashion standards of the day, one finds certain clothes beautiful, others frumpy, and the choice of wardrobe seems, introspectively, as free as any choice. There is no escaping, however, the fact that what is in fashion has a huge effect on what we find beautiful, and this affects not only choice in clothes, but also such things as aesthetic judgment regarding plumpness or slenderness of the female body. Baseball hats worn backward have been in fashion for about ten years and are considered to look good, but from another perspective, most people look less attractive if wearing a backward baseball cap.

Social psychologists have produced dozens of examples that further muddy the waters, but a simple one will convey the point. On a table in a shopping mall, experimenters placed ten pairs of identical panty hose, and asked shoppers to select a pair, and then briefly explain their choice. Choosers referred to color, denier, sheerness, and so forth as their rationale. In fact, there was a huge position effect: shoppers tended to pick the panty hose in the rightmost position on the table. None of them considered this to be a factor, none of them referred to it as a basis for choice, yet it clearly was so. The ten pairs of panty hose were, after all, identical to one another. Other examples of priming, subliminal perception, and emotional manipulation also suggest that an appeal to introspection to solve our problem, about which behavior is in our control and which is not, is unlikely to go very far.[6]

1.3.4   Could have done otherwise

In a different attack on the problem, philosophers have explored the idea that if the choice were free, the agent *could have chosen otherwise*; that is, in some sense, the agent had the power to do something else.[7] Certainly this idea does comport with conventional expectations about voluntary behavior, and insofar as it is appealing. Lyndon Johnson, historians say, could have done otherwise regarding Vietnam. He could have decided to stop the war in Vietnam in 1965 when he correctly judged it to be unwinnable. I could have decided not to get coffee, and perhaps to have water instead. Nobody *forced* me or coerced me; the desire for coffee was mine. So far so good. The weakness in the strategy shows up when we ask further, "what exactly does *that* mean?" If all behavior has antecedent causes, then "could have done otherwise" seems to boil down to "would have done otherwise if antecedent conditions had been different." Accepting that equivalence means the criterion is too *weak* to distinguish between the shouted insults of a Touretter, whose utterances include such random and undirected outbursts as "idiot, idiot, idiot," and those of a member of parliament responding to an honorable member's proposal, "idiot, idiot, idiot." In both cases, had the antecedent conditions been different, obviously the results would have been different. Nevertheless, we hold the parliamentarian responsible, but not the Touretter. So the proposed criterion seems not so much wrong, as unhelpful in revealing the nature of the difference between the causes of voluntary behavior and the causes of *non*voluntary behavior.

The further problem here is a lurking circularity. Testing for whether an agent could have done otherwise seems exactly the same as testing whether the behavior was voluntary. Hence specifying what counts as voluntary behavior by referring to the possibility that the agent might have done otherwise just goes around in a small circle. It does not seem to get us anywhere.

1.4   Prototypes and responsibility

In our legal as well as our daily practice, the pattern is to accept certain prototypical conditions as excusing a person from responsibility, but to assume him responsible unless a definite exculpatory condition obtains. In other words, responsibility is the default condition; excuse from and mitigation of responsibility has to be positively established. The set of conditions regarded as exculpatory can be modified as we learn more about behavior and its etiology. A different but related issue concerns what to do with someone who harms others but has diminished responsibility.

Aristotle (384–322 BC) in his great work, *The Nicomachean Ethics*, was the first to articulate the responsible-unless-exculpating-reasons principle. The wisdom of the principle is still reflected in much of human practice, including current legal practice. In his systematic and profoundly sensible way, Aristotle pointed out that for an agent to be held responsible, it is a necessary condition (but not a sufficient condition) that the cause be internal to the agent. In addition, he characterized as involuntary, actions produced by coercion and actions produced in certain kinds of ignorance. As Aristotle well knew, however, no simple rule demarcates cases here. Clearly, some ignorance is not considered excusable, when it may be fairly judged that the agent *should* have known. Additionally, in some cases of coercion, the agent is expected to resist the pressure, given the nature of the situation. A captured soldier is supposed to resist giving information to the enemy. As Aristotle illustrates in his own discussion of such complexities, we seem to proceed to deal with these cases by judging their similarity to uncontroversial and well-worn prototypes, which is perhaps why precedent law is so useful.[8]

Increasingly, it seems unlikely that there is a *sharp* distinction – brain-based or otherwise – between the voluntary and the involuntary – between being in control and being out of control – either in terms of behavioral conditions or in terms of the underlying neurobiology. This does not imply that there is *no* distinction, but only that whatever the distinction, it is not sharp; that is, it is not like the distinction between having a valid California driver's license and *not* having one. It is rather more like categories with a prototype structure, for example being a good sled dog, being a navigable river, being a fertile valley. These sorts of categories are useful even though we cannot specify necessary and sufficient conditions for membership in the category. We teach the category by citing prototypical instances, along with contrasting prototypical *non*instances.

Once we consider *being in control* in this light, we instantly recognize the degrees and nuances typical of freedom of choice. An agent's decision to change television channels may be more unconstrained than his decision to pay for his child's college tuition, which may be more unconstrained than his decision to marry his wife, which may be more unconstrained than his decision to turn off the alarm clock. Some desires or fears may be very powerful, others less so, and we may have more self-control in some circumstances than in others. Prolonged sleep deprivation makes it extremely hard to stay awake, even when the need to do so is great. Hormonal changes, for example in puberty, make certain behavior patterns highly likely, and in general, the neurochemical milieu has a powerful effect on the strength of desires, urges, drives, and feelings.

These considerations motivate thinking of control as coming in degrees, and hence as falling along a spectrum of possibilities. Toward opposite ends of the self-control spectrum are prototypical cases that contrast sufficiently in behavioral and internal features to provide a foundation for a basic, if somewhat rough-hewn, fuzzy-bordered distinction between being in control and not, between being responsible and not. In fact, as we consider various points on the spectrum, it seems likely that there are in fact *many* parameters relevant to being in control. Consequently, we should upgrade the simple one-dimensional notion of a *spectrum* to a multi-dimensional *parameter space*, where the dimensions of the parameter space reflect the primary determinants of in-control behavior.

In our current state of knowledge, we do not know how to specify all those parameters, nor how to weigh their significance. Nor are the relations between the parameters likely to be linear. We can, nevertheless, make a start. We do know now that activity patterns in certain brain structures, including the anterior cingulate cortex, hypothalamus, insula, and ventromedial frontal cortex are important. For example, large bilateral lesions to anterior cingulate abolish voluntary movement.[9] One fortunate patient recovered some voluntary function. She also had good memories of her symptomatic period, during which, she explained "nothing mattered" and that she "had nothing to say."[10] Smaller lesions to the anterior cingulate are associated with severe depression and anxiety[11] (Figure 1.1).

Functional subdivisions of the cingulate cortex

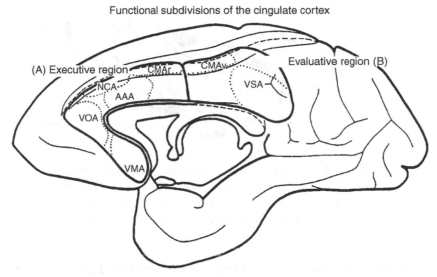

Figure 1.1 Functional division of the cingulate cortex of the rhesus monkey brain. The executive region (A) and the evaluative region (B) are the two major divisions. Subdivisions in (A): visceromotor (VMA); vocalization (VOA); nociceptive (pain) (NCA); rostral cingulate motor (CMAr); and attention to action (AAA). Subdivisions in (B) ventral cingulate motor (CMAv) and visuospatial (VSA) (based on Vogt, Finch, & Olson, 1992).

If the middle area of the cingulate is where the lesion occurs, patients may show loss of voluntary control over a hand. In *alien hand syndrome*, as this deficit is called, the hand behaves as though it has a will of its own. To the consternation of the patient, the hand may grab cookies, or behave in socially inappropriate ways. One patient discovered he could regain some control over his misbehaving alien hand if he yelled at it, "stop that!"

Imaging data implicate the anterior cingulate gyrus in the exercise of self-control over sexual arousal. In a functional magnetic imaging resonance (fMRI) study, male subjects were first exposed to erotic pictures, and then were asked to inhibit their feelings of sexual arousal. Comparisons between the two conditions show that when subjects are responding normally to erotic pictures, limbic areas show increased activation. When subjects engage in inhibition of sexual arousal, this activation disappears, and the right anterior cingulate gyrus and the superior frontal gyrus become more highly activated.[12]

The anterior cingulate again emerges as a player in autism. One undisputed finding is that autistics have deficits in analyzing affective signals. Because limbic structure play a central role in affect, a leading hypothesis claims the primary basis in autism to reside in defective affective evaluation, resulting from structural abnormalities in the limbic system.[13] This hypothesis has been

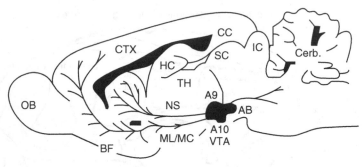

Figure 1.2 The central dopamine pathways, a crucial part of the reward system.
The pathways originate in the brainstem, in the substantia nigra (NS) and the ventral
tegmental area (VTA). The latter projection is very broad, and reaches areas cortically and
subcortically, including the basal forebrain (BF), orbitofrontal cortex (OB), and amygdala.

tested by comparing the microstructure of normal and autistic brains. Using
whole-brain serial sections, the brains of nine deceased autistic subjects were
examined. The only cortical structure to show abnormalities was the anterior
cingulate gyrus, where the cells were smaller and the packing density greater.
There were similar abnormalities in limbic subcortical structures including the
hypothalamus, amygdala, and mammillary bodies. Abnormalities in the cerebellum were also seen.[14]

Additionally, it is known that levels of neuromodulators such as serotonin
and dopamine; neurotransmitters such as norepinephrine and acetylcholine; as
well as various hormones such as estrogen and testosterone are highly pertinent
parameters in the well-tuned decision-making neural organization. For example, obsessive-compulsive pathologies and depressive pathologies involving loss
of motivation can be greatly modified by up-regulated serotonin levels
(Figure 1.2). It is also known that subjects with Klinefelter's syndrome (that is,
with XXY chromosomes) have poor long-term judgment and impulse control,
even when they are cognitively capable. Yet the judgmental capacities of
Klinefelter's subjects improve markedly when they are given constant administration of testosterone through a skin patch. Tourette's syndrome is much
more controlled when patients are given serotonin agonists; the subjects just do
not feel the same desire to engage in their customary *ticcing* behavior. Since the
anterior cingulate has been implicated in voluntary behavior, it is noteworthy
that both the dopamine projections and the norepinephrine projections can
influence the processing of the anterior cingulate, and thus have an influence
on executive and attentional functions.[15]

Appetite is a particularly promising parameter to consider in discovering the
brain-based differences between being and not being *in control*. Gluttony is,

allegedly, one of the seven deadly sins; overeating, we are repeatedly reminded, can be controlled by sheer will power. The discovery of the role of the protein leptin in eating, and particular in overeating, has provoked reconsideration of just how much freedom of choice to push back from the table the very obese actually have, and whether leptin-related interventions will give them greater control.[16]

Leptin is a hormone released by fat cells. It acts on neurons in the hypothalamus that regulate feelings of hunger and satisfaction. Experiments on normal mice show that when the mouse has had an adequate meal, the leptin levels *increase*, and the mice leave the food for other pleasures. Some mice are different. They are obese, and they continue to eat even when their leptin levels rise. Genetic analysis shows that the receptor to which leptin binds can have a variety of mutations, and that the specific mutation predicts how overweight the animal is. For example, if the mouse has the *tu* mutation it is somewhat tubby, relative to normals, and has *twice the leptin levels of normals*; if it has *db* mutation, is truly obese, and has ten times the leptin levels. There is something *very* different about the appetite regulation of the mutant animals.

If one is born with the *db* mutation of the leptin-receptor gene, and if, in consequence, one feels as ravenous at the end of dinner as at the beginning, it seems inevitable that one will overeat. More precisely, it seems reasonable to assume that such a person will have less control over his eating behavior than a person with the standard version of the leptin-receptor. He may have perfectly normal self-control when it comes to other matters, such as sex, alcohol, or gambling, but for food, his situation is markedly different because his leptin-receptors in the hypothalamus are markedly different. The suggestion, therefore, is that the leptin-receptor and its possible variations constitute yet another component in the complex neurobiological profile of "in control" subjects, at least where food is concerned.

Many neural details remain to be uncovered, needless to say, but identifying the major neurochemical players is a profoundly important beginning. Beginnings such as these inspire the vision that ultimately neuroscience might be able specify a range of optimal values for the relevant parameters, such that behavior falling within that range is behavior we consider in the control of the agent. A contrasting range that is clearly suboptimal, where the behavior is considered out of the agent's control, will then be mirror-specifiable. In between, there may be gray areas where control is neither clearly normal nor clearly abnormal.[17]

Research from basic neuroscience as well as from lesions studies and scan studies will be needed to transform this speculative parameter space into a substantial, detailed, testable account of the features of the landscape that are typical of "in control" subjects. These properties may be quite abstract, for "in control" individuals may have different temperaments and different cognitive strategies.[18] As Aristotle put it, there are different ways to harmonize the soul.

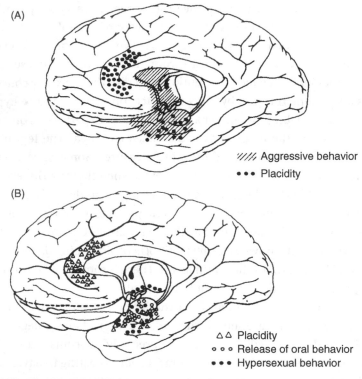

(A)

/// Aggressive behavior
• • • Placidity

(B)

△ △ Placidity
○ ○ ○ Release of oral behavior
• • • Hypersexual behavior

Figure 1.3   Localized lesions in limbic structures lead to specific behavioral changes. (A) Lesions resulting in increases in aggressive behavior and in placidity. (B) Lesions resulting in a release of oral behavior and in hypersexuality (from Poeck, 1969).

Nevertheless, the prediction is that, at the very least, some such general features probably are specifiable. It is relatively easy to see that dynamical-systems properties do distinguish between brains that perform well or poorly in certain tasks such as walking. What I am proposing here is that more abstract skills, characterizable behaviorally, such as being a successful shepherd dog or a competent lead sled dog can also be specified in terms of dynamical-systems properties, dependent as they are on neural networks and neurochemical concentrations. My hunch is that human skills in planning, preparing, and co-operating can likewise be specified. Not now, not next year, but in the fullness of time as neuroscience and experimental psychology develop and flourish (Figure 1.3).

In the next sections, we shall consider in more detail some of the evidence that speaks in favor of this general approach.

1.5   Learning self-control

Aristotle would have us add here the point that there is an important relation between self-control and habit formation. A substantial part of learning

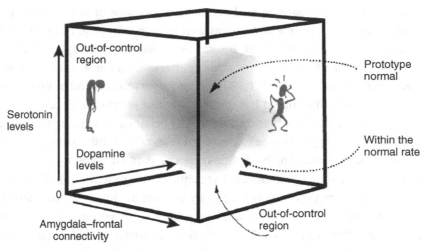

Figure 1.4 A cartoon sketch to illustrate the concept of an in-control parameter space. Although there are undoubtedly many more than three dimensions, for simplicity the cartoon depicts only three – serotonin levels, dopamine levels, and amygdala–frontal connectivity. The boundary between the "in-control" volume and the "no-in-control" volume is depicted as fuzzy, thus conveying the idea that the boundary between these capacities is not sharp but fuzzy. The cartoon should show, but cannot, that there are nonlinear interactions between the parameters.

to cope with the world, defer gratification, show anger and compassion appropriately, to have courage when necessary, involves acquiring appropriate *decision-making habits*. In the metaphor of dynamical systems, this is interpreted as contouring the terrain of the neuronal state space so that behaviorally appropriate trajectories are "well-grooved" or strongly attractive. Clearly, we have much to learn about what this consists of, both at the behavioral and at the neuronal level. We do know, however, that if an infant has damage in some of the critical regions, such as the ventromedial frontal cortex or amygdala, then typical acquisition of the proper "Aristotelian" contours may be next to impossible, and more direct intervention may sometimes be necessary to achieve what normal children routinely achieve as they grow up (Figure 1.4).

The characterization of a choice or an action as *rational* carries a strongly normative component; insofar it is not sheerly descriptive, in contrast, for example, to describing the action as performed hurriedly or with a hammer. Claiming an action as rational often carries the implication that the choice was conducive in some significant way to the agent's interests or well-being or to those of kith and kin; that it properly took into account the consequences of the action, both long and short term; thus the evaluative component. Though a brief dictionary definition can capture some salient aspects of what it means to be rational and reasonable, it hardly does justice to the real complexity of the concept.

As children, we learn to evaluate actions as more or less rational by being exposed to prototypical examples, as well as to prototypical examples of foolish or unwise or irrational actions. Insofar as we learn by example, learning about rationality is like learning to recognize patterns in general, whether it be recognizing what is a dog, what is food, or when a person is afraid or embarrassed or weary. As Paul Churchland has argued, we also learn ethical concepts such as "fair" and "unfair," "kind" and "unkind," by being shown prototypical cases, and slowly learning to generalize to novel but relevantly similar situations.[19]

Peer and parental feedback fine-tune the pattern recognition networks so that over time they come closely to resemble the standard upheld in the wider community. Nevertheless, as Socrates was fond of showing, articulating those standards is awesomely difficult, even when a person successfully uses the expression "rational," case by case. Discriminating the reasonable from the unreasonable may be a skill, like discriminating whether the river is now navigable by canoe, or whether and how attacking an enemy's position will succeed. With the benefit of hindsight, we can see how Scott's skill in conducting his Antarctic exploration was pitiful, while Amundsen's was superb. Making "rational" precise in a way that fulfills the conditions for an algorithm is almost certainly impossible. The failure to program computers to conform even roughly to common sense, or to understand what is relevant, is an indication of the nonalgorithmic, *skill-based* nature of rationality.

This is important, because most philosophers regard the evaluative dimension of ethical concepts to imply that their epistemology must be entirely different from that of descriptive concepts. What appears to be special about learning some concepts, such as "rational," "impractical" and "fair," is that the basic wiring for feeling the appropriate emotion must be intact. That is, the prototypical situation of something's being impractical or shortsighted typically arouses unpleasant feelings of dismay and concern; the prospect of something's being dangerous arouses feelings of fear, and these feelings, along with perceptual features, are probably an integral part of what is learned in perceptual pattern recognition.

Frankly dangerous situations – crossing a busy street, encountering a grizzly with cubs – can likely be learned as dangerous without the relevant feelings. At least that is suggested by the evidence based on patient S who, as a result of amygdala destruction, has no feelings of fear. Although she can identify which *simple* situations are dangerous, this seems for her to be a purely cognitive, nonaffective judgment. Where her recognition is poor, however, is when she needs to detect the menace or hostility or pathology in complex social or marketing situations, where no simple formula for identifying danger is available. As suggested earlier, the appropriate feelings may be necessary for skilled application of a concept, if not for fairly routine applications. This is perhaps why the fictional Mr. Spock, lacking emotions as he is, is plausibly poor at predicting what will provoke strong sympathy or dread or embarrassment in humans.

Stories, time-honored as well as those passing as local gossip, provide a basic core of scenarios where children imagine and feel, if vicariously, the results of various choices such as failing to prepare for future hard times (*The Ant and The Grasshopper*) or failing to heed warnings (*The Boy Who Cried Wolf*), of being conned by a smooth talker (*Jack and the Beanstalk*), of vanity in appearance (*Narcissus*). As children, we can vividly feel and imagine the foolishness of trying to please everybody (*The Old Man and His Donkey*), of not caring to please anybody (Scrooge in Dickens' *A Christmas Carol*), and of pleasing the "wrong" people (the prodigal son). Many of the great and lasting stories, for example by Shakespeare, Ibsen, Tolstoy, Aristophanes, are rife with moral ambiguity, reflecting the fact that real life is rife with conflicting feelings and emotions, and that simple foolishness is far easier to avoid than great tragedy.

Buridan's dithering ass was just silly;[20] Hamlet's ambivalence and hesitation was deeply tragic and all too understandable. In the great stories is also a reminder that our choices are always made amidst a deep and unavoidable ignorance of many of the details of the future, where coping with that very uncertainty is something about which one can be more or less wise. For all decisions save the trivial ones, there is no algorithm for making a wise choice. For matters such as choosing a career or a mate, having children or not, moving to a certain place or not, deciding the guilt or innocence of a person on trial, deciding whether to surrender or press on, and so on, these are usually complex constraint satisfaction problems.

As we deliberate about a choice, we are guided by our reflection on past deeds, our recollection of pertinent stories, and our imagining the sequence of effects that would be brought about by choosing one option or another. Antonio Damasio calls the feelings generated in the imagining–deliberating context "secondary emotions" to indicate that they are a response not to external stimuli, but to internally generated representations and recollections.[21] As we learn and grow up, we come to associate certain feelings with certain types of situation, and this combination can be reactivated when a similar set of conditions arises. Often a moral dilemma cannot easily be labeled, and instead we draw analogies between types of dilemmas: "this is like the time my father got lost in the blizzard and built a quinze"; "this is like the time Clarence Darrow defended a teacher's right to teach evolutionary biology," and so on. Recognition of a present situation as relevantly like a certain past case has of course a cognitive dimension, but it also evokes feelings that are similar to those evoked by the past case, and this is important in aiding the cortical network to relax into a solution concerning what to do next.

1.6   Uncaused choice considered again

Much of this chapter has focused on the emerging account of the neurobiology of decision-making. The hypothesis on offer is that there are systematic neurobiological differences between being *in control* and being *out of control*, and that these differences can be characterized in terms of fuzzy-bordered subvolumes of the multi-dimensional parameter space. The "in control" subvolume of the space may be relatively large, allowing for the fact that in-control humans have different habits, cognitive styles, emotional tone, and so forth. Similarly, the "out of control" subvolume may be very large, reflecting the fact that dysfunction to the reward system may yield an out-of-control profile that is very different from that of a dysfunctional anterior cingulate cortex which in turn is different from that of a degenerating basal ganglia.

As noted in earlier (p. 5) there are spirited defenses of a totally different hypothesis, namely that decisions made by "in control" subjects are actually *uncaused* decisions, whereas decisions made by "out of control" subjects are *caused*. The most modern variation defends the idea that quantum indeterminacy is at the root, somehow, of uncaused choice. Though briefly introduced earlier, it is time now to reconsider the idea that real choice requires a break in causality milliseconds prior to the emergence of the brain state that constitutes the choice. An empirical hypothesis, it deserves to be weighed and evaluated as an empirical hypothesis and compared to the rather different picture of the brain discussed above.

Hume and his arguments aside, the credibility of the noncausal-choice hypothesis depends on whether it can mesh with what is known so far about neurons and nervous systems. Defenders of the hypothesis want it to be *consistent* with existing well-established neurobiological data, not openly clash with the data. The hypothesis is just that among the many details neuroscience has not yet discovered is this fact: for quantum mechanical reasons, voluntary choice is uncaused. Our task here is to ask whether, given what *is* well-established neurobiologically, this appears to be a plausible hypothesis with promising research prospects. As usual, we can begin by raising questions to which the hypothesis should have some noncontrived answers.

Why and how does a break in causality occur just for those particular brain events that supposedly are paradigm cases of choice? How does the brain work such that a simple behavior in conformity with good habit – routinely putting on my seat belt, for example – *is* caused, whereas choosing a latte rather than a cappuccino after dithering is *not* caused? What prevents the noncausal events from occurring when a nicotine addict reaches for another cigarette or a child sucks his thumb or a highly trained but off-duty spy surveys his fellow passengers for assassins? If, as is entirely likely, the brain events constituting choice are distributed across many neurons, how is the noncausality (quantum indeterminacy) orchestrated across the relevant population? If the brain events constituting choice are uncaused, then what precisely *are* their relations to background desires, beliefs, habits, emotions, and so forth? Philosophical fantasies floated in abstraction from the tough and detailed constraints of the real world have an in-a-single-bound-Jack-was-free quality. Flippant answers to empirically informed questions are of course always possible: "it just works like that" or "magic!" Unless the hypothesis can interdigitate with neurobiology and cognitive science, however, to come up with nonfrivolous answers to these questions, it will continue to look nakedly ad hoc.

Before the hypothesis can be taken seriously, it will have to garner some empirical confirmation and survive empirical tests. If uncaused choice is a quantum-level effect, as may be supposed, the aforementioned questions, as well as those raised on pp. 6–8, demand empirical answers: Under *exactly what conditions* do the supposed noncaused events occur? Does noncausal choice exist only when I am dithering or agonizing between two equally good – or perhaps equally bad – alternatives? How do quantum-level effects know (so to speak) when to occur and when not? Beyond the business of *decisions*, do quantum-level indeterminacies exist with respect to such processes as the generation of *desires*? Or *beliefs*? Why not? How is it they come into play with only some conscious decisions but not others? Does this break in causality occur at the synapse? If advocates of the noncaused decision-making are serious, they will have to do more than wave the flag of quantum-level indeterminacy and claim that in a single bound the choice is free. They will have to get into the business of empirical confirmation.

1.7   What happens to the concept of responsibility?

We need now to return to the dominant background question motivating this chapter: If choices and decisions are caused, is anyone ever really responsible for his actions? One very general conclusion is provoked by the foregoing discussion. "Responsible" is not a property like weighing 40 pounds or absorbing light at 640 nm. Rather, it has a cultural dimension, reflecting the assumptions regarding the social role of punishment and reward. On the whole, it seems to be assumed, social groups work best when individuals are presumed to be responsible agents. Consequently, as a matter of practical life, it is probably wisest to hold mature agents responsible for their behavior and for their habits. That is, it is probably in everyone's interest if we match up assignment of responsibility with being in control, and adopt the default assumption that agents have control over their actions. Barring clear evidence that an agent's behavior was in the out-of-control subvolume of parameter space, in general, agents are liable to punishment and praise for their actions. This is of course a highly complex and subtle issue, but the basic idea is that *feeling* the social consequences of one choices is a critical part of socialization – of learning to be in the give-and-take of the group. It is part of acquiring the appropriate Aristotelean habits.[22] *Feeling* those consequences is necessary for contouring the parameter space landscape in the appropriate way, and that means *feeling* the approval and disapproval meted out.

A child must learn about the physical world by interacting with it and bearing the consequences of its actions, or by watching others engage the world, or by hearing about how others engage the world. Similarly, learning about the social world involves cognitive–affective learning, directly or indirectly, about the nature of the social consequences of a choice. This must of course be consistent with reasonably protecting the developing child, and with compassion, kindness, and understanding. In short, I do not want the simplicity of the general conclusion to mask the tremendous subtleties of child-rearing. Nevertheless, if the only known way for "social decency" circuitry to develop requires that the subject generate the relevant feelings pursuant to social pattern recognition, then the responsibility assumption may be preferable to any version of a thorough-going paternalist assumption.

This of course leaves it open that under special circumstances agents should be excused from responsibility or be granted diminished responsibility. In general, the law courts are struggling, case by case, to make reasonable judgments about what those circumstances are, and no simple rule really works. Neuropsychological data are clearly relevant here as, for example, in cases where the subjects' brains have lesions that impair impulse control and the capacity to evaluate consequences. Quite as obviously, however, the data do *not* show that no one is ever really responsible and that no one is really deserving of punishment or praise. Nor do they show that when life is hard, one is entitled to avoid responsibility. To most of us, the "Twinkie defense" seems a travesty of justice, but so does ignoring someone's massive lesion in the ventromedial frontal cortex.

Is direct intervention in the circuitry morally acceptable? This too is a hugely complex issue. My personal bias is twofold: First, that in general, at any level, be it ecosystem or immune system, intervening in biology always requires immense caution. When the target is the nervous system, then caution by another order of magnitude is wanted. Still, not taking action is still doing something, and *acts of omission can be every bit as consequential as acts of commission.*

Second, the movie, *Clockwork Orange*, typically conjured up by the very idea of direct intervention by the criminal law, probably had a greater impact on the collective amygdaloid structures than it deserves to have. Certainly some kinds of direct intervention are morally objectionable. So much is easy. But *all* kinds? Even pharmacological? Is it possible that some forms of nervous system intervention might be more humane than lifelong incarceration or death? I do not wish to propose specific guidelines to allow, or disallow, any form of direct intervention. Nevertheless, given what we now understand about the role of emotion in decision-making, perhaps the time has come to give direct interventions a calm and thorough reconsideration. Approaching these questions with a careful Aristotelian determination to be as wise as possible, may be preferable to giving free rein to unreflective self-righteousness. Ideological fervor, on the right or on the left, can often do greater harm than unhurried common sense.

Notes

Much of this chapter is drawn from Chapter 5 of my book, *Brain-Wise: Studies in Neurophilosophy* (2002).

1. See Campbell (1957), Kane (1996).
2. In his anonymously published, *A Treatise on Human Nature*.
3. See Hume (1739), p. 411.
4. See, for example, Kane (1996) and Stapp (1999). For more discussion, see also Walter (2000).
5. See also Dennett, *Freedom Evolves* (2003).
6. See also Wegner, *The Illusion of Conscious Will* (2002).
7. See Taylor (1992), Van Inwagen (1975).
8. See more extended explanations in Churchland (1995).

9. This syndrome is also known as *akinetic mutism.* For a review paper, see Vogt et al. (1992).
10. See Damasio and Van Hoesen (1983).
11. See Ballantine *et al.* (1987).
12. For this study, see Beauregard *et al.* (2001).
13. For a fuller discussion, see Hobson (1993).
14. See Bauman and Kemper (1995).
15. For a review paper on the ascending projection systems, see Robbins and Everitt (1995).
16. This was first pointed out to me by Carmen Carillo in a paper for my class, and was subsequently discussed in an editorial

in *Nature Neuroscience, Fat and free will* (2000), **3**, 1057.
17. See also Walter (2000).
18. See Kagan, *Galen's Prophecy* (1994).
19. Churchland (1995) from a different perspective. See also Casebeer (2003).
20. Recall that Buridan's ass was placed midway between two bales of hay, and could not decide which to approach first, and so died of starvation.
21. See Damasio (1999).
22. This view can also be found in the classic essays of Hobart (1934) and Schlick (1939).

References

Aristotle (1955). *The Nichomachean Ethics.* Trans. J. A. K. Thompson. Harmondsworth: Penguin Books.

Ballantine, H. T., Jr., Bouckoms, A. J., and Thomas, E. K. (1987). Treatment of psychiatric illness by stereotactic cingulotomy. *Biological Psychiatry,* **22**, 807–19.

Bauman, M. L. and Kemper, T. L. (1995). Neuroanatomical observations of the brain in autism. In J. Panksepp, ed., *Advances in Biological Psychiatry.* New York: JAI Press, pp. 1–26.

Beauregard, M., Lévesque, J., and Bourgouin, P. (2001). Neural correlates of conscious self-regulation of emotion. *Journal of Neuroscience*, **21**, 1–6.

Campbell, C. A. (1957). Has the self "free will"? *On Selfhood and Godhood*, London: Allen and Unwin; and New Jersey: Humanities Press Inc., pp. 158–79.

Casebeer, W. (2003). *Natural Ethical Facts: Evolution, Connectionism, and Moral Cognition*. Cambridge, MA: MIT Press.

Churchland, P. M. (1995). *The Engine of Reason, The Seat of the Soul*. Cambridge, MA: MIT Press.

Churchland, P. S. (2002). *Brain-Wise: Studies in Neurophilosophy*. Cambridge, MA: MIT Press.

Crick, F. H. C. (1994). *The Astonishing Hypothesis*. New York: Scribner's.

Damasio, A. R. (1999). *The Feeling of What Happens*. New York: Harcourt Brace.

Damasio, A. R. and Van Hoesen, G. (1983). Emotional disturbances associated with focal lesions of the limbic frontal lobe. In K. Heilman and P. Satz, eds., *Neuropsychology of Human Emotion*. New York: Guilford, pp. 268–99.

Dennett, D. C. (2003). *Freedom Evolves*. New York: Basic.

Hobart, R. E. (1934). Free will as involving determinism and inconceivable without it. *Mind*, **43**, 1–27.

Hobson, J. A. (1993). Understanding persons: the role of affect. In S. Baron-Cohen, H. Tager-Flusberg, and D. J. Cohen, eds., *Understanding Other Minds: Perspectives from Autism*. Oxford: Oxford University Press, pp. 204–27.

Hume, D. [1739] (1962). *A Treatise of Human Nature*. Ed. Norman Kemp Smith. Oxford: Oxford University Press.

Kagan, J. (1994). *Galen's Prophecy: Temperament in Human Nature*. New York: Basic Books.

Kane, R. (1996). *The Significance of Free Will*. Oxford: Oxford University Press.

Robbins, T. W. and Everitt, B. J. (1995). Arousal systems and attention. In M. Gazzaniga, ed., *The Cognitive Neurosciences*, Cambridge, MA: MIT Press, pp. 703–20.

Schlick, M. (1939). When is a man responsible? *Problems of Ethics*. New York: Prentice-Hall, pp. 143–56.

Stapp, H. P. (1999). Attention, intention and will in quantum physics. In B. Libet, A. Freeman, and K. Sutherland, eds., *The Volitional Brain: Towards a Neuroscience of Free Will*. New York: Academic Press, pp. 143–74.

Taylor, R. (1992). *Metaphysics*, 4th edn. Englewoods Cliffs, NJ: Prentice-Hall.

Van Inwagen, P. (1975). The incompatibility of free will and determinism. *Philosophical Studies*, **27**, 185–99. Reprinted in G. Watson, ed., *Free Will*. Oxford: Oxford University Press, pp. 46–58.

Vogt, B. A., Finch, D. M., and Olson, C. R. (1992). Functional heterogeneity in the cingulate cortex: the anterior executive and the posterior evaluative regions. *Cerebral Cortex*, **2**, 435–43.

Walter, H. (2000). *Neurophilosophy of Free Will: From Libertarian Illusions to a Concept of Natural Autonomy*. Cambridge, MA: MIT Press.

Wegner, D. M. (2002). *The Illusion of Conscious Will*. Cambridge, MA: MIT Press.

PART I HIGHER ORDER PERCEPTION

Overview of higher order visual perception

MICHAEL I. POSNER

The three chapters that follow this introduction all deal with aspects of visual perception related to the processing of scenes and the recognition of objects. There was a time when it was clear that higher order visual perception meant processing that took place in brain areas beyond the primary visual cortex. The primary visual cortex was thought to perform simple computations, each covering a small separate part of the visual world (receptive field) and hard wired in the sense that little could be done by learning or attention to modify them. This view stressed hierarchical processing among visual areas, particularly those from primary visual cortex V1 to the anterior temporal areas. Evidence for the hierarchical view is thoroughly summarized in the chapter by Kastner, De Weerd, and Ungerleider. However, all the three chapters deal in rather different ways with qualification to the hierarchical view of visual areas driven passively from the *bottom up*, based upon the influence of context, attention, and task demands.

In his chapter, Charles Gilbert describes the research work of his group, which has changed the view of how the primary visual cortex works. The older view gave rise to the hope that studies of primary visual cortex might provide the basic immutable building blocks from which it might be possible to launch an analysis of the remaining functions grouped under the title of higher perception. Gilbert argues that the primary visual cortex is "dynamic" in that receptive field organization can be changed by learning all through life. It can also be modified moment to moment by task instruction. According to this view, even the earliest cortical brain areas are modified by attention, motivation, and past experience that form much of the basis of psychology. Many psychologists hoped that by studying the brain they could avoid the hard problems of perception, but this route does not take us even as far as the primary visual cortex. If

Topics in Integrative Neuroscience: From Cells to Cognition, ed. James R. Pomerantz. Published by Cambridge University Press. © Cambridge University Press 2008.

even primary visual cortex is a part of higher visual perception, what is left of the building blocks from which higher perception was to be attacked.

Fortunately, Gilbert shows how a combination of behavioral studies using psychophysical research methods and cellular recording might help us understand the transformations supplied by the primary visual cortex. Gilbert believes that knowledge of the nature of the visual world in which humans are raised allows us to understand the organization of context-dependent effects within the visual cortex. In psychology, Gibson (1979) and later Shepard (1994) used this same argument as a reason not to bother with detailed physiological studies of sensory systems. Gibson and Shepard thought that so complete was the adaptability of the sensory systems that if we could describe in mathematical detail the properties of the visual world to which all humans had to adapt, we would know all that was needed to understand visual function. Although there are many in psychology who would agree with this view, it seems more likely that the combined method of cognitive and neuroscience studies described in these chapters provides a much larger and more fruitful perspective.

The reader should keep in mind that Gilbert is not saying that all aspects of processing by the primary visual cortex are equally subject to context and attentional effects. In fact, these higher order effects may be limited to the horizontal fibers that allow communication across receptive fields. The horizontal connections may allow receptive field properties of primary cortical neurons to be "dynamic," first of all by providing a source for contextual influences, and secondly allowing those influences to change with experience according to the task.

Perhaps the classical receptive field in the absence of contextual influences from the horizontal fibers is more like the hard-wired local system originally thought to be the role of primary visual cortex. With attention the receptive field might prove to be flexible and dynamic, but with attention directed elsewhere the classical receptive field might still serve as a basic building block of neural activity driven by input and without the contextual influences provided by the horizontal fibers.

The neuroimaging methods, so beautifully described and imaginatively employed by Kastner, DeWeerd and Ungerledier in their chapter, allow us to view activation in all parts of the brain involved in the perception of visual input. The early part of the chapter deals with activity along the ventral visual pathway, starting with area V1, described by Gilbert, and moving into the temporal lobe. They describe evidence for the hierarchical nature of this system as well as the role of this ventral visual pathway in the recognition of visual objects. While their chapter allows for higher level influences in V1, it emphasizes the operations that take place in later visual areas.

Kastner *et al.* show, both from cellular and neuroimaging studies, that the extrastriate visual areas are important sites for the manifestation of attention. Attention serves to highlight objects and assemble the features of color and shape, which are processed within the separate visual areas that follow the striate cortex. Just as Gilbert describes attentional effects in V1, Kastner *et al.* are able to show its influences in sites throughout the visual system. Indeed the size of the attentional effects appears to increase as one moves toward higher levels of the visual system. The chapter stresses the importance of attention in resolving conflict within the receptive field of neurons found in these extra-striate areas. The authors conclude that attention acts to boost the contrast of the target, allowing its perception to win over distracters.

Kastner *et al.* also show how closely the monkey physiology, so well described by Gilbert in V1, fits with the new results being obtained from humans using functional imaging. This is very fortunate since there are many tasks only humans can perform and even when tasks can be learned by monkeys they do not show the flexibility and swift adaptation which language allows in human subjects. The use of both human and monkey studies is a strong feature of current work on visual attention.

In V1, where receptive fields are very small, attention might be most important in integrating related information that crosses classic receptive field boundaries, while where receptive fields are quite large, such as in V4, the main role of attention may be to allow differentiation among objects, all of which are within the classic receptive field. The fMRI and cellular recording described in these two chapters should eventually allow us to delineate the full range of visual areas involved in object recognition and describe their detailed computations. Kastner *et al.* also mention briefly the use of scalp electrical activity to obtain the time course of attentional activations (Hillyard & Anllo-Vento, 1998). The addition of scalp electrical methods provides some promise for being able to observe the subtle interactions between brain regions as information is shared between them in complex perceptual tasks such as reading (Nikolaev *et al.*, 2001).

Toward the end of their chapter Kastner *et al.* describe brain areas that become active even before the visual system responds to the sensory input. These areas correspond to what Jin Fan and I call the "orienting network," which represents one of the three networks that we regard as being important sources of attentional influences. Our chapter serves to correct some early mistakes made in the identification of the function of selected areas within this orienting network. Although orienting to sensory input has been the most frequently studied area for integrating psychological and neuroscience questions, we discuss in our chapter an executive attentional network by which humans manifest control over their thoughts, actions, and emotions. This network is implicated in allowing for the kind of task-specific effect of instruction for which humans are noted and that Gilbert finds to influence processing even within primary visual cortex of monkeys.

There has been less research devoted to understanding the detailed anatomy and cellular mechanisms for this fronto-striatal executive network than has been the case for the more posterior areas related to visual perception. However, research on this network is starting to develop and is likely to be of great importance for the future of the field. We see the executive network as operating along with the orienting network to serve as major sources of attention within the human brain (Posner & Petersen, 1990).

The main novel aspect of our chapter is an effort to deal with individual differences in the development of these networks. Because of recent developments in molecular genetics, understanding the detailed mechanisms that underlie differences among people in cognitive processes is an important new area for research. We argue that the development of attention in infants and young children indicates the importance of the executive attention network in achieving the kind of self-regulation needed for socialization into a culture. Individual differences in these control networks arise as a result of both genetics and experience, and we attempt to use studies of the basis of these differences to help illuminate both normal attention and its pathologies.

The three chapters provide differing levels of analysis which are closely related to the methods used by the authors. Gilbert's chapter emphasizes analysis at the level of the detailed inter-cellular communication related to visual input. Kastner *et al.* concentrate on imaging of the human brain, but they also make a great effort to develop explicit links to cellular levels. Fan and I deal primarily with behavior, but attempt to link it to imaging, cellular, and genetic mechanisms. All three of the chapters reflect the new reality that attention, learning, and context can influence visual input at least from the striate cortex through the rest of the visual system. This situation makes discriminating higher and lower perception more difficult because of the anatomical and temporal overlap between the two. However, since the physical structure of V1 is better understood and more accessible than other structures the evidence of its involvement in higher processes provides new opportunities for experimental analysis of the detailed circuitry by which learning and instruction influence visual computations. Because of their differing levels and viewpoints, the chapters together provide the reader a snapshot of current research into systems and cognitive neuroscience in general, and perception and attention in particular.

References

Gibson, J. J. (1979). *The Ecological Approach to Visual Perception.* Boston: Houghton-Mifflin.

Hillyard, S. A. and Anllo-Vento, L. (1998). Event related brain potentials in the study of visual selective attention. *Proceedings of the National Academy of Sciences USA*, **95**, 781–7.

Nikolaev, A. R., Ivanitsky, G. A, Ivanitsky, A. M., Posner, M. I., and Abdullaev, Y. G. (2001). Short-term correlation between frontal and Wernicke's areas during word association: an event-related potential analysis in human subjects. *Neuroscience Letters*, **298**, 107–10.

Posner, M. I. and Petersen, S. E. (1990). The attention system of the human brain. *Annual Review of Neuroscience*, **13**, 25–42.

Shepard, R. N. (1994). Perceptual-cognitive universals as reflections of the world. *Psychonomic Bulletin & Review*, **1**, 2–28.

2

Attention as an organ system

MICHAEL I. POSNER AND JIN FAN

2.1   Introduction

Attention is relatively easy to define subjectively as in the classical definition of William James (1890) who said: "Everyone knows what attention is. It is the taking possession of the mind in clear and vivid form of one out of what seem several simultaneous objects or trains of thought."

However, this subjective definition does not provide hints that might lead to an understanding of attentional development or pathologies. The theme of our chapter is that it is now possible to view attention much more concretely as an organ system. We follow the *Webster* dictionary definition of an organ system: "An organ system may be defined as differentiated structures in animals and plants made up of various cell and tissues and adapted for the performance of some specific function and grouped with other structures into a system."

We believe that viewing attention as an organ system aids in answering many perplexing issues raised in cognitive psychology, psychiatry, and neurology. Neuroimaging studies have systemically shown that a wide variety of cognitive tasks can be seen as activating a distributed set of neural areas, each of which can be identified with specific mental operations (Posner & Raichle, 1994, 1998). Perhaps the areas of activation have been more consistent for the study of attention than for any other cognitive system. We can view attention as involving specialized networks to carry out functions such as achieving and maintaining the alert state, orienting to sensory events, and controlling thoughts and feelings.

In Section 2.2, we examine the functional anatomy of the network involved in alerting and orienting to sensory events. Studies involved with orienting to

Topics in Integrative Neuroscience: From Cells to Cognition, ed. James R. Pomerantz. Published by Cambridge University Press. © Cambridge University Press 2008.

sensory events provide the most active model system for the study of attention within neuroscience. Section 2.3 considers attention in the sense of exercising voluntary control over thoughts, feelings, and actions. In this section, we examine a frontal network involved in this form of cognitive and emotional control. In Sections 2.4 and 2.5, we consider the development of attentional networks in normal individuals. The final two sections consider the impact of viewing attention as an organ system on questions in cognition (Section 2.6) and neuropsychology (Section 2.7).

2.2   Orienting to sensory events

The vast majority of studies on attention have involved orienting to sensory events, particularly visual events. The findings of these studies provide the basis for our limited understanding of how to approach brain mechanisms of attention. In this field, a basic distinction is between those brain areas which are influenced by acts of orienting (*sites*) and those which are parts of the orienting network itself, thus the *sources* of the orienting influence (see Figure 2.1).

Function	Structures	Modulator	Sites
Orient	Superior parietal	Acetylcholine	V1, A1, S1
	Temporal parietal junction		
	Frontal eye fields		
	Superior collicutus		
Alert	*Locus coruleus*	Norepinephrine	Orient system
	Right frontal and parietal cortex		
Exec. Attn.	Ant. Cingulate	Dopamine	All brain areas
	Lateral ventral		
	Prefrontal		
	Basal ganglia		

Figure 2.1   Brain structures that are networks found active in studies of the three functions of attention, dominant neuromodulators and the sites where that function has its influence.

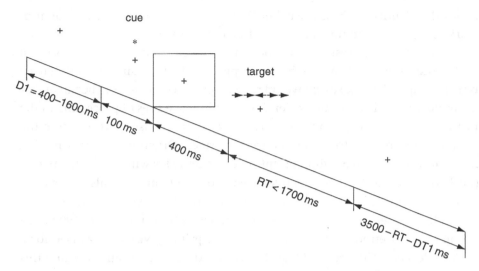

Figure 2.2 The attention network test. The cue provides information of when and where the target will occur. The target is a central arrow that indicates a left or right response surrounded by congruent or incongruent flankers.

Although our discussion is limited to vision, we believe that the sources of the attention effects are similar in other modalities (Macaluso *et al.*, 2000).

2.2.1   Sites and sources

Normally, all sensory events act both to contribute to a state of alertness and to orient attention. In order to distinguish the brain areas that are involved in orienting from the sites at which they operate, it is useful to separate the presentation of a cue indicating where a target will occur from the presentation of the target requiring a response (Corbetta *et al.*, 2000; Posner, 1978). This methodology has been used for behavioral studies with normal people (Posner, 1978), patients (Posner, 1988), monkeys (Marrocco & Davidson, 1998), and in studies using scalp electrical recording and event-related neuroimaging (Heinze *et al.*, 1994). A recent version of the cueing approach embedded in the attention network test (ANT) is shown in Figure 2.2 (Fan *et al.*, 2002). Two types of cues are of interest. Some cues provide information on when the target will occur. These warning signals lead to changes in a network of brain areas related to alerting. Other cues provide information on aspects of the target such as where it will occur and lead to changes in the orienting network.

Studies using event-related fMRI have shown that following the presentation of the cue and before the target is presented, a network of brain areas become active (Corbetta *et al.*, 2000; Kastner *et al.*, 1999). There is widespread agreement about the identity of these areas but there remains a considerable amount of work to do in order to understand the function of each area.

When a target is presented in isolation at the cued location, it is processed more efficiently than if no cue had been presented. The brain areas influenced by orienting will be those that would normally be used to process the target. For example, in the visual system orienting can influence sites of processing in the primary visual cortex, or in a variety of extra striate visual areas where the computations related to the target are performed. Orienting to target motion influences area MT (V5) while orienting to target color will influence area V4 (Corbetta *et al.*, 1991). This principle of activation of brain areas also extends to higher-level visual input as well. For example, attention to faces modifies activity in the face sensitive area of the fusiform gyrus (Wojciulik *et al.*, 1998). The finding that attention can modify activity in primary visual areas (see for a review, Posner & Gilbert, 1999) has been of particular importance because this brain area has been more extensively studied than any other.

When multiple targets are presented, they tend to suppress the normal level of activity, which they would have produced if presented in isolation (Kastner *et al.*, 1999). One important role of orienting to a particular location is to provide a relative enhancement of the target at that location in comparison with other items presented in the visual field.

2.2.2   Functional anatomy

Work with stroke patients shows that lesions of many brain areas result in difficulty shifting attention to locations or objects that were conveyed directly to the damaged hemisphere (Rafal, 1998). In neurology, these patients would be said to be suffering from extinction. Experimental studies suggested that we could define different forms of extinction due to lesions of the parietal lobe, the midbrain, or the thalamus (Posner, 1988) (see Figure 2.3). These results suggest that lesions to different areas produce a loss of particular mental operations. By mental operation, it is meant a component or subroutine of an overall act. For example, in order to shift attention to a new object, one first has to disengage attention from its current focus and move it to the new location where the target can be engaged. Data in the 1980s suggested that operations of disengage (parietal lobe), move (superior colliculus), and engage (pulvinar) were computed in different brain areas that formed a vertical network that together performed the task of orienting (for a recent review, see Losier & Klein, 2001). The idea of localization of mental operations in separate brain areas was appealing because it suggested a solution to the old problem of how there could be localization when widely separated damage could produce the same general behavioral effect (e.g., extinction). It suggested that to perform an integrated

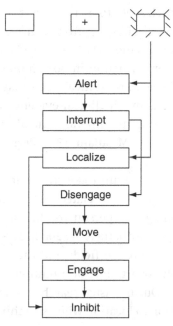

Figure 2.3 A view of orienting of attention proposed in the 1980s. In this view the superior parietal lobe was involved in the operation of disengaging attention, the colliculus in moving it, and the pulvinar in engaging the target (Posner, 1988). More recent views discussed in this chapter indicate that the superior parietal areas seem related to voluntary movements of attention, while disengaging to handle novel inputs appears to involve the temporal–parietal junction.

task the brain had to orchestrate a distributed network of brain areas, yet the computations underlying a single mental operation were local.

More recent studies involving both patient and imaging studies seem to support this general approach to localization, but suggest somewhat different separation of the operations involved. As new methods of neuroimaging have become available, they have been applied to the problem of orienting to sensory (often visual input). The results have helped to clarify how operations are localized. A paradox of the lesion studies in the early 1980s was that the superior parietal lobe seemed to be the area most related to producing a difficulty in disengaging from a current focus of attention. Yet most clinical data seemed to support the idea that clinical extinction arose from more inferior lesions in the temporal–parietal junction and/or superior temporal lobe.

Event-related imaging studies have served to reconcile this difference. There seem to be two separate regions, both of which can produce difficulty in shifting attention in contralesional space, but for quite different reasons. Lesions of the temporal–parietal junction or superior temporal lobe are important when a novel or unexpected stimulus occurs (Friedrich *et al.*, 1998; Karnath *et al.*, 2001). When functioning normally, this area allows disengaging from a current focus of attention to shift to the new event. This area is most critical in producing the core elements of the syndrome of neglect or extinction in both humans and monkeys although the exact location of the most critical area may differ between the two species. In addition, there is much clinical evidence that in the human there is lateralization in that the right-temporal parietal junction may be more important to the deficit than the left (Mesulam, 1981; Perry & Zeki, 2000).

A different region, the superior parietal lobe, seems to be critical for voluntary shifts of attention following the cue. In one event-related fMRI study, this region was active following a cue informing the person to shift attention covertly (without eye movement) to the target (Corbetta *et al.*, 2000). The region is part of a larger network that includes frontal eye fields and the superior colliculus that appears to orchestrate both covert shift of attention and eye movements toward targets (Corbetta, 1998). During visual search when people voluntarily move their attention from location to location while searching for a visual target this brain area is also active.

There is evidence from groups other than stroke patients also indicating brain areas involved in shifting attention. For example, patients with Alzheimer's disease, involving degeneration in the superior parietal lobe, have difficulty in dealing with central cues that inform them to shift their attention (Parasuraman *et al.*, 1992). There is also evidence that lesions of the superior colliculus may be involved in the preference for novel locations rather than locations to which one has already oriented (Sapir *et al.*, 1999). Patients with lesions of the thalamus (most likely the pulvinar) also show subtle deficits in visual orienting tasks that may be related to the access of the ventral information-processing stream. It seems that a vertical network of brain areas related to voluntary eye movements and to processing novel input are critical elements of orienting, but a precise model including a role for all of these areas is still lacking.

The methods of neuroimaging have proven critical to testing the general proposition that mental operations involved in a given task were widely distributed among brain areas (Posner & Raichle, 1998). In fact, the very first papers using positron emission tomography suggested that visual and auditory words were analyzed by a distributed network of brain areas, each of which performed an operation (Posner *et al.*, 1988). In the fifteen years since that time studies have shown that many tasks produce networks of widely spaced activation that most often were interpreted as carrying out particular operations.

It is likely that we still do not have the final answer as to the exact operations that occur at each location even in a relatively simple act like shifting attention to a novel event. Nonetheless, the imaging data provide reconciliation between clinical observations and imaging studies. The results of attentional studies, as with many other areas of cognition, support the general idea of localization of component operations.

2.2.3   Transmitters

It is very important to be able to link the neurosystem results that suggest brain areas related to attention, with cellular and synaptic studies that provide more details as to the local computations. One strategy for doing so is to study the pharmacology of each of the attention networks. To carry out these tests in is important to be able to study monkeys who, like humans, are able to use cues to direct attention to targets. Fortunately, cueing studies can be run successfully in monkeys.

A series of pharmacological studies with alert monkeys have related each of the attentional networks we have discussed with specific chemical neuro-modulators (Davidson & Marrocco, 2000; Marrocco & Davidson, 1998). Alerting is thought to involve the cortical distribution of the brain's norepinepherine (NE) system arising in the locus coeruleus of the midbrain. Drugs like clonidine and guanfacine act to block NE, reduce or eliminate the normal effect of warning signals on reaction time, but have no influence on orienting to the target location (Marrocco & Davidson, 1998).

Cholinergic systems arising in the basal forebrain play a critical role in orienting. Lesions of the basal forebrain in monkeys interfere with orienting attention (Voytko et al., 1994). However, it does not appear that the site of this effect is in the basal forebrain. Instead, it appears to involve the superior parietal lobe. Injections of scopolamine directly into the lateral interparietal area of monkeys – a brain area containing cells which are influenced by cues about spatial location – have been shown to have a large effect on the ability to shift attention to a target. Systemic injections of scopolamine have a smaller effect on covert orienting of attention than do local injections in the parietal area. Cholinergic drugs do not affect the ability of a warning signal to improve performance, and thus appear to be a double dissociation that relates NE to the alerting network and Ach (acetylcholine) to the orienting network. These observations in the monkey have also been confirmed by similar studies in the rat (Everitt & Robbins, 1997). Of special significance in the rat, comparisons of the cholinergic and dopaminergic mechanisms have shown that only the former influence the orienting response (Everitt & Robbins, 1997; Stewart et al., 2001).

The evidence relating Ach to the orienting network and NE to the alerting network provides strong evidence of dissociation between the different attentional networks. In the next section, we examine the frontal executive network and show that it is closely related to dopamine as a neural modulator.

2.3   Executive network

Executive control is most needed in situations, which involve planning or decision-making, error detection, novel responses, and in overcoming habitual actions. While these concepts are somewhat vague, a more explicit version of the idea of executive attention has recently been developed which stresses the role of attention in monitoring and resolving conflict between computations occurring in different brain areas (Botwinick *et al.*, 2001). While this view may not be adequate to explain all of the existing data, it provides a useful model for summarizing much of what is known.

2.3.1   *Functional anatomy*

A very large number of functional imaging studies have examined tasks that involve executive attention. These "thinking" tasks often activate a wide range of frontal and often posterior areas. Moreover, manipulations of the content of material have often shown that the same areas may be active irrespective of whether the stimuli are spatial, verbal, or visual objects. This has led some to conclude that the frontal lobes may be an exception to the specific identification of brain areas with mental operations that we have discussed for orienting (Duncan & Owen, 2000; Goldberg, 2001).

A frontal network including the anterior cingulate and lateral prefrontal cortex has been active in different tasks that involve attention when conflict is present and producing a nonhabitual response is required. One important study (Duncan *et al.*, 2000) examined a wide range of verbal, spatial, and object tasks selected from intelligence tests that had in common a strong loading on the factor of general intelligence (g). These items were contrasted with perceptually similar control items that did not require the kind of attention and thought involved in general intelligence. This subtraction led to differential activity in two major areas: one was the anterior cingulate and the second was lateral prefrontal cortex.

Many imaging studies have been conducted using either the Stroop task or variants of it that involved conflict among elements (Bush *et al.*, 2000). The Stroop task requires the person to respond to the color of ink (e.g., red) when the target is a competing color word (e.g., blue). Another frequently used conflict task is the target tasks illustrated in Figure 2.2. In this flanker task (Eriksen & Eriksen, 1974), the person is required to respond to a central stimulus (e.g., an arrow pointing left) when it is surrounded by flankers that either point in the

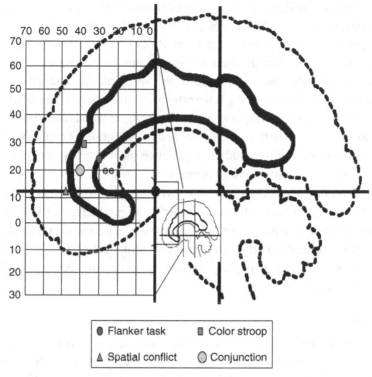

Figure 2.4   View of the anterior cingulate. Small dot indicates Flanker task, triangle indicates spatial conflict task, rectangle indicates color Stroop task, and large circle indicates the conjunction of the three conflict tasks.

same direction (congruent) or in the opposite direction (incongruent). Recently, we examined three conflict tasks using the same subjects and scanner to determine areas of activation (Fan, Flombaum *et al.*, 2003). We found that all three tasks activated areas of the anterior cingulate some of which were unique, but had a common focus (see Figure 2.4). In addition, all activated some areas of the prefrontal cortex.

An event-related fMRI study of the Stroop effect used cues to separate presentation of the task instruction from reaction to the target (MacDonald *et al.*, 2000). Lateral prefrontal areas were responsive to cues indicating whether the task involved naming the word or dealing with the ink color. The cue did not activate the cingulate. When the task involved naming the ink color, the cingulate was more active on incongruent than congruent trials. This result reflects the general finding that lateral areas are involved in representing specific information over time (working memory), while medial areas are more related to the detection of conflict.

Another cue to the functional activity in these areas comes from studies of generating the use of a word. In a typical version of this task, subjects are shown a series of 40 simple nouns (e.g., hammer) (Raichle *et al.*, 1994). In the experimental condition, they indicate the use of each noun (e.g., hammer -> pound). In the control condition, they simply read the word aloud. The difference in activation between the two tasks illustrates what happens in the brain when subjects are required to develop a very simple thought; in this case, how to use a hammer. Results illustrate that the anatomy of this high-level cognitive activity is similar enough among individuals to produce focal average activations that are both statistically significant and reproducible.

One area that is more strongly activated when generating the use of a word is on the midline of the frontal lobe in the anterior cingulate gyrus. Two additional areas of cortical activation that are more active in the generate condition are in the left lateral prefrontal cortex and posterior temporal cortex. Both of these areas have been shown to be involved in many tasks dealing with processing the meaning of words or sentences.

2.3.2   Circuitry

To examine the time course of these activations, it is possible to use a large number of scalp electrodes to obtain scalp signatures of the generators found active in imaging studies (Abdullaev & Posner, 1998). When subjects obtain the use of a noun, there is an area of positive electrical activity over frontal electrodes starting about 150 ms after the word appears. This early electrical activity is generated by the large area of activation in the anterior cingulate.

A left prefrontal area (anterior to and overlapping classical Broca's area) begins to show activity about 200 ms after the word occurs. In our initial data, we identified this area with semantic processing because it was active in tasks such as classifying the word into categories, obtaining an association, or treating one type of word (e.g., animal names) as a target, but not in reading words aloud. These empirical findings have proven to be true in much subsequent work (for a review, see Abdullaev & Posner, 1998). However, the finding that frontal areas appear involved in working memory and the finding that the time course of the activation of the lateral frontal area was early both make it likely that this lateral frontal area is related to operations such as holding the lexical item in a brief store during the time needed to which to look up the associated word use. The left posterior brain area found to be more active during the processing of the meaning of visual words did not appear until a much later time (500 ms). This activity is near the classical Wernicke's area – lesions of which are known to produce a loss of understanding of meaningful speech. We found evidence of the transfer of information from left frontal electrodes to the posterior area at about 450 ms into the task. Since the response time for this task was about 1100 ms, this would leave time for the generation of related associations needed to solve the task.

Practice on a single list of words reduces the activation in the cingulate and lateral cortical areas (Raichle et al., 1994). Thus the very same task, when it is highly over learned, avoids the circuits involved in thought and relies upon an entirely different circuitry.

These studies provide a start in understanding the functional roles of different brain areas in carrying out executive control. The medial frontal area appears most related to the executive attention network and is active when there is conflict among stimuli and responses. It may be serving as a monitor of conflict, but it is possible that it plays other roles as well. The lateral prefrontal area seems to be important in holding in mind the information relevant to the task. Even when a single item is presented, it may still be necessary to hold it in some temporary area while other brain areas retrieve information relevant to the response. Together these two areas are needed to solve nearly any problem, which depends upon retrieval of stored information. Both of these areas could be related to attention, or one might identify only the medial area with attention and the lateral one with working memory. In either case, they begin to give us a handle on how the brain parses high-level tasks into individual operations that are carried out in separate parts of the network.

2.3.3   Lesion studies

Classical studies of strokes of the frontal midline including the anterior cingulate showed a pervasive deficit of voluntary behavior (Damasio, 1994; Kennard, 1955). Patients with akinetic mutism can orient to external stimuli and follow people with their eyes, but they do not initiate voluntary activity. Recent studies of patients with small lesions of the anterior cingulate (Ochsner et al., 2001; Turken & Swick, 1999) show deficits in conflict-related tasks, but these patients frequently recover from their deficits suggesting that other areas may also be involved. In some cases, lesions of the mid-frontal area in children and adults may produce permanent loss of future planning and appropriate social behavior (Damasio, 1994). Early-childhood damage in this area can produce permanent deficits in decision-making tasks that require responses based on future planning (Anderson et al., 2000).

2.3.4   Cellular mechanisms

The anterior cingulate and lateral frontal cortex are target areas of the ventral tegmental dopamine system. All of the dopamine receptors are expressed in layer V of the cingulate.

The association of the anterior cingulate with high-level attentional control may seem rather odd because this is clearly a phylogenetically old area of the brain. Although the anterior cingulate is an ancient structure, there is evidence that it has evolved significantly in primates. Humans and great apes appear to have a unique cell type found mainly in layer V of the anterior cingulate and insula, a cell type not present in other primates (Nimchinsky et al., 1999). These cells also undergo a rather late development in line with the findings that executive control systems develop strongly during childhood (Allman, 2001) (see also next section). Although the precise function of this cell is not known, high correlations between its volume and encephalization suggest a likely role in higher cortical functioning. The proximity of these cells to vocalization areas in primates led Nimchinksy and colleagues to speculate that these cells may link emotional and motor areas, ultimately resulting in vocalizations that convey emotional meaning. Although there is as yet no direct evidence linking the cellular architecture of the anterior cingulate to cingulate activity detected during neuroimaging studies, the importance of this area for emotional and cognitive processing (Bush et al., 2000) makes further exploration compelling.

Several replicated human genetic studies demonstrate an association of one of the dopamine receptor genes D4 (DRD4) located on chromosome 11p15.5 and an attentional disorder common in childhood (attention deficit/hyperactivity disorder or ADHD). About 50% of the ADHD cases have a 7-repeat allele whereas only about 20% ethnically matched control subjects have a 7-repeat allele. However, a direct comparison of children with ADHD who either have or do not have the 7-repeat allele suggests that attentional abnormalities are more common in those children without the 7-repeat allele (Swanson et al., 2000). The authors suggest that there are different routes to ADHD only some of which involve a specific reduction in cognitive ability.

The anterior cingulate is strongly activated by a wide variety of tasks that create conflict between elements (Bush et al., 1998). For example, if people are asked to respond to the number of items in the visual field and the items are digits whose name differs from the number of objects present, conflict exists between the digit name and the desired numerical response. This counting Stroop task, like many other conflict tasks studied by neuroimaging, produces activation of the anterior cingulate (Bush et al., 1998). Adult subjects who suffer from ADHD have been studied in the numerical Stroop. While they perform only slightly worse than normal persons, they appear to activate an entirely different network of brain areas than do the normals. Where normals activate the anterior cingulate, the ADHD adults seem to rely on the anterior insula, which is usually associated with responses in more routine tasks not involving conflict (Bush et al., 1999). The insula is active when reading words but not in generating new uses unless they are well practiced, thus this area may represent a more primitive pathway allowing for less effortful control over the task.

Washburn (1998) demonstrated the effects of conflict in rhesus monkeys by first training them to appreciate the quantity of a digit by pairing digits with appropriate amounts of reward. The monkeys were then asked to indicate which of two displays contained the larger number of items. When the items were digits, the number in the display could either be congruent (larger number of objects was also the larger digit) or incongruent (smaller number of objects was the larger digit). Monkeys performed this task and showed greater difficulty in errors and RT in the incongruent condition. Moreover, despite hundreds of trials at the task, monkeys continued to produce many more errors on incongruent trials than do humans. Monkeys appeared to have a reduced capacity to avoid interference despite extensive training.

Washburn and his associates noticed that mastery of complex tasks, such as the Stroop by Rhesus monkeys, led to a reduction of aggression and an improvement in their social behavior. They suggested that the Rhesus monkey might serve as a model of ADHD in humans. The existence of animals' models for the Stroop (Washburn, 1998) opens up the possibility of cellular studies for examining the role of the cingulate in attention.

Schizophrenia is another disorder that produces a disruption of attentional control in addition to other emotional and cognitive problems. Benes (1999) reports subtle abnormalities of the anterior cingulate in postmortem analyses of schizophrenic brains. She argues that schizophrenic brains may be dysfunctional due to a shift in dopamine regulation from pyramidal to nonpyramidal cells. These effects involve the D2 receptor and are strongest within layer II of the anterior cingulate. Her theory provides a possible cellular level explanation for anterior cingulate dysfunction in a second abnormality noted for its attentional deficits.

In this section, we have examined imaging, cellular, and genetic studies that illustrate the physical basis of the executive attention network. While attention deficit disorder and schizophrenia are striking examples of pathologies related to this network, it is clear that attention also differs between normal individuals. The next section examines studies on this topic.

2.4   Individual differences

Almost all studies of attention have been concerned with either the general abilities involved or with the effects of brain injury or pathology on attention. However, it is clear that normal individuals differ in their ability to

Network measurement		Average value*	Heritability**
Executive	$RT_{Incongruent} - RT_{Congruent}$	84	0.89
Alerting	$RT_{Double\ cue} - RT_{No\ cue}$	47	0.18
Orienting	$RT_{Valid\ cue} - RT_{Central\ cue}$	51	0.0

* As measured from 40 normal subjects (Fan *et al.*, 2001).

** From a study of 26 pairs of monozygotic and 26 pairs of same-sex dyzygotic twins (Fan *et al.*, 2001).

Figure 2.5 Subtraction used to obtain values for the three networks. Average refers to the mean value for 40 normal persons. Heritability refers to the results of a twin study described in the text.

attend to sensory events and even more clearly in their ability to concentrate for long periods on internal trains of thought.

To study these individual differences, we have developed an attention network test (ANT) (see Figure 2.2) that examines the efficiency of the three brain networks we have described (Fan *et al.*, 2002). We used reaction times derived from the task shown in Figure 2.2 to make subtractions shown in Figure 2.5. The data provide three numbers that represent the skill of each individual in the alerting, orienting, and executive networks. In a sample of 40 normal persons, we found each of these numbers to be reliable over repeated presentations. In addition, we found no correlation among the numbers. An analysis of the reaction times found in this task showed large main effects for cue type and for the type of target. There were only two small interactions indicating some lack of independence among the networks. One of these interactions was that orienting to the correct target location tended to reduce the influence of the surrounding flankers (Rob *et al.*, 2001). In addition, omitting a cue, which produces relatively long reaction times, also reduces the size of the flanker interference. Presumably, this is because some of the conflict is reduced during the time the subject is preparing to process the target location.

The ability to measure differences in attention among adults raises the question of the degree to which attention is heritable. In order to deal with this issue, we used our attention network test to study 26 pairs of monozygotic and 26 pairs of dyzygotic same sex twins (Fan *et al.*, 2001). We found strong correlations between the monozygotic twins for both the executive and alerting networks. For the alerting network, we found a similar, although somewhat smaller, correlation among the dizygotic twins, but for the executive network the dyzygotic twins were only slightly correlated. This led to a high heritability of the executive network. Because of the small sample, it is not possible to determine heritability very exactly, nonetheless, these data support a role for genes in the executive and possibly in the alerting network.

We have used the association of the alerting and executive network with the neuromodulators NE and DA as a way of searching for candidate genes that might relate to the efficiency of these networks (Fossella *et al.*, 2002). To do this, we have so far run 100 persons in the ANT and taken buccal swabs to examine frequent polymorphisms in genes related to their respective neuromodulators. So far we have obtained very preliminary evidence of the association of the DRD4 and MAOA gene alone or in combination with the executive network. We have also seen some relation of MAOA and COMT with the alerting network. At this time, we are continuing the search both in normal subjects and in patient populations for which abnormalities may be in attentional networks (see addendum Page 54).

2.5   Development of attentional networks

A major advantage of viewing attention as an organ system is to trace the ability of children and adults to regulate their thoughts and feelings. Over the first few years of life, the regulation of emotion is a major issue of development. Panksepp (1998) lays out anatomical reasons why the regulation of emotion may pose a difficult problem for the child as follows:

> One can ask whether the downward cognitive controls or the upward emotional controls are stronger. If one looks at the question anatomically and neurochemically the evidence seems overwhelming. The upward controls are more abundant and electrophysiologically more insistent: hence one might expect they would prevail if push came to shove. Of course, with the increasing influence of cortical functions as humans develop, along with the pressures for social conformity, the influences of the cognitive forces increase steadily during maturation. We can eventually experience emotion without sharing them with others. We can easily put on false faces, which can make the facial analysis of emotions in real-life situations a remarkably troublesome business. (Panksepp, 1998, 319)

The ability of attention to control distress can be traced to early infancy (Harman *et al.*, 1997). In infants as young as three months, we have found that orienting to a visual stimulus provided by the experimenter produces powerful if temporary soothing of distress. One of the major accomplishments of the first few years is for infants to develop the means to achieve this regulation on their own.

An early sign of the control of cognitive conflict is found in the first year of life. For example, in A-not-B tasks, children are trained to reach for a hidden object at location A, and then tested on their ability to search for the hidden object at a new location B. Children younger than 12 months of age tend to look in the previous location A, even though they see the object disappear behind location B. After the first year, children develop the ability to inhibit the pre-potent response toward the trained location A, and successfully reach for the new location B (Diamond, 1991). During this period, infants develop the ability to resolve conflict between line of sight and line of reach when retrieving an object. At 9 months of age, line of sight dominates completely. If the open side of a box is not in line with the side in view, infants will withdraw their hand and reach directly along the line of sight, striking the closed side (Diamond, 1991). In contrast, 12-month-old infants can simultaneously look at a closed side while reaching through the open end to retrieve a toy.

The ability to use context to reduce conflict can be traced developmentally using the learning of sequences of locations. Infants as young as 4 months anticipate the location of a stimulus, provided the association in the sequence are unambiguous. In unambiguous sequences, each location is invariably asso-ciated with another location (e.g., 123) (Clohessy et al., 2001). Because the loca-tion of the current target is fully determined by the preceding item, there is only one type of information that needs to be attended and therefore no conflict (e.g., location 3 always follows location 2). Adults can learn unambiguous sequences of spatial locations implicitly even when attention is distracted by a secondary task (Curran & Keele, 1993).

Ambiguous sequences (e.g., 1213) require attention to the current association in addition to the context in which the association occurs (e.g., location 1 may be followed by location 2, or by location 3). Ambiguous sequences pose conflict because for any association there exist two strong candidates that can only be disambiguated by context. When distracted, adults are unable to learn both ambiguous sequences of length six (e.g., 123213) (Curran & Keele, 1993), a finding that demonstrates the need for higher-level attentional resources to resolve this conflict. Even simple ambiguous associations (e.g., 1213) were not learned by infants until about 2 years of age (Clohessy et al., 2001).

Developmental changes in executive attention were found during the third year of life using a spatial conflict task (Gerardi-Caulton, 2000). Because children of this age do not read, location and identity rather than word meaning and ink color served as the dimensions of conflict (spatial conflict task). Children sat in front of two response keys, one located to the child's left and one to the right. Each key displayed a picture, and on every trial a picture identical to one of the pair appeared on either the left or right side of the screen. Children were rewarded for responding to the identity of the stimulus, regardless of its spatial compatibility with the matching response key (Gerardi-Caulton, 2000). Reduced accuracy and slowed reaction times for spatially incompatible relative to spatially compatible trials reflect the effort required to resist the prepotent response and resolve conflict between these two competing dimensions. Performance on this task produced a clear interference effect in adults and activated the anterior cingulate (see Figure 2.4). Children of 24 months of age tended to fix on a single response, while 36-month-old children perform at high accuracy levels, but like adults responded more slowly and with reduced accuracy to incompatible trials.

At 30 months, when toddlers were first able to successfully perform the spatial conflict task, we found that performance on this task was significantly correlated with the same toddlers' ability to learn the ambiguous associations in the sequence learning task described above (Rothbart et al., 2003). This finding, together with the failure of 4-month-olds to learn ambiguous sequences, holds out the promise of being able to trace the emergence of executive attention during the first years of life.

The importance of being able to study the emergence of executive attention is enhanced because cognitive measures of conflict resolution in these laboratory tasks have been linked to aspects of children's self control in naturalistic settings. Children relatively less affected by spatial conflict also received higher parental ratings of temperamental effortful control and higher scores on laboratory measures of inhibitory control (Gerardi-Caulton, 2000).

Questionnaires have shown the effortful control factor, defined in terms of scales measuring attentional focusing, inhibitory control, low intensity pleasure, and perceptual sensitivity (Rothbart et al., 2001) to be inversely related to negative affect. This relation is in keeping with the notion that attentional skill may help attenuate negative affect, while also serving to constrain impulsive approach tendencies.

Empathy is also strongly related to effortful control, with children high in effortful control showing greater empathy. To display empathy toward others requires that we interpret their signals of distress or pleasure. Imaging work in normals shows that sad faces activate the amygdala. As sadness increases, this activation is accompanied by activity in the anterior cingulate as part of the attention network (Blair et al., 1999). It seems likely that the cingulate activity represents the basis for our attention to the distress of others. Cingulate activity is related to regulation of positive as well as negative affects. The effort to control arousal to a sexually stimulating movie also show specific activation of this brain network (Beauregard et al., 2001).

Developmental studies find the two routes to successful socialization. A strongly reactive amygdala would provide the signals of distress that would easily allow empathic feelings toward others. These children are relatively easy to socialize. In the absence of this form of control, the development of the cingulate would allow appropriate attention to what signals are provided by amygdala activity. Consistent with its influence on empathy, effortful control also appears to play a role in the development of conscience. The internalization of moral principles appears to be facilitated in fearful preschool-aged children, especially when their mothers use gentle discipline (Kochanska, 1995). In addition, internalized control is facilitated in children high in effortful control (Kochanska *et al.*, 1996). Two separable control systems, one reactive (fear) and one self-regulative (effortful control), appear to regulate the development of conscience.

Individual differences in effortful control are also related to some aspects of metacognitive knowledge, such as theory of mind (i.e., knowing that people's behavior is guided by their beliefs, desires, and other mental states) (Carlson & Moses, 2001). Moreover, tasks that require the inhibition of a prepotent response correlate with theory of mind tasks even when other factors, such as age, intelligence, and working memory are factored out (Carlson & Moses, 2001). Inhibitory control and theory of mind share a similar developmental timecourse, with advances in both arenas between the ages of 2 and 5.

One function that has been traced to the anterior cingulate is monitoring of error. One form of conflict was studied by having children play a Simple Simon game, which asked them to execute a response command given by one puppet while inhibiting commands given by a second puppet (Jones *et al.*, 2003). Children of 36–38 months showed no ability to inhibit their response and no slowing following an error, but at 39–41 months children showed both an ability to inhibit and slowing of reaction time following an error. These results suggest that between 38 and 39 months performance changes based upon detecting an error response. Because error detection has been studied using scalp electrical recording (Gehring *et al.*, 1993; Luu *et al.*, 2000) and shown to originate in the anterior cingulate (Bush *et al.*, 2000), we now have the means to examine the emergence of this cingulate functioning in children.

We have examined the ANT network tests in children of 7 years of age using a version specifically adapted to them (see Figure 2.6). The results for children of this age are remarkably similar to those found for adults using the version of the task shown in Figure 2.2. The child reaction times are much longer but they show similar independence between the three networks. Children have larger scores for alerting and conflict than adults, suggesting that they have trouble in maintaining the alert state when not warned of the new target and in resolving conflict.

This age (7 years) is amenable to neuroimaging using MRI. Children aged 5 to 16 years show a significant correlation between the volume of the area of the right anterior cingulate and the ability to perform tasks requiring focal

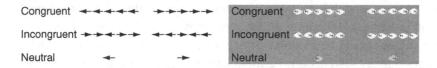

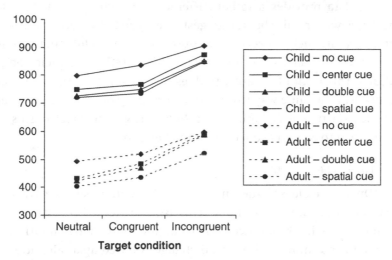

Figure 2.6 Upper panel shows the stimuli used for 7-year-old children in the ANT. Bottom panel compares adults and children R.T. both using this version of the ANT.

attention (Casey *et al.*, 1997a). In a functional MRI study, performance of children ages 7–12 and adults were studied in a go/no-go task. In comparison with a control condition in which children responded to all stimuli, the condition requiring inhibitory control activated prefrontal cortex in both children and adults. Also, the number of false alarms in this condition correlated significantly with the extent of cingulate activity (Casey *et al.*, 1997b).

These studies provide evidence for the development of an executive network during early childhood. Moreover, the development of executive attention contributes to the socialization process by increasing the likelihood of learning important behaviors related to self-regulation and understanding the cognition and emotion of others. It seems likely that understanding normal development of this system will illuminate pathologies of attention.

2.6   Cognitive science problems

2.6.1   *Modularity*

There has been a great deal of discussion in the cognitive psychology literature of the concept of modularity. These discussions have often defined modularity in a way which required a system to be unaffected by top-down (attentional) influences. According to this view, only a very few vertical sensory and motor systems could be modular (Fodor, 1983). However, the evidence that even primary sensory systems can be modulated by attention makes it unlikely that any higher-level brain system will meet the criterion of modularity so defined.

Imaging data provides a rather different perspective on modularity. The material reviewed in this chapter suggests that even brain networks that reflect voluntary activity such as executive attention may be modular in the sense that very specific brain areas perform computations reflecting their component operations. This form of modularity does not suggest that these mechanisms will operate in the same way irrespective of strategy or context. However, they do provide a starting place for linking cellular and genetic mechanisms to brain areas and then to cognitive operations and behavior.

2.6.2   Early and late selection

One of the oldest issues in the field of attention is how early in processing can attention influence input. This issue arose before there was much discussion of specific brain mechanisms of attention. Many empirical studies were done to determine if attentional changes showed up as alterations in the beta (decision) parameter of a signal detection analysis or whether instead they involved changes in the d' (sensory) parameter (Hawkins et al., 1990). Although many elegant studies were conducted attempting to clarify this issue, there has been no final resolution (although it seems likely that both parameters can be varied by some experimental conditions) (Hawkins et al., 1990).

The early vs. late question can be resolved into three somewhat interdependent issues. (1) How early in the nervous system can attention influence stimulus input? The results suggest that it can be as early as V1 (Posner & Gilbert, 1999) under some conditions, but more often attention influences extrastriate visual areas (Kastner et al., 1999). (2) How quickly after input can attention influence information processing? Again, the cellular and physiological data indicate that it can be about as early as clear evidence of cortical processing can be obtained, although in many situations the influence is not present until 80–100 ms after stimulus onset (Martinez et al., 2001). The timing issue is of particular importance because activation of a particular brain area may be either along the input pathway or could be due to feedback from higher areas. (3) What does early selection mean for the processing of information both selected and unselected? Here the answer is more complex. It seems to mean that certain aspects of complex scenes may be available for conscious report while other aspects will only be available if they succeed in producing reorienting of attention. Unattended objects, however, may still be processed to fairly high levels and the processing itself may summon attention. The depth of cognitive processing of unattended objects and the possibility of attention to higher level codes suggest that early selection does not have the cognitive consequence originally implied. Selecting one stimulus over others does not mean that unselected items will not produce a reorienting of attention or still influence behavior (McCormick, 1997).

2.6.3   Priming

Priming refers to the influence of one event on the processing of subsequent events. Behavioral studies suggested that reaction time could be improved to a target by the presentation of a stimulus (prime) that shares a part of the same pathway. Priming can occur in either of two ways. In one way, a stimulus activates a pathway automatically and a second stimulus that shares the same pathway is improved in performance (Posner, 1978). These effects can occur even when the prime is presented and masked so that subjects are not able to report its identity. A second way that priming can occur is if a person attends to some feature that will be shared by the target. For example, if people are taught that the word "animal" should be interpreted as a body part, the target finger will be primed. The priming is from the subjects' attention to body part not from automatic activation of finger by the prime animal.

Data from imaging studies of priming by input and by attention support this distinction by showing very different effects on neural activity in the primed area. If priming occurs automatically by input, the target shows reduced activation of the primed cells. On the other hand, attending to an area will enhance neural activity and increase the effect of the target (Corbetta et al., 1991).

The imaging data shows the reality of the distinction between automatic priming and priming by attention. However, it is not at all clear how the brain brings about similar changes in performance sometimes by reducing and sometimes by increasing the activity of the target. This puzzle remains to be explained by future studies.

2.7   Relation to neuropsychology

The ability to image the human brain has also provided new perspectives for neuropsychologists in their efforts to understand, diagnose, and treat insults to the human brain that might occur as the result of stroke, tumor, traumatic injury, degenerative disease, or errors in development (Fernandez-Duque & Posner, 2001).

As we have argued, attention networks have anatomical and functional independence, but that they also interact in many practical situations. Damage to a node of these networks, irrespective of the source, produces distinctive neuropsychological deficits. This principle has been best established with respect to damage to the parietal lobe. Studies have shown that damage to parietal neurons that occur in stroke, due to degeneration in Alzheimer disease, blocking of cholinergic input, due to lesions of nucleus bassalis, temporary damage from transcranial magnetic stimulation, direct injections of scopolamine, or closed head injury all lead to difficulties in using cues to process targets in the visual field opposite the insult. Recently, normal persons who have one or two copies of the APOE4 gene, which increases the risk of Alzheimer's disease, have also been shown to have increased difficulty in orienting attention and in adjusting the spatial scale of attention, however, they had no difficulty with maintaining the alert state (Greenwood *et al.*, 2000). Additional evidence for a common effect of damage to a node is reviewed in some detail elsewhere (Fernandez-Duque & Posner, 2001).

In one sense, the convergence between imaging, lesions, and pharmacology in terms of cognitive effect is obvious. If computations of parietal neurons lead to shifts of visual attention, damage to these neurons should produce difficulties. Yet there has been the notion in neuropsychology that localization is not so important as the cause of the lesion. Moreover, there has also been the argument that imaging does not provide a good account of the computations that can predict the effect of damage (Uttal, 2001). Here we see that the imaging results provide clear evidence of the importance of areas of the parietal lobe in shifts of attention and damage to these areas regardless of cause interfering with orienting.

In addition, efforts to better understand the nature of brain disorder there have been efforts to adopt ideas related to the physical basis of attention for rehabilitation. Some recent studies have tried to rehabilitate specific attentional networks (Robertson, 1999; Sohlberg *et al.*, 2000; Strum *et al.*, 1997). These studies suggest that rehabilitation procedures should focus on the particular attentional operations of the lesioned area, while at the same time considering the contribution of those deficits to other attentional functions.

In one study (Strum *et al.*, 1997), a computerized rehabilitation program was designed to try to enhance specific attentional networks. The authors concluded from these findings that vigilance and alertness are the most fundamental functions in the hierarchy, and that selective attention and divided attention recruit these functions for their normal operation. Another study that utilized a practice-oriented therapy (attention process therapy) with brain-injured patients showed an overall improvement in performance (Sohlberg *et al.*, 2000). In some tasks, the group that had relatively high vigilance scores showed better effects of the therapy in agreement with the Strum idea.

A third rehabilitation study tested the possible interaction between vigilance and orienting by training patients to increase their self-alertness, and exploring whether the rehabilitation of self-alertness had an impact on patients' neglect (i.e., orienting deficit) (Robertson *et al.*, 1995). Exogenous alertness was used as a basis for training patients to be self-alert. External warning signals were presented, and patients were instructed to generate a self-alertness signal in response to it. Exogenous alertness, as produced by a loud noise, depends on a thalamo-mesencephalic path and is relatively unimpaired in right parietal patients. After the training procedure was explained, the patient started the task and at variable intervals the experimenter knocked on the table while at the same time saying "Attend!" in a loud voice. At the next stage in the training, it was the patient who shouted "Attend!" each time the experimenter knocked on the table. Later, the patient would do both the knocking and the vocal command, first loudly, then subvocally, and finally mentally. Patients were encouraged to try this self-alertness method in their everyday life. This rehabilitation training not only improved patients' self-alertness, but also reduced the extent of their spatial neglect.

The availability of imaging as a means of examining brain networks prior to and following rehabilitation should provide new opportunities for research that could fine-tune both behavioral and pharmacological intervention methods. Genetic analysis could also aid in an understanding of who might benefit from particular forms of therapy. Taken together these methods and the analysis of attention networks described in this and subsequent chapters in this part could provide significant new approaches to rehabilitation following brain injury.

Addendum

The pace of research in cognitive neuroscience has been very fast so that in the time since the original meeting at which this paper was presented there have been many new developments. In this brief addendum, we try to describe some of the most critical of these new findings.

The attention network task has now been studied using event-related fMRI to examine the brain areas associated with alerting, orienting, and executive attention (Fan *et al.*, 2005). For the most part, the results confirm the brain areas illustrated in Figure 2.1. The main difference is new findings with respect to the role of a warning of when the target will occur on activity in the cortex. While sustained vigilance involves mainly areas of the right cerebral hemisphere, considerable fMRI evidence has shown that phasic changes in alertness following warning signals tend to operate through left hemisphere sites (Coull *et al.*, 2001). However, norepinepherine still appears to be crucial to these changes (Beane & Marrocco, 2004).

Event-related fMRI studies of orienting were well summarized by Corbetta and Shulman (2002). They identify a dorsal system including the interparietal sulcus and frontal eye fields as being involved in volitional shifts of attention. A more ventral parietal frontal network serves as a circuit breaker leading to shifts of attention particularly to novel stimuli. They regard the more ventral system as being the major factor in producing neglect from cortical lesions. This and many other summaries included in new books on imaging of visual cognition and attention (Kanwisher & Duncan, 2004; Posner, 2004) suggest considerable agreement on the cortical areas that orchestrate shifts of attention toward sensory information. There is also considerable agreement with the functions of these areas described by Corbetta and Shulman (2002). However, imaging studies have generally been less successful in identifying the subcortical areas described in Figure 2.1.

What it is still unclear is exactly how information in the brain areas that forms the source of the orienting network influences sensory information. There has been progress on this front; Duncan (2004) summarizes the competition within visual areas when multiple potential targets are activated and argues persuasively that attention works to resolve the suppression of neural activity between potential targets.

There has been considerable theoretical work attempting to define the exact role of areas like the anterior cingulate and lateral prefrontal cortex. Several researchers (Cohen *et al.*, 2004) have argued that the cingulate involves a monitoring function, while lateral prefrontal areas act more directly to suppress neural activity in unselected areas. While there is considerable agreement on the brain areas illustrated in Figure 2.1 under executive attention, whether they operate as a whole or can be divided into specific operations and, if so, which ones remains an area of active discussion (Posner, 2004).

In our paper, we described our initial work on the molecular genetics of attention. There were then, essentially no published papers in this field. No wonder our very preliminary evidence described in the paper was met with some skepticism. This has changed dramatically. Not only have our papers now been published describing evidence on the role of MAOA, COMT, DRD4, and DAT1 genes on conflict scores of the ANT (Fan, Fossella *et al.*, 2003; Fossella *et al.*, 2002), but major studies from a large group at NIH have confirmed the role of COMT in attention (Blasi *et al.*, 2005) and shown important evidence of the role of genes in memory (Egan *et al.*, 2003). In addition, papers have shown two cholinergic genes that are involved in individual differences in the orienting network (Parasuraman *et al.*, 2005). There have also been studies showing how neuroimaging can be used to explore the anatomy of these genetics differences (Egan *et al.*, 2003; Fan, Fossella *et al.*, 2003). The area of cognitive genetics has become a large one and has brought the study of individual differences in attentional efficiency down to the molecular level (Goldberg & Weinberger, 2004).

In our paper, we stressed the importance of child development in the study of attention as an organ system. At the time, we did not have strong evidence on the development of executive attention. But in the last 5 years, we have come to identify its development with the increased degree of self-regulation found in children between 2.5 and 7 years of age (Rueda *et al.*, 2004a, b). This research has helped to shape our effort to examine how the combination of experience and genetics serves to produce the executive attention network and the consequences for the development of children (Posner & Rothbart, 2005).

Despite these many changes, the very general framework of our paper of attention as an organ system with specific networks carrying its basic functions seems to us to be even sounder than it was a few years ago. This framework points the way to linking molecular, neural systems, and cognitive studies into an overall view of attention that can illuminate its role both in the development of children and in the performance of adults.

Acknowledgment

This paper was presented at the De Lange Conference, March 2001. This research was supported by a grant NSF BCS9907831 and from a 21st Century Research Grant from the James S. McDonnell Foundation to the Sackler Institute and the University of Oregon. We are grateful to our colleagues at the Institute and to Mary K. Rothbart for their help in the research reported here.

Notes

This research was supported by NSF grant BCS9907831 and by a 21st Century Grant from the James S. McDonnell Foundation. The second author held a DeWitt Clinton Readers Digest Grant while carrying out this research. The authors wish to thank members of the Sackler Institute for their assistance with the research reported here.

References

Abdullaev, Y. G. and Posner, M. I. (1998). Event-related brain potential imaging of semantic encoding during processing single words. *Neuroimage*, **7**, 1–13.

Allman, J. (2001). The anterior cingulate cortex: the evolution of an interface between emotion and cognition. In A. Damasio *et al.* (eds.), *Unity of Knowledge. Annals of New York Academy of Science*, **935**, 107–17.

Anderson, S. W., Damasio, H., Tranel, D., and Damasio, A. R. (2000). Long-term sequelae of prefrontal cortex damage acquired in early childhood. *Developmental Neuropsychology*, **18**(3), 281–96.

Beane, M. and Marrocco, R. T. (2004). Cholinergic and noradrenergic inputs to the parietal cortex modulate the components of exogenous attention. In Posner, M. I. (ed.), *Cognitive Neuroscience of Attention*, New York: Guilford, pp. 313–28.

Beauregard, M., Levesque, J., and Bourgouin, P. (2001). Neural correlates of conscious self-regulation of emotion. *Journal of Neuroscience*, **21**, RC165:1–6.

Benes, F. (1999). Model generation and testing to probe neural circuitry in the cingulate cortex of postmortem schizophrenic brains. *Schizophrenia Bulletin*, **24**, 219–29.

Blair, R. J. R., Morris, J. S., Frith, C. D., Perrett, D. I., and Dolan, R. J. (1999). Dissociable neural responses to facila expression of sadness and anger. *Brain*, **1222**, 883–93.

Blasi, G., Mattay, V. S., Bertolino, A., *et al.* (2005). Effects of Catecol-O-Methyltransferase val[158] met genotype on attentional control. *Journal of Neuroscience*, **25**, 5038–45.

Botwinick, M. M., Braver, T. S., Barch, D. M., Carter, C. S., and Cohen, J. D. (2001). Conflict monitoring and cognitive control. *Psychological Review*, **108**, 624–52.

Bush, G., Frazier, J. A., Rauch, S. L., *et al.* (1999). Anterior cingulate cortex dysfunction in attention deficit/hyperactivity disorder revealed by fMRI and the counting Stroop. *Biological Psychiatry*, **45**, 1542–52.

Bush, G., Luu, P., and Posner, M. I. (2000). Cognitive and emotional influences in the anterior cingulate cortex. *Trends in Cognitive Science*, **4/6**, 215–22.

Bush, G., Whalen, P. J., Rosen, B. R., *et al.* (1998). The counting Stroop: An interference task specialized for functional neuroimaging – validation study with functional MRI. *Human Brain Mapping*, **6**, 270–82.

Carlson, S. M. and Moses, L. J. (2001). Individiual differences in inhibitory control and children's theory of mind. *Child Development*, **72**, 1032–53.

Casey, B. J., Trainor, R., Giedd, J., *et al.* (1997a). The role of the anterior cingulate in automatic and controlled processes: a developmental neuroanatomical study. *Developmental Psychobiology*, **3**, 61–9.

Casey, B. J., Trainor, R. J., Orendi, J. L., *et al.* (1997b). A developmental function MRI study of prefrontal activation during performance of a go-no-go task. *Journal of Cognitive Neuroscience*, **9**, 835–47.

Clohessy, A. B., Posner, M. I., and Rothbart, M. K. (2001). Development of the functional visual field. *Acta Psychologica*, **106**, 51–68.

Cohen, J. D., Aston-Jones, G., and Gilzenrat, M. S. (2004). Guided activation, adaptive gating and conflict monitoring, and exploitation versus exploration. In Posner, M. I. (ed.), *Cognitive Neuroscience of Attention*, New York: Guilford, pp. 71–90.

Corbetta, M., Kincade, J. M., Ollinger, J. M., McAvoy, M. P., and Shulman, G. (2000). Voluntary orienting is dissociated from target detection in human posterior parietal cortex, *Nature Neuroscience*, **3**, 292–7.

Corbetta, M. (1998). Frontoparietal cortical networks for directing attention and the eye to visual locations: Identical, independent, or overlapping neural systems? *Proceedings of the National Academy of Sciences USA*, **95**, 831–8.

Corbetta, M. and Shulman, G. L. (2002). Control of goal-directed and stimulus-driven attention in the brain. *Nature Reviews Neuroscience*, **3**(3), 201–15.

Corbetta, M., Miezin, F. M., Dobmeyer, S., Shulman, G. L., and Petersen, S. E. (1991). Selective and divided attention during visual discriminations of shape, color, and speed: Functional anatomy by positron emission tomography. *Journal of Neuroscience*, **11**, 2383–402.

Coull, J. T., Nobre, A. C., and Frith, C. D. (2001). The noradrenergic alph2 agonist clonidine modulates behavioural and neuroanatomical correlates of human attentional orienting and alerting. *Cerebral Cortex*, **11**(1), 73–84.

Curran, T. and Keele, S. W. (1993). Attentional and non-attentional forms of sequence learning. *Journal of Experimental Psychology: Learning, Memory and Cognition*, **19**, 189–202.

Damasio, A. (1994) *Descartes Error: Emotion, Reason and the Brain*. New York: G. P. Putnam.

Davidson, M. C. and Marrocco, R. T. (2000). Local infusion of scopolamine into intraparietal cortex slows cover orienting in rhesus monkeys. *Journal of Neurophysiology*, **83**, 1536–49.

Diamond, A. (1991). Neuropsychological insights into the meaning of object concept development. In S. Carey and R. Gelman (eds.), *The Epigenesis of Mind: Essays on Biology and Cognition*, Hillsdale, NJ: Lawrence Erlbaum Associates, pp. 67–110.

Duncan, J. (2004). Selective attention in distributed brain systems. In Posner, M. I. (ed.), *Cognitive Neuroscience of Attention*, New York: Guilford, pp. 105–13.

Duncan, J. and Owen, A. M. (2000). Common regions of the human frontal lobe recruited by diverse cognitive demands. *Trends in Neurosciences*, **23**, 475–83.

Duncan, J., Seitz, R. J., Kolodny, J., *et al.* (2000). A neural basis for general intelligence. *Science*, **289**, 457–60.

Egan, M. F., Kojima, M., Callicott, J. H., *et al.* (2003). The BDNF val66met polymorphism affects activity-dependent secretion of BDNF and human memory and hippocampal function. *Cell*, **112**, 257–69.

Eriksen, B. A. and Eriksen, C. W. (1974). Effects of noise letters upon the identification of a target letter in a nonsearch task. *Perception & Psychophysics*, **16**, 143–9.

Everitt, B. J. and Robbins, T. W. (1997). Central cholinergic systems and cognition. *Annual Review of Psychology*, **48**, 649–84.

Fan, J., Flombaum, J. I., McCandliss, B. D., Thomas, K. M., and Posner, M. I. (2003). Cognitive and brain consequences of conflict. *Neuroimage*, **18**, 42–57.

Fan, J., Fossella, J. A., Summer, T., and Posner, M. I. (2003). Mapping the genetic variation of executive attention onto brain activity. *Proceedings of the National Academy of Sciences USA*, **100**, 7406–11.

Fan, J., McCandliss, B. D., Fossella, J., Flombaum, J. I., and Posner, M. I. (2005). The activation of attentional networks. *Neuroimage*, **26**, 471–9.

Fan, J., McCandliss, B. D., Sommer, T., Raz, M., and Posner, M. I. (2002). Testing the efficiency and independence of attentional networks. *Journal of Cognitive Neuroscience*, **3**(14), 340–7.

Fan, J., Wu, Y., Fossella, J., and Posner, M. I. (2001). Assessing the heritability of attentional networks. *BioMed Central Neuroscience*, **2**, 14.

Fernandez-Duque, D. and Posner, M. I. (2001). Brain imaging of attentional networks in normal and pathological states. *Journal of Clinical and Experimental Neuropsychology*, **23**, 74–93.

Fodor, J. (1983). *Modularity of Mind*. Cambridge, MA: MIT Press.

Fossella, J., Sommer, T., Fan, J., *et al.* (2002). Assessing the molecular genetics of attention networks. *BMC Neuroscience*, **3**, 14.

Friedrich, F. J., Egly R., Rafal, R. D., and Beck, D. (1998). Spatial attention deficits in humans: A comparison of superior parietal and temporal-parietal junction lesions. *Neuropsychology*, **12**(2), 193–207.

Gehring, W. J., Gross, B., Coles, M. G. H., Meyer, D. E., and Donchin, E. (1993). A neural system for error detection and compensation. *Psychological Science*, **4**, 385–90.

Gerardi-Caulton, G. (2000). Sensitivity to spatial conflict and the development of self-regulation in children 24–36 months of age. *Developmental Science*, **3/4**, 397–404.

Goldberg, E. (2001). *The Executive Brain*. New York: Oxford.

Goldberg, T. E. and Weinberger, D. R. (2004). Genes and the parsing of cognitive processes. *Trends in Cognitive Sciences*, **8**(7), 325–35.

Greenwood, P. M., Sunderland, T., Friz, J. L., and Parasuraman, R. (2000). Genetics and visual attention: Selective deficits in healthy adult carriers of the epsilon 4 allele of the apolipoprotein E gene. *Proceedings of National Academy of Sciences USA*, **97**, 11661–6.

Harman, C., Rothbart, M. K., and Posner, M. I. (1997). Distress and attention interactions in early infancy. *Motivation and Emotion*, **21**, 27–43.

Hawkins, H. L., Hillyard, S. A., Luck, S. J., *et al.* (1990). Visual attention modulates signal detection. *Journal of Experimental Psychology: Human Perception & Performance*, **16**, 802–11.

Heinze, H. J., Mangun, G. R., Burchert, W., *et al.* (1994). Combined spatial and temporal imaging of brain activity during visual selective attention in humans. *Nature*, **372**, 543–6.

James, W. (1890). *Principles of Psychology*. New York: Holt.

Jones, L., Rothbart, M. K., and Posner, M. I. (2003). Development of inhibitory control in preschool children. *Developmental Science*, **6**, 498–504.

Kanwisher, N. and Duncan, J. (eds.) (2004). *Attention and Performance XX*, Oxford University Press, pp. 505–28.

Karnath, H.-O., Ferber, S., and Himmelbach, M. (2001). Spatial awareness is a function of the temporal not the posterior parietal lobe. *Nature*, **411**, 95–953.

Kastner, S., Pinsk, M. A., De Weerd, P., Desimone, R., and Ungerleider, L. G. (1999). Increased activity in human visual cortex during directed attention in the absence of visual stimulation. *Neuron*, **22**, 751–61.

Kennard, M. A. (1955). The cingulate gyrus in relation to consciousness. *Journal of Nervous Mental Disorders*, **121**, 34–9.

Kochanska, G. (1995). Children's temperament, mothers' discipline, and security of attachment: Multiple pathways to emerging internalization. *Child Development*, **66**, 597–615.

Kochanska, G., Murray, K., Jacques, T. Y., Koenig, A. L., and Vandegeest, K. A. (1996). Inhibitory control in young children and its role in emerging internationalization. *Child Development*, **67**, 490–507.

Losier, B. J. W. and Klein, R. (2001). A review of the evidence for a disengage deficit following parietal damage. *Neuroscience and Biobehavioral Reviews*, **25**, 1–13.

Luu, P., Collins, P., and Tucker, D. M. (2000). Mood, personality and self-monitoring: Negative affect and emotionality in relation to frontal lobe mechanisms of error-detection. *Journal of Experimental Psychology General*, **129**, 43–60.

Macaluso, E., Frith, C. D., and Driver, J. (2000). Modulation of human visual cortex by crossmodal spatial attention. *Science*, **289**, 1204–8.

MacDonald, A. W., Cohen, J. D., Stenger, V. A., and Carter, C. S. (2000). Dissociating the role of the dorsolateral prefrontal and anterior cingulate cortex in cognitive control. *Science*, **288**, 1835–8.

Marrocco, R. T. and Davidson, M. C. (1998). Neurochemistry of attention. In R. Parasuraman (ed.), *The Attentive Brain*. Cambridge, MA: MIT Press, pp. 35–50.

Martinzez, A., DiRusso, F., Anllo-Vento, L., *et al.* (2001). Putting spatial attention on the map: Timing and localization of stimulus selection processing striate and extrastriate visual areas. *Vision Research*, **41**, 1437–57.

McCormick, P. A. (1997). Orienting without awareness. *Journal of Experimental Psychology: Human Perception & Performance*, **23**, 168–80.

Mesulam, M.-M. (1981). A cortical network for directed attention and unilateral neglect. *Annals of Neurology*, **10**, 309–25.

Nimchinsky, E. A., Gilissen, E., Allman, J. M., *et al.* (1999). A neuronal morphologic type unique to humans and great apes. *Proceedings of the National Academy of Sciences*, **96**, 5268–73.

Ochsner, K. N., Kossyln, S. M., Cosgrove, G. R., *et al.* (2001). Deficits in visual cognition and attention following bilateral anterior cingulotomy. *Neuropsychologia*, **39**, 219–30.

Panksepp, J. (1998). *Affective Neuroscience*. New York: Oxford.

Parasuraman, R., Greenwood, P. M., Haxby, J. B., and Grady, C. L. (1992). Visuospatial attention in dementia of the Alzheimer type. *Brain*, **115**, 711–33.

Parasuraman, R., Greenwood, P. M., Kumar, R., and Fossella, J. (2005). Beyond heritability: Neurotransmitter genes differentially modulate visuospatial attention and working memory. *Psychological Science*, **16**, 200–7.

Perry, R. J. and Zeki, S. (2000). The neurology of saccades and covert shifts of spatial attention. *Brain*, **123**, 2273–93.

Posner, M. I. (1978). *Chronometric Explorations of Mind*. Hillsdale, NJ: Lawrence Erlbaum Associates.

Posner, M. I. (1988). Structures and functions of selective attention. In T. Boll and B. Bryant (eds.), *Master Lectures in Clinical Neuropsychology and Brain Function: Research, Measurement, and Practice*, American Psychological Association, pp. 171–202.

Posner, M. I. (ed.) (2004). *Cognitive Neuroscience of Attention*. New York: Guilford.

Posner, M. I. and Gilbert, C. D. (1999). Attention and primary visual cortex. *Proceedings of the National Academy of Sciences of the USA*, **96/6**, 2585–7.

Posner, M. I. and Raichle, M. E. (1994). *Images of Mind*. Scientific American Books.

Posner, M. I. and Raichle, M. E. (eds.) (1998). Neuroimaging of Cognitive Processes. *Proceedings of the National Academy of Sciences of the USA*, **95**, 763–4.

Posner, M. I. and Rothbart, M. K. (2005). Influencing brain networks: Implications for education. *Trends in Cognitive Science*, **9**, 99–103.

Posner, M. I., Petersen, S. E., Fox, P. T., and Raichle, M. E. (1988). Localization of cognitive functions in the human brain. *Science*, **240**, 1627–31.

Rafal, R. (1998). Neglect. In R. Parasuraman (ed.), *The Attentive Brain*. Cambridge, MA: MIT Press, pp. 711–33.

Raichle, M. E., Fiez, J. A., Videen, T. O., *et al.* (1994). Practice-related changes in the human brain: Functional anatomy during nonmotor learning. *Cerebral Cortex*, **4**, 8–26.

Rob, H. J., Lubbe, V., and Keuss, P. J. G. (2001). Focused attention reduces the effect of lateral interference in multi-element arrays. *Psychological Research*, **65**, 107–18.

Robertson, I. H., Tegnér, R., Tham, K., Lo, A., and Nimmo-Smith, I. (1995). Sustained attention training for unilateral neglect: Theoretical and rehabilitation implications. *Journal of Clinical and Experimental Neuropsychology*, **17**(3), 416–30.

Robertson, I. H. (1999). Cognitive rehabilitation, attention and neglect. *Trends in Cognitive Neuroscience*, **3**, 385–93.

Rothbart, M. K., Ahadi, S. A., Hershey, K. L., and Fisher, P. (2001). Investigations of temperament at three to seven years: The Children's Behavior Questionnaire. *Child Development*, **72**, 1394–408.

Rothbart, M. K., Ellis, L. K., Rueda, M. R., and Posner, M. I. (2003). Developing mechanisms of effortful control. *Journal of Personality*, **71**, 1113–43.

Rueda, M. R., Fan, J., Halparin, J., *et al.* (2004a). Development of attention during childhood, *Neuropsychologia*, **42**, 1029–40.

Rueda, M. R., Posner, M. I., and Rothbart, M. K. (2004b). Attentional control and self-regulation. In R. F. Baumeister and K. D. Vohs (eds.), *Handbook of Self-Regulation: Research, Theory, and Applications*, New York: Guilford Press, **14**, 283–300.

Sapir, A., Soroker, N., Berger, A., and Henik, A. (1999). Inhibition of return in spatial attention: Direct evidence for collicular generation. *Nature Neuroscience*, **2**(12), 1053–4.

Sohlberg, M. M., McLaughlin, K. A., Pavese, A., Heidrich, A., and Posner, M. I. (2000). Evaluation of attention process therapy training in persons with acquired brain injury. *Journal of Clinical and Experimental Neuropsychology*, **22**, 656–76.

Stewart, C., Burke, S., and Marrocco, R. (2001). Cholinergic modulation of covert attention in the rat. *Psychopharmocology*, **155**(2), 210–18.

Strum, W., Willmes, K., Orgass, B., and Hartje, W. (1997). Do specific attention effects need specific training. *Neurological Rehabilitation*, 81–103.

Swanson, J., Oosterlaan, J., Murias, M., *et al.* (2000). ADHD children with 7-repeat allele of the DRD4 gene have extreme behavior but normal performance on critical neuropsychological tests of attention. *Proceedings of the National Academy of Sciences USA*, **97**, 4754–9.

Turken, A. U. and Swick, D. (1999). Response selection in the human anterior cingulate cortex. *Nature Neurosceince*, **2**(10), 920–4.

Uttal, W. R. (2001). *The New Phrenology: The Limits of Localizing Cognitive Processes in the Brain*. Cambridge, MA: MIT Press.

Voytko, M. L., Olton, D. S., Richardson, R. T., *et al.* (1994). Basal forebrain lesions in monkeys disrupt attention but not learning and memory. *Journal of Neuroscience*, **14**(1), 167–86.

Washburn, D. A. (1998). Stroop-like effects for monkeys and humans: Processing speed or strength of association? *Psychological Science*, **5**, 375–9.

Wojciulik, E., Kanwisher, N., and Driver, J. (1998). Covert visual attention modulates face-specific activity in the human fusiform gyrus: fMRI study. *Journal of Neurophysiology*, **79**(3), 1574–8.

3

Cortical dynamics and visual perception

CHARLES GILBERT

3.1 Introduction

The primary visual cortex is the first cortical stage at which the visual world is analyzed. It has classically been thought to be a passive filter, only deriving information about local contrast and orientation, and passing that on to later cortical stages for the more complex task of object recognition. But a very different view is now emerging, showing that V1 plays a central role in much more complex processes involving intermediate level vision, integrating contours and parsing the visual world into surfaces belonging to objects and their backgrounds. The higher order properties of cortical neurons are reflected in the dependence of their responses on the context within which features of the visual stimulus are embedded. In addition, the properties of neurons in V1 reflect an ongoing process of experience-dependent modification, known as "perceptual learning." This process begins early in life, incorporating the structural properties of the visual world into the functional properties of neurons. It continues throughout adulthood, encoding information about different shapes with which individuals become familiarized. Superimposed upon the influence of context and experience is a powerful top-down modification of neuronal function, such that the properties exhibited by neurons change according to attentional state, expectation, and perceptual task.

3.2 The receptive field and cortical circuitry: contextual influences

The central functional element of sensory systems is the receptive field, the portion of the sensory surface (retina) or environment (visual field) within which a stimulus will cause a cell to fire. Even in some of the original work on the receptive field, however, it was known that cell responses could be modulated

Topics in Integrative Neuroscience: From Cells to Cognition, ed. James R. Pomerantz. Published by Cambridge University Press. © Cambridge University Press 2008.

over a larger area, and that these more extended regions needed to be incorporated in the definition of the receptive field (Kuffler, 1953). The way in which one defines the receptive field is highly dependent on the nature of the stimulus used to measure it. As a consequence, the characterization of the receptive field has undergone radical change along with the use of complex stimuli and the exploration of contextual influences. One cannot predict the response of cells to complex patterns from their responses to individual line segments placed in different parts of the visual field – cells are highly nonlinear in their responses to the combination of multiple elements in the visual scene. However, these nonlinearities show a clear relationship with perceptual rules governing contour saliency and psychophysical measures of contour interactions.

The contextual interactions observed at both the perceptual and the receptive field levels also show a close relationship with the geometry of cortical circuits. In fact, some of the original evidence that neurons in V1 integrated information over a large area of visual space came from intracellular injections, which revealed a plexus of long-range connections extending for many millimeters parallel to the cortical surface. Because of the orderly visual topography within V1, these connections enable cells to integrate information over an area of visual cortex representing a relatively large area of visual space (Gilbert and Wiesel, 1979, 1983; Rockland and Lund, 1982; Martin and Whittcridge, 1984). The discovery of these connections was surprising since their extent seemed larger than the receptive field as mapped by conventional methods. The resolution for this seeming contradiction is that the horizontal connections have a modulatory influence, and, under normal circumstances, the longest range connections cannot by themselves activate their targets. Their influence, however, can be considerable when activated together with other inputs.

A distinctive feature of the horizontal connections is the clustered distribution of the axon collaterals. This clustering gives the intrinsic horizontal connections considerable specificity, whereby the pattern of connections is registered with the columnar functional architecture of the cortex. Cells in V1 are selective for the orientation of line segments lying within their receptive fields, and cells with similar orientation preference are distributed in columns extending from the cortical surface to the white matter. As one moves across the cortical surface, there is a regular clockwise shift in the preferred orientation of the columns one encounters, with roughly a 0.75 mm to 1 mm periodicity. The clusters of the horizontal connections have the same periodicity, and the horizontal connections link columns of similar orientation preference (Gilbert and Wiesel, 1989; Malach et al., 1993; Weliky et al., 1995; Bosking et al., 1997). This iso-orientation rule of anatomical interactions mirrors the specificity of contextual interactions, and, as will be described below, the Gestalt rules of contour saliency.

Lateral cortical interactions lead to a number of perceptual consequences and are responsible for a range of receptive field properties. The perceived brightness of a line segment is influenced by the presence of a second, collinear line segment placed nearby. One can detect the target line at 40% lower contrast when the second line is present than when the target is presented in isolation (Dresp, 1993; Polat and Sagi, 1993, 1994; Kapadia et al., 1995). Similarly, the response of cells in the superficial layers of V1 to a line placed within the receptive field core is facilitated when a second, collinear line is placed outside the receptive field (Kapadia et al., 1995). The second line, when presented by itself, elicits no response, yet when presented along with the line inside the receptive field can increase the cell's response two or threefold (Figure 3.1). The brightness induction effect measured psychophysically and the contextual line facilitation obey the same dependencies on the relative positions and orientations of the paired lines: the effects are maximal when the lines are of the same orientation, collinear and close together. As one pulls the lines apart, offsets them from collinearity, or changes their relative orientations, the effect gradually disappears. The spatial scale of the perceptual and physiological effects, when compared at the same visual field eccentricity, are the same. Moreover, the scale closely matches the extent of the intrinsic long-range horizontal connections in primary visual cortex, and the dependency on orientation reflects the clustered nature of these connections, linking columns of similar orientation preference.

This highlights the problem of how the receptive field is defined. One way of mapping the receptive field uses a procedure known as the "minimum response field technique," where one places an appropriately oriented line segment in different parts of the visual field to define the edges of the responsive region. Another way is to make length-tuning measurements, increasing the size of the stimulus until the response plateaus, or, in the case of end-inhibited cells, until it begins to drop when the line extends into the inhibitory regions. The optimum length is dependent on stimulus characteristics such as contrast (Kapadia et al., 1999, 2000; Sceniak, 1999), or on the presence of other elements within the visual scene (Kapadia et al., 1999), therefore giving different measures of the receptive field size depending on the stimulus used. The responses of V1 neurons depend as much on the global characteristics of contours extending well beyond the receptive field core as the attributes of local line elements centered within the receptive field.

The ability of neurons to signal information about foreground/background relationships and contour shape demonstrates the perceptual consequences of contextual influences. If a line, centered in the receptive field, is embedded in a complex background of randomly oriented and positioned line elements, the response of the cell is greatly inhibited by the surrounding pattern, even if the central line is at the cell's optimum orientation. As one shifts the surrounding lines

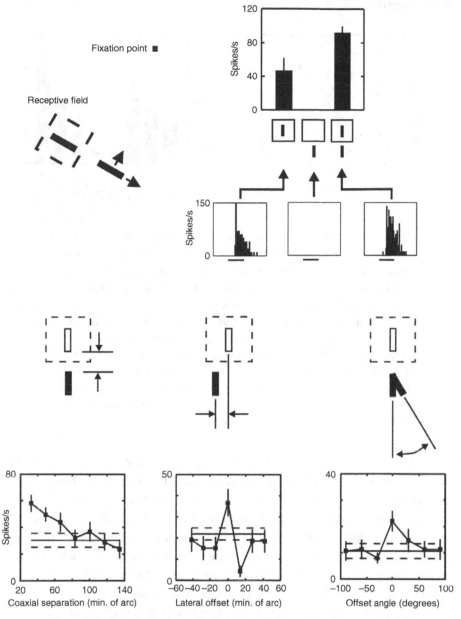

Figure 3.1 Facilitation by contextual stimuli. Recordings from superficial layer cells in the behaving Macaque monkey show that stimuli outside the minimum response field can increase cells' responses severalfold to stimuli presented inside the receptive field. The top shows this high degree of nonlinearity in the response, where the line segment centered in the receptive field gives a response, the one placed outside gives no response, but when presented together will increase the response over twofold. This facilitation is dependent on the precise geometric relationship of the two line segments, diminishing as the line segments are separated, offset from collinearity or changed in relative orientation. Similar effects, operating over the same spatial scales, are seen psychophysically, where flanking lines increase the perceived brightness of target lines (adapted from Kapadia *et al.*, 1995).

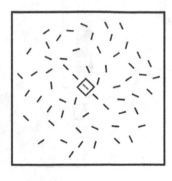
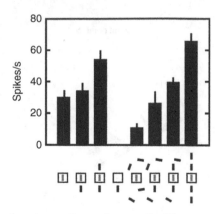

Figure 3.2 Contextual facilitation and contour saliency. As a result of the nonlinearities illustrated in Figure 3.1, the responses of neurons in visual cortex are as dependent on the global characteristics of contours extending beyond the receptive field as they are on the attributes of local features centered within the receptive field. This property gives cells sensitivity to salient contours in the visual environment. When an appropriately oriented line segment is presented in the receptive field (left bar in histogram) one gets a good response, but that response is greatly attenuated when the line segment is embedded in a complex background of randomly placed and oriented line segments. As line elements are shifted into positions of collinearity with the receptive field, this inhibition is eliminated and one gets a further facilitation of the response to a level higher than that seen with the single bar alone (from Kapadia *et al.*, 1995).

into alignment with the receptive field, forming a line extending well beyond the minimum response field, the inhibition is gradually lifted, and one obtains larger responses than those elicited by the single line in isolation (Kapadia *et al.*, 1995; Figure 3.2). The saliency of a contour is dependent on the placement of the line elements from which the contour is formed, obeying the Gestalt rule of "good continuation." Contours that are more salient have elements that have similar orientations and that are collinear (Wertheimer, 1938; Ullman, 1990; Field *et al.*, 1993). This, again, is reflected in the geometry of the long-range horizontal connections and the facilitatory effects of receptive field surrounds. Though one might expect salient contours to extend for longer distances than the visuotopic representation of the cortical area spanned by horizontal connections, the effects of these connections can cascade over multiple steps. Though such a cascade can only operate when the gaps between the segments from which a contour is made do not go above a certain distance, it does enable the horizontal connections to play a role in perceptual interactions operating over relatively large distances in visual space.

One can see long-range contextual influences operating along all three dimensions in space. These interactions are observed in "interaction fields,"

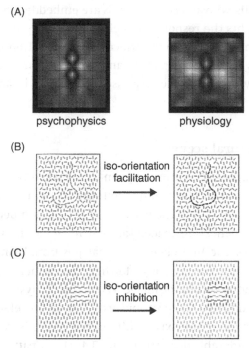

Figure 3.3 Contextual interactions in two dimensions. (A) Contextual interactions were measured psychophysically using the tilt illusion as a probe (left), and physiologically using a measure of facilitation of responses (right). In the psychophysical experiments, when contextual lines are presented in a collinear configuration, but tilted 5° relative to a centrally placed target line, the target line appears tilted in the same direction as the contextual lines (blue). When the contextual lines are presented in a side-by-side configuration, the apparent tilt reverses (red). A similar distribution of interactions is seen physiologically, where iso-orientation facilitation occurs along the orientation axis of the neuron, and iso-orientation inhibition predominates along the orthogonal axis. These interactions are proposed to play a role in contour saliency. (B) bringing out the responses from neurons with receptive fields aligned with salient contours in complex visual environments, and in surface segmentation (C) bringing out the responses from neurons with receptive fields aligned with surface boundaries (for color image please see www.cambridge.org/9780521143400).

where one measures the influence of lines flanking a central line in different positions. Facilitation is maximal along the orientation axis of the central line, inhibition strongest when the flankers are in a side-by-side configuration with the central line. The facilitatory effects play a role in contour integration and the inhibitory effects play a role in surface segmentation, as schematized in Figure 3.3 (Kapadia *et al.*, 2000). The facilitation brings out the responses of cells whose receptive fields are distributed along salient contours. Inhibition suppresses the responses of cells whose receptive fields are embedded in fields of uniform texture, but highlights the responses of cells whose receptive fields are located at texture discontinuities, signaling surface boundaries. Depth cues also play an important role in contour integration and surface segmentation, and global depth cues strongly influence the responses of neurons in area V2 (Bakin *et al.*, 2000).

3.3   Gestalt rules and natural scenes

The higher order properties of neurons in primary visual cortex reflect the structural regularities present in the world. Contours in natural scenes possess a simple geometry. This is seen in the patterns of correlation between line elements of which these scenes are made. Take an image and, at each position, find the orientation of the line element at that position. Using one line segment as a reference, find the probability of other line elements of the same orientation at other positions within the image. When this analysis is done for thousands of images, one finds that the probability of finding line elements of similar orientation is highest along the axis of collinearity, and this increase in probability extends for a considerable distance (Figure 3.4). Other patterns are seen for line elements of different orientation. Perpendicular lines are found, for example, along 45° axes from the reference line. All of these relationships obey a simple geometric rule, a rule of cocircularity. That is, the most likely arrangement of lines within contours is one where the contours maintain a constant radius of curvature (Sigman *et al.*, 2000; Geisler *et al.*, 2001).

The contextual influences measured in the two-dimensional interaction fields of neurons obey the same arrangement: facilitation between similarly oriented lines is seen along the collinear axis. Facilitation between perpendicular lines has been seen along the 45° axes. The implication of this finding is that the cortex is designed to assimilate the probable correlations present in the natural world. In the visual system, it helps the process of parsing the world into contours and surfaces belonging to objects and background. Linking one element in a scene with another is an ill-posed problem, unless one takes into account the likeliest solutions, based on experience of the way the world is put together. The structure of receptive fields is designed to signal which of the most probable correlations or forms are present in a given part of a scene.

3.4   Perceptual learning and top-down control

Contextual influences can be modified by experience, even in the adult visual cortex. This represents a sea change in our thinking about cortical

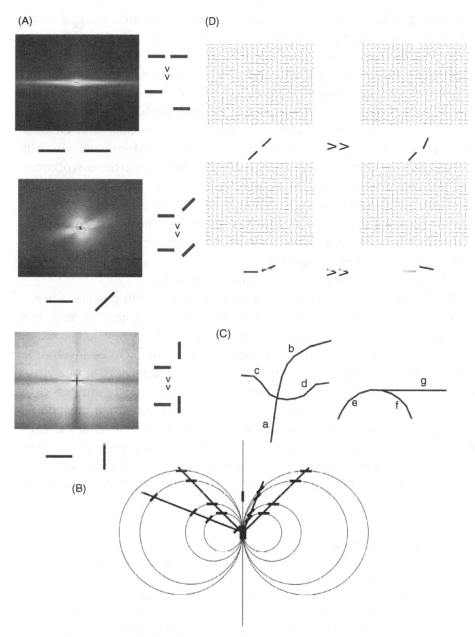

Figure 3.4 Relationship between contextual interactions, the geometry of natural scenes, and the Gestalt rule of good continuation. (A) From a library of natural scenes, the local orientation of contours at each location was determined, and correlated with the distribution of other line elements within the scenes. The most probable relationships occur between similarly oriented line elements, which extend for long distances along the same axis of orientation (*top panel*, brighter blue and red areas). Relationships of line elements of different relative orientation are shown in the other

plasticity. It is known that certain receptive field properties, such as ocular dominance, are altered by abnormal visual experience during a limited period in the first few months or years of life. The existence of this critical period led many to expect that all properties in primary visual cortex, and all connections, should be fixed in adulthood. But this idea was turned upside down by the finding that following CNS lesions, cortical areas are capable of changing their topography, with cells shifting their receptive fields. Following binocular retinal lesions, the area of cortex representing the lesioned area, the cortical scotoma, is initially silenced, but over time becomes remapped, with a shrinkage in the area of cortex representing the lesioned part of the retina and an expansion in the representation of the surrounding area (Gilbert *et al.*, 1990; Gilbert and Wiesel, 1992; Kaas *et al.*, 1990; Heinen and Skavenski, 1991). Associated with the remapping of cortex is a sprouting of the horizontal connections into the cortical scotoma (Darian-Smith and Gilbert, 1994), changing these inputs from a modulatory role, as described above, into a suprathreshold, driving influence.

The fact that cortical circuits can be modified in the adult provides a useful mechanism for functional recovery following stroke and neurodegenerative disease. But the underlying mechanisms undoubtedly evolved for processes occurring under normal visual experience. They are likely to be involved in different forms of learning, where we assimilate components of our visual experience, learning to recognize shapes and to discriminate differences in visual attributes. In the visual modality, the storage of information about object identity is thought to involve the temporal lobe – lesions of which can lead to an inability to recognize faces, a syndrome known as "prosopagnosia." But there are other forms of learning that are unconscious, known as "implicit learning," including improvement in one's ability to discriminate attributes such as line

---

Caption for Figure 3.4   (cont.)

panels. (B) All of these relationships fit within a single geometric rule – collinearity and cocircularity (adapted from Sigman *et al.*, 2001). Iso-oriented line segments occur collinearly, line segments of different orientation tend to fall along circles of constant radius of curvature. (C) This provides a mathematical basis for the Gestalt rule of "good continuation." The linkage of line elements tend to follow perceptual rules – lines (a) and (b), and lines (e) and (f) are seen as belonging to the same object, but not lines (a) and (d) or (e) and (g) (adapted from Wertheimer, 1923). (D) The geometric relationships shown in (A) and (B) are reflected in the salience of contours. One can readily see the line at top left or the circle at bottom left because the arrangement of their line elements follow collinearity and cocircularity. Putting jitter in the orientation of consecutive line elements breaks these rules and the contours are no longer visible (from Gilbert *et al.*, 2001) (for color image please see www.cambridge.org/9780521143400).

position or orientation. This is known as "perceptual learning." Implicit learning may be represented in a large number of cortical areas outside the temporal lobe, including primary sensory cortex (for review, see Gilbert *et al.*, 2001).

Perceptual learning has properties suggestive of the involvement of early stages in cortical processing. It is specific for the trained location in visual space and for the orientation of the stimuli used, pointing toward its representation in areas that have small receptive fields, that are visuotopically mapped and that show the sharpest orientation tuning, such as primary visual cortex. One plausible mechanism for perceptual learning is cortical recruitment, similar to what one observes following retinal lesions, a change in the magnification factor of cortex in the trained region. This relies on the idea of probability summation, where one improves signal-to-noise if there are more neurons involved in making the discrimination. However, other aspects of the specificity of perceptual learning mitigate against this idea. In one model of perceptual learning, three-line bisection, subjects are asked to report whether the central line of 3 parallel lines is located closer to the one on the left or the one on the right (Crist *et al.*, 1997; Figure 3.5). Above a threshold offset from the central position, subjects can consistently report one direction or the other. This threshold decreases by as much as a factor of 3 with repeated performing of the task, over a period of weeks. The task fails to transfer to other tasks involving the same line in the same visual field location, ones where the target line is the same but the context is different. For example, training on three-line bisection does not transfer to a vernier discrimination task where the context is a collinear line rather than two side-by-side flanking lines. One therefore has to look to other changes in receptive field properties that may underlie the learning.

Animals trained on the task showed improvement similar to that observed in humans. When comparing cortical properties in the hemisphere representing the trained location of the visual field with the hemisphere representing untrained locations, a number of properties were unchanged. The cortical maps in the two hemispheres were nearly identical, showing that cortical recruitment was in fact not the mechanism underlying the improvement in performance. The receptive fields had the same size and orientation selectivity, indicating that the properties related to the tuning to simple attributes and simple stimuli were also unchanged. There was a dramatic change, however, in the contextual tuning of the cells in the trained hemisphere. The change was specific to an attribute related to the task – the tuning to the separation between lines, one within the receptive field and a second, parallel line placed at varying distances from the first (Crist *et al.*, 2001; Figure 3.6).

But the most notable and dramatic aspect of this change is that it is task-dependent. That is, the increased modulation by the flanking line is seen only

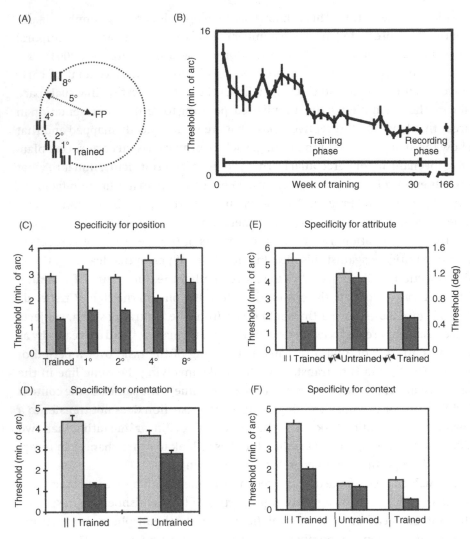

Figure 3.5 Perceptual learning – psychophysics. (A) Subjects were trained to discriminate the position of the central element of an array of three parallel lines in one visual field position, and were tested at that and several other positions. (B) The threshold in the task showed marked improvement, by up to a factor of 3. (C) The improvement was relatively specific for visual field location, (D) for the orientation of the lines, (E) for the trained attribute (position vs. orientation), and (F) for the same attribute but for a different context – a collinear line as opposed to lines in a side-by-side configuration.

when the animal is performing the trained task. The increased modulation disappeared when the animal performed an unrelated task, detecting the dimming of a spot at the fixation point. The contextual tuning for another attribute, the modulation in response by a collinear line placed at different offsets from

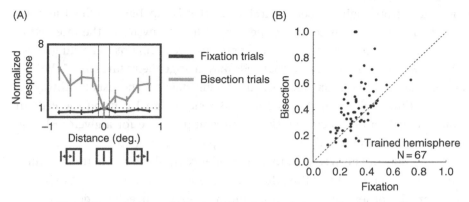

Figure 3.6 Perceptual learning – physiological changes in primary visual cortex. Recordings were made from alert animals trained on the three-line bisection task and on an unrelated task, detecting the dimming of a fixation spot. No changes were observed in the cells' receptive field size, orientation tuning, or in the visuotopic maps of the cortical areas representing the trained region of visual space. There was, however, a pronounced change in the tuning to a contextual stimulus related to that involved in the task: the modulation in the response to a line within the receptive field by a second parallel line outside the receptive field. Under fixation trials, the second line had an inhibitory influence (as was typically seen in the 2D contextual maps of untrained animals shown in Figure 3.3A). In trials where the animal was performing the three-line bisection task, however, the influence of the second line switched from being inhibitory to being facilitatory, and there was much more modulation in the response as the separation between the lines was changed. The effect of training selectively influenced an aspect of contextual tuning related to the trained task, and this influence was task–dependent, only being present when the animal was performing the trained task.

the central line, was unaffected. Taken together, the results show that there is a long-term change in receptive field properties in primary visual cortex resulting from perceptual learning, that the change operates in the domain of contextual influences, and that the change is gated on a trial-by-trial basis according to the perceptual task that the animal is currently performing. This level of top-down control shows how cells can multiplex their function by, in effect, loading a different program according to the immediate perceptual requirements.

At this stage, one can only speculate on the mechanisms of the functional correlates of perceptual learning in terms of the underlying circuitry. Because of the push–pull nature of the horizontal connections, altering the balance between excitation and inhibition in the horizontally evoked synaptic potentials for laterally placed inputs at different separations from the recorded cell can produce the modulation in the tuning to lines of different separation. Superimposed on this change, however, is a top-down control, possibly mediated by feedback

connections from higher order cortical areas, that is capable of gating the influence of the intrinsic horizontal connections. The biophysics of the interaction
between intrinsic inputs and feedback inputs to a cell remains to be studied. An
implication of this interaction is that cells may change their "line label," the way
in which their firing is interpreted by subsequent stages in the visual pathway. At
the same time that the higher order areas send a signal causing the cells in
primary visual cortex to change their tuning appropriate for a given task, the
signal emitted from these cells must be interpreted accordingly.

The relationship between contextual influences and the geometry of natural
scenes on the one hand and the effects of perceptual learning in primary visual
cortex on the other suggests a continuum of experience-dependent cortical
plasticity beginning early in postnatal life and continuing throughout adulthood. Early experience encodes the correlations existing in the natural world,
reflecting fundamental statistical regularities that are common to the experience of all individuals. Studies in children show that the ability to link elements
of the visual scene into global contours progresses over many years (Kovacs *et al.*,
1999; Kovacs, 2000). We continue this process throughout our lives to encode
information about shapes that have to be processed rapidly and in parallel. The
neural response properties appropriate to a given shape are likely to be unique
to each individual, depending on one's unique experiences and the particular
use to which we put a given set of visual stimuli.

These findings suggest that the kind of information represented by a given
cortical area may not be fixed, and that learning in part involves a shift in the
distribution of areas over which the learned information is represented. The
involvement of top-down influences in the representation of learned information suggests that perceptual learning involves an interaction between circuits,
including local circuits at early cortical stages and feedback connections coming
from higher order cortical areas.

References

Bakin, J. S., Nakayama, K., and Gilbert, C. D. (2000). Visual responses in monkey areas
V1 and V2 to three-dimensional surface configurations. *Journal of Neuroscience*, **20**,
8188–98.

Bosking, W. H., Zhang, Y., Schofield, B., and Fitzpatrick, D. (1997). Orientation
selectivity and arrangement of horizontal connections in tree shrew striate
cortex. *Journal of Neuroscience*, **17**, 2112–27.

Crist, R. E., Kapadia, M., Westheimer, G., and Gilbert, C. D. (1997). Perceptual learning
of spatial localization: specificity for orientation, position and context. *Journal of
Neurophysiology*, **78**(6), 2889–94.

Crist, R. E., Li, W., and Gilbert, C. D. (2001). Learning to see: experience and attention in primary visual cortex. *Nature Neuroscience*, **4**, 519–25.

Darian-Smith, C. and Gilbert, C. D. (1994). Axonal sprouting accompanies functional reorganization in adult cat striate cortex. *Nature*, **368**, 737–40.

Dresp, B. (1993). Bright lines and edges facilitate the detection of small line targets. *Spatial Vision*, **7**, 213–25.

Field, D. J., Hayes, A. and Hess, R. F. (1993) Contour integration by the human visual system: evidence for a local "association field." *Vision Research*, **33**, 173–93.

Geisler, W. S., Perry, J. S., Super, B. J., and Gallogly, D. P. (2001). Edge co-occurrence in natural images predicts contour grouping performance. *Vision Research*, **41**, 711–24.

Gilbert, C. D., Hirsch, J. A., and Wiesel, T. N. (1990). Lateral interactions in visual cortex. *Cold Spring Harbor Symposia on Quantitative Biology*, **55**, 663–77.

Gilbert, C. D., Sigman, M., and Crist, R. E. (2001). Neural basis of perceptual learning. *Neuron*, **31**, 681–97.

Gilbert, C. D. and Wiesel, T. N. (1979). Morphology and intracortical projections of functionally characterised neurones in the cat visual cortex. *Nature*, **280**, 120–5.

Gilbert, C. D. and Wiesel, T. N. (1983). Clustered intrinsic connections in cat visual cortex. *Journal of Neuroscience*, **3**, 1116–33.

Gilbert, C. D. and Wiesel, T. N. (1989). Columnar specificity of intrinsic horizontal and corticocortical connections in cat visual cortex. *Journal of Neuroscience*, **9**, 2432–42.

Gilbert, C. D. and Wiesel, T. N. (1992). Receptive field dynamics in adult primary visual cortex. *Nature*, **356**, 150–2.

Heinen, S. J. and Skavenski, A. A. (1991). Recovery of visual responses in foveal V1 neurons following bilateral foveal lesions in adult monkey. *Experimental Brain Research*, **83**, 670–4.

Kaas, J. H., Krubitzer, L. A., Chino, Y. M., et al.. (1990). Reorganization of retinotopic cortical maps in adult mammals after lesions of the retina. *Science*, **248**, 229–31.

Kapadia, M. K., Ito, M., Gilbert, C. D., and Westheimer, G. (1995). Improvement in visual sensitivity by changes in local context: parallel studies in human observers and in V1 of alert monkeys. *Neuron*, **15**, 843–56.

Kapadia, M. K., Westheimer, G., and Gilbert, C. D. (1999). Dynamics of spatial summation in primary visual cortex of alert monkeys. *Proceedings of the National Academy of Sciences USA*, **96**, 12073–8.

Kapadia, M. K., Westheimer, G., and Gilbert, C. D. (2000). Spatial distribution of contextual interactions in primary visual cortex and in visual perception. *Journal of Neurophysiology*, **84**, 2048–62.

Kovacs, I. (2000). Human development of perceptual organization. *Vision Research*, **40**, 1301–10.

Kovacs, I., Feher, A., and Benedek, G. (1999). Late maturation of visual spatial int. *Proceedings of the National Academy of Sciences USA*, **96**, 12204–9.

Kuffler, S. W. (1953) Discharge patterns and functional organization of mammalian retina. *Journal of Neurophysiology*, **16**, 37–68.

Malach, R., Amir, Y., Harel, M., and Grinvald, A. (1993). Relationship between intrinsic connections and functional architecture revealed by optical imaging and in vivo targeted biocytin injections in primate striate cortex. *Proceedings of the National Academy of Sciences*, **90**, 10469–73.

Martin, K. A. C. and Whitteridge, D. (1984). Form, function and intracortical projections of spiny neurones in the striate visual cortex of the cat. *Journal of Physiology*, **353**, 270–92.

Polat, U. and Sagi, D. (1993). Lateral interactions between spatial channels: suppression and facilitation revealed by lateral masking experiments. *Vision Research*, **33**, 993–9.

Polat, U. and Sagi, D. (1994). The architecture of perceptual spatial interactions. *Vision Resarch*, **28**, 115–32.

Rockland, K. S. and Lund, J. S. (1982). Widespread periodic intrinsic connections in the tree shrew visual cortex. *Brain Research*, **169**, 19–40.

Sceniak, M. P., Ringach, D. L., Hawken, M. J., and Shapley, R. (1999). Contrast's effect on spatial summation by macaque V1 neurons. *Nature Neuroscience*, **2**, 733–9.

Sigman, M., Cecchi, G., Gilbert, C. D., and Magnasco, M. (2001). On a common circle: natural scenes and Gestalt rules. *Proceedings of the National Academy of Sciences USA*, **98**(1), 935–1940.

Ullman, S. (1990). Three-dimensional object recognition. *Cold Spring Harbor Symposia on Quantitative Biology*, **55**, 889–98.

Weliky, M., Kandler, K., Fitzpatrick, D., and Katz, L. (1995). Patterns of excitation and inhibition evoked by horizontal connections in visual cortex share a common relationship to orientation columns. *Neuron*, **15**, 541–52.

Wertheimer, M. (1938). *Laws of Organization in Perceptual Forms*, London: Harcourt, Brace and Jovanovich.

4

Cortical mechanisms of visuospatial attention in humans and monkeys

SABINE KASTNER, PETER DE WEERD, AND LESLIE G. UNGERLEIDER

4.1   Introduction

In everyday life, the scenes we view are typically cluttered with many different objects. However, the capacity of the visual system to process information about multiple objects at any given moment in time is limited (Broadbent, 1958; Neisser, 1967; Schneider & Shiffrin, 1977; Tsotsos, 1990). This limited processing capacity can be exemplified in a simple experiment. If subjects are presented with two different objects and asked to identify two different attributes at the same time (e.g., color of one and orientation of the other), the subjects' performance is worse than if the task had been performed with only a single object (Duncan, 1980, 1984; Treisman, 1969). Hence, multiple objects present at the same time in the visual field compete for neural representation due to limited processing resources.

How can the competition among multiple objects be resolved? One way is by bottom-up, stimulus-driven processes. For example, in Figure 4.1A, the vertical line among the multiple distracter lines is effortlessly and quickly detected because of its salience in the display, which biases the competition in favor of the vertical line. Stimulus salience depends on various factors, including simple feature properties such as line orientation or color of the stimulus (Treisman & Gelade, 1980; Treisman & Gormican, 1988), perceptual grouping of stimulus features by Gestalt principles (Driver & Baylis, 1989; Duncan, 1984; Lavie & Driver, 1996; Prinzmetal, 1981), and the dissimilarity between the stimulus and nearby distracter stimuli (Duncan & Humphreys, 1989, 1992; Nothdurft, 1993).

In the display depicted in Figure 4.1B, the competition among the multiple lines is not resolved by salience, and one must actively search through the

Topics in Integrative Neuroscience: From Cells to Cognition, ed. James R. Pomerantz. Published by Cambridge University Press. © Cambridge University Press 2008.

(A)   (B)   (C)

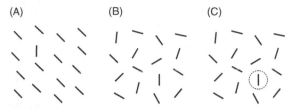

Figure 4.1   *Cluttered visual scenes.* Multiple stimuli present simultaneously in the visual field compete for neural representation due to the limited processing capacity of the visual system. This competition can be biased in several ways. One way is by bottom-up stimulus-driven factors, such as the salience of a stimulus (A). In a condition, in which the competition is not biased by stimulus salience (B), it can be biased by top-down processes such as directing attention to a particular stimulus location (depicted by the dashed circle in C). Processing of stimuli occurring at the attended location will be facilitated.

display to identify the vertical line (Treisman & Gelade, 1980; Wolfe *et al.*, 1989; Wolfe, 1994). In such cases, where target salience is low, it is possible to bias the competition among the multiple lines by top-down processes, such as spatially directed attention. For example, if one is spatially cued to attend to the target location, as depicted by the dashed circle in Figure 4.1C, the identification of the vertical line in that location will be facilitated (Bashinski & Bacharach, 1980; Posner, 1980). This result suggests that spatially directed attention enhances information processing at the attended location. In effect, attention operates to filter out irrelevant information from nearby distracters.

Selective attention to a spatial location has been shown to improve the accuracy and speed of subjects' responses to target stimuli that occur in that location (e.g., Posner, 1980). Attention also increases the perceptual sensitivity for the discrimination of target stimuli (Lu & Dosher, 1998), reduces the interference caused by distracters (Shiu & Pashler, 1995) and improves acuity (Carrasco & Yeshurun, 1998). In this review, we will describe mechanisms of selective attention that operate in the human and monkey visual cortex and may account for many of the known behavioral effects of attention. In particular, we will emphasize results from functional brain imaging studies in humans as they relate to results from single-cell recording studies in monkeys in the context of a biased competition model of attention (Bundesen, 1990; Desimone, 1998; Desimone & Duncan, 1995; Duncan, 1996, 1998; Harter & Aine, 1984). In the following sections, we will first describe the evidence for competition among multiple visual stimuli for neural representation. Second, we will describe mechanisms of attentional top-down modulation of sensory-evoked activity in visual cortical areas. Third, we will present evidence that visual cortical areas are sites where competition is resolved through top-down attentional modulation. And finally we will turn to the potential sources for generating and controlling these attentional top-down mechanisms.

4.2   The neural basis of competition for representation

4.2.1   *Organization of visual cortex*

Most of our knowledge about the organization of visual cortex comes from behavioral, anatomical, and physiological studies in monkeys. These studies have shown that the monkey cortex contains more than 30 separate visual areas (Felleman & Van Essen, 1991), which are organized into two functionally specialized processing pathways (Desimone & Ungerleider, 1989; Ungerleider, 1995; Ungerleider & Mishkin, 1982). Both pathways orginate in the primary visual cortex (V1) and both are composed of multiple areas beyond V1. The occipitotemporal pathway, or ventral stream, is crucial for the identification of objects, whereas the occipitoparietal pathway, or dorsal stream, is crucial for the appreciation of the spatial relations among objects as well as the visual guidance of movements toward objects in space (Goodale & Milner, 1992; Ungerleider & Mishkin, 1982).

Results from single-cell recordings from areas within the ventral and dorsal streams are consistent with this model of functional specialization. Thus, neurons in areas V4, TEO, and TE of the ventral stream show response selectivities for stimulus attributes important for object vision, such as shape, color, and texture (Desimone & Ungerleider, 1989). By contrast, neurons in area MT (middle temporal area) and further stations of the dorsal stream are not tuned for these stimulus attributes, but rather show response selectivity for the speed and direction of stimulus motion, consistent with the role of these areas in visuospatial function (Goldberg & Colby, 1989; Newsome & Salzman, 1990).

Within the ventral stream, or object vision pathway, the processing of information is largely hierarchical (Figure 4.2). For example, the processing of object features begins with simple spatial filtering by cells in V1, but by the time the inferior temporal cortex (area TE) is activated the cells respond selectively to global object features, such as shape, and some cells are even specialized for the analysis of faces (Desimone & Ungerleider, 1989). Likewise, the average receptive field (RF) size increases as one moves along the pathway toward the temporal lobe; at parafoveal eccentricities, RFs of neurons are about 1.5 degrees in V1, and about 4 degrees in V4, whereas neurons in area TE have a median RF size of 26 degrees $\times$ 26 degrees (Gattass *et al.*, 1981, 1988; Desimone & Ungerleider, 1989). It thus appears that large RFs in later areas are built up from smaller ones in earlier areas. Viewed in this way, it is possible to consider much of the neural mechanisms for object vision as a bottom-up process.

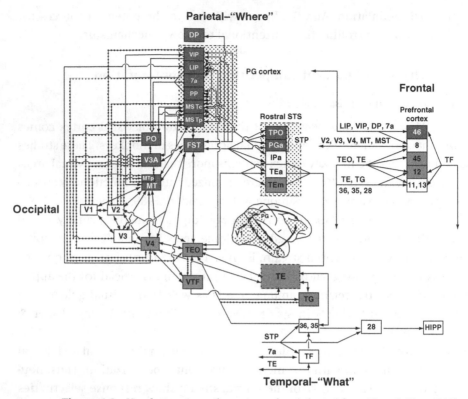

Figure 4.2 *Visual processing pathways in monkeys* (adapted from Ungerleider, 1995). Each box represents a functionally distinct visual area, based on differential architecture, patterns of connections, and physiological properties of neurons, and lines connecting boxes indicate interconnections between the areas. Solid lines indicate connections arising from both central and peripheral visual field representations; dotted lines indicate connections restricted to peripheral field representations. Light grey boxes indicate ventral stream areas related primarily to object vision; dark grey boxes indicate dorsal stream areas related primarily to spatial vision; and white boxes indicate areas not clearly allied with either stream. Closed arrowheads indicate feedforward projections from lower-order to higher-order visual areas, whereas open arrowheads indicate feedback projections from higher-order to lower-order visual areas. A line with two closed arrowheads indicates a connection between areas at the same level of the visual hierarchy. Dotted region on the lateral view of the brain represents the extent of the cortex included in the diagram.

Like the ventral stream, the early stations of the dorsal stream also have a hierarchical organization. For example, the processing of moving stimuli begins with simple direction-of-motion selectivity in V1 cells, but in the higher order areas of the parietal cortex the cells respond selectively to complex patterns of motion, such as rotation, and to the optic flow patterns produced when one moves through the environment (Andersen *et al.*, 1990; Duffy & Wurtz, 1991;

Tanaka & Saito, 1989). At the same time, the hierarchy probably gives way to parallel processing among numerous small cortical areas at the later stations of this pathway (Figure 4.2).

Anatomical studies reveal that virtually all connections between successive pairs of areas within both the ventral and dorsal streams are reciprocally connected, that is, projections from one area to the next are reciprocated by projections from the second area back onto the first (Felleman & Van Essen, 1991). Additionally, there exist other "feedback" projections to these two processing streams from prefrontal cortex (Cavada & Goldman-Rakic, 1989; Ungerleider et al., 1989; Webster et al., 1994). Feedback projections both within a processing stream and from areas beyond it may form the anatomical basis for top-down influences on visual perception. One prime example of a top-down influence is the effect of attention on object perception, that is, the selection of relevant objects in the visual scene for further processing. In this connection, it is noteworthy that feedback projection to the ventral stream arise from both prefrontal and parietal cortex.

Functional brain imaging studies have begun to reveal a remarkably similar organization within the human visual cortex. Functional brain imaging measures hemodynamic changes, blood flow in the case of positron emission tomography and blood oxygenation in the case of functional magnetic resonance imaging (fMRI), and these can be used as indirect measures of neural activity (Bandettini et al., 1992; Fox & Raichle, 1986; Kwong et al., 1992; Ogawa et al., 1992). The existence of separate processing streams has been tested by having subjects perform object identity and spatial localization tasks analogous to the tasks that have been used in monkeys (Haxby et al., 1994; Ungerleider & Haxby, 1994). These studies demonstrated regions activated in the ventral occipitotemporal cortex in the object identity tasks and regions activated in the dorsal occipitoparietal cortex in the spatial localization tasks, in agreement with the organization of the monkey cortex. Individual processing areas within the two streams have been identified on retinotopic or functional grounds, as outlined in the next section. These areas include V1, V2, V3, V3A, V4, and the middle temporal area (MT), many of which appear to be homologous to monkey visual areas (DeYoe et al., 1996; Engel et al., 1997; Schneider et al., 1993; Sereno et al., 1995; Tootell et al., 1995). Studies that have measured brain activation in tasks requiring the perception of color and faces tend to find foci in the vicinity of V4, as well as in more anterior ventral stream areas (Beauchamp et al., 1999; Hadjikhani et al., 1998; Halgren et al., 1999; Haxby et al., 1994; Kanwisher et al., 1997; Kleinschmidt et al., 1996; McCarthy et al., 1997; McKeefry & Zeki, 1997; Sakai et al., 1995; Zeki et al., 1991), all of which contain neurons selective for these features in the monkey (Desimone, 1991; Schein & Desimone, 1990; Zeki,

1978). Studies that have measured activation during perception of motion often find foci in areas associated with the dorsal stream, particularly in a region that seems homologous to monkey MT (Tootell *et al.*, 1995; Watson *et al.*, 1993; Zeki *et al.*, 1991), an area that contains a high proportion of neurons selective for visual motion (Desimone & Ungerleider, 1986; Maunsell & Van Essen, 1983; Zeki, 1974).

Functional brain imaging data in humans, like physiological data in monkeys, also argue for an increase in the complexity of processing as activity proceeds anteriorly through the ventral stream into the temporal lobe. Whereas posterior regions in the cortex are preferentially activated during the processing of object attributes, such as colors or scrambled objects and faces, more anterior regions are activated selectively during the processing of intact objects and faces (Grill-Spector *et al.*, 1998; Haxby *et al.*, 1994; Kanwisher *et al.*, 1997; Puce *et al.*, 1996). In addition, as described below, the RF sizes of neurons in human visual cortex have been shown to increase progressively from V1 to TEO, an area in the posterior inferior temporal cortex (Kastner *et al.*, 2001). Thus, like the monkey visual cortex, the visual cortex of humans appears to be organized hierarchically.

4.2.2   Sensory interactions among multiple visual stimuli

What are the neural correlates for competitive interactions among multiple objects in the visual field? Single-cell recording studies in the monkey have shed light on this question by comparing responses to a single visual stimulus presented alone in a neuron's RF with the responses to the same stimulus when a second one is presented simultaneously within the same RF (Moran & Desimone, 1985; Recanzone *et al.*, 1997; Reynolds *et al.*, 1999). This is illustrated in Figure 4.3A, where the responses of neurons in area V4 are shown under two different presentation conditions. In the first condition, a horizontal bar stimulus was presented alone to the neuron's RF eliciting a strong response. In the second condition, a second bar stimulus was presented simultaneously with the same horizontal bar within the RF; the resulting response to the paired stimuli was much smaller than to the single bar stimulus. This result indicates that two stimuli present at the same time within a neuron's RF are not processed independently, for, if they were, the responses to the two stimuli when presented together would have summed. Rather, the reduced response to the paired stimuli suggests that the two stimuli within the RF interacted with each other in a mutually suppressive way. Such sensory suppressive interactions have been shown in ventral stream areas including V4 and inferior temporal cortex (Miller *et al.*, 1993; Moran & Desimone, 1985; Reynolds *et al.*, 1999; Rolls & Tovee, 1995; Sato, 1989), and also in dorsal stream areas, including the

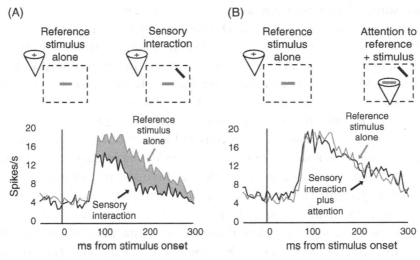

Figure 4.3 *Sensory suppression is counteracted by directed attention* (courtesy of J. Reynolds & R. Desimone, unpublished data). Single-cell recordings from area V4 (population responses). (A) Responses to a bar stimulus presented alone in a neuron's receptive field (RF – dashed rectangle) and to the same stimulus when it was presented with a second bar stimulus. The responses evoked by the paired stimuli were much smaller than the responses evoked by the single stimulus, suggesting sensory suppressive interactions between the two stimuli. (B) Reponses from the same population of neurons recorded during the same sensory stimulation conditions. However, this time the monkey directs attention to one of the stimuli (as indicated by the "focus of attention") and performs an orientation discrimination task. During directed attention to one of the two stimuli the responses were as large as if the attended stimulus had been presented alone, suggesting that attention eliminated the suppressive influence of the second stimulus in the RF.

MT and MST, the medial superior temporal area (Recanzone *et al.*, 1997). In MT/MST, the responses to an object moving in the preferred direction were smaller when it was paired with another object that was presented within the same RF and moved in a nonpreferred direction (Recanzone *et al.*, 1997). In both ventral and dorsal stream areas, it appears that the responses to the paired stimuli are best described as a weighted average of the responses to the individual stimuli when presented alone (Recanzone *et al.*, 1997; Reynolds *et al.*, 1999). Sensory suppressive interactions among multiple stimuli have been interpreted as an expression of competition for neural representation.

Based on hypotheses derived from these monkey physiology studies, we examined sensory suppression among multiple stimuli in the human cortex using fMRI (Kastner *et al.*, 1998, 2001). In these studies, hemodynamic changes as measured by fMRI were used as indirect measures of neural activity (Bandettini *et al.*, 1992; Kwong *et al.*, 1992; Ogawa *et al.*, 1992). Complex, colorful visual stimuli, known to evoke robust responses in ventral visual areas of the monkey brain, were presented in four nearby locations of the upper right quadrant of the visual field, while subjects maintained fixation (Kastner *et al.*, 1998). Having the subjects count the occurrences of Ts or Ls at fixation, an attentionally demanding task, ensured fixation. The stimuli were presented under two different presentation conditions, simultaneous and sequential. In the sequential presentation condition, a single stimulus appeared in one of the four locations, then another appeared in a different location, and so on, until each of the four stimuli had been presented in the different locations. In the simultaneous presentation condition, the same four stimuli appeared in the same four locations, but they were presented together. Thus, integrated over time, the physical stimulation parameters were identical in each of the four locations in the two presentation conditions. However, sensory suppression among stimuli within RFs could take place only in the simultaneous, not in the sequential, presentation condition. Based on the results from monkey physiology, we predicted that the fMRI signals would be smaller during the simultaneous than during the sequential presentation condition due to the presumed mutual suppression induced by the competitively interacting stimuli.

The visual areas that were consistently activated in striate and extrastriate cortex during visual stimulation as compared to blank periods were in the calcarine sulcus (Brodmann area [BA] 17), the lingual gyrus (BA 18), the fusiform gyrus (BA 19 and 37), the superior occipital gyrus (BA 19), and the lateral occipital sulcus (BA 19) of the left hemisphere. Activated voxels were assigned to retinotopically organized areas V1, V2, V4, TEO, V3A, and the MT complex (hereafter called area MT) by means of meridian mapping or upper and lower visual field topography, respectively, in a blocked design. Briefly, areas V1, V2, and VP were identified by determining the alternating representations of the vertical (VM) and horizontal (HM) meridians, which form the borders of these areas (e.g., Sereno *et al.*, 1995). Because the representations of the HM, forming the anterior border of V2, and the VM, forming the anterior border of VP, were overlapping in some of the subjects, it was difficult to separate V2 and VP in these subjects. Therefore, the activity was averaged across the two areas in all subjects; the combined region will be referred to as V2. Areas V4 and TEO were identified by their characteristic upper (UVF) and lower visual field (LVF) topography. The UVF and the LVF are separated in V4 and located medially and laterally, respectively, on the fusiform gyrus. This separation is not seen in the region just anterior to V4, which we term TEO (Kastner *et al.*, 1998, 2001). Area V4 in this study likely corresponds to area V4 of McKeefry and Zeki (1997) and

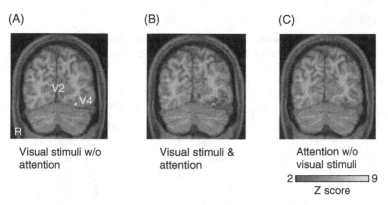

(A) (B) (C)

Visual stimuli w/o
attention

Visual stimuli &
attention

Attention w/o
visual stimuli

2 ▬▬▬▬▬ 9
Z score

Figure 4.4 *Activation in visual cortex during unattended, attended, or expected visual stimuli.*
Coronal brain slice of a single subject at a distance of 25 mm from the posterior pole
with overlaid functional activity. The subject was tested under three different conditions in the same scanning session. (A) Visual stimuli were presented to the periphery of
the visual field while the subject performed a letter counting task at fixation (unattended peripheral visual presentations). (B) Activations evoked by the same visual
stimuli used in the unattended condition, but when the subject covertly attended to
one of the peripheral stimuli performing a pattern discrimination task (attended peripheral visual presentations). A significantly larger brain volume was activated within
area V4. (C) Activation evoked by directing attention to a peripheral target location in
the expectation of stimulus onset. Area V4 is activated even in the absence of visual
stimulation. R indicates right hemisphere (for color image please see
www.cambridge.org/9780521143400).

appears to overlap with V4v and V0 described by Hadjikhani *et al.* (1998).
Activations in area V3A were identified on the basis of their location in dorsal
extrastriate cortex, where the UVF is represented among LVF representations of
other visual areas (Tootell *et al.*, 1997). Activations in area MT were identified
based on the characteristic anatomical location of this area at the junction of the
ascending limb of the inferior temporal sulcus and the lateral occipital sulcus
(e.g., Watson *et al.*, 1993). Activations for a single subject are illustrated on a
coronal section in Figure 4.4A.

As predicted by our hypothesis that stimuli presented together interact in a
mutually suppressive way, simultaneous presentations evoked weaker responses
than sequential presentations for single subjects in areas V4 and TEO and for all
subjects, as revealed in the group analysis, in all activated visual areas, as shown
by the averaged time series of fMRI signals (Figure 4.5A). The difference in activations between sequential and simultaneous presentations was smallest in V1 and
increased in magnitude toward ventral extrastriate areas V4 (Figure 4.5A) and
TEO, and dorsal extrastriate areas V3A and MT. This increase in magnitude of the
sensory suppression effects across visual areas suggests that the sensory interactions were scaled to the increase in RF size of neurons within these areas. That is,

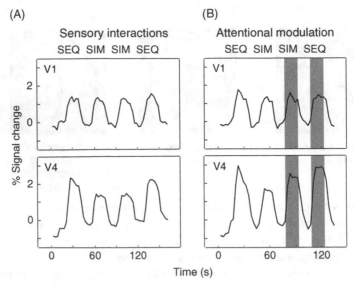

Figure 4.5 *Sensory suppression and attentional modulation in human visual cortex* (from Kastner *et al.*, 1998). (A) Sensory suppression in V1 and V4. As shown by the time series of fMRI signals, simultaneously presented stimuli evoked less activity than sequentially presented stimuli in V4, but not in V1. This finding suggests that sensory suppressive interactions were scaled to the receptive field size of neurons in visual cortex. Presentation blocks were 18 seconds. (B) Attentional modulation of sensory suppression. The sensory suppression effect in V4 was replicated in the unattended condition of this experiment, when the subjects' attention was directed away from the stimulus display (unshaded time series). Spatially directed attention (gray-shaded time series) increased responses to simultaneously presented stimuli to a larger degree than to sequentially presented ones in V4. Presentation blocks were 15 seconds.

the small RFs of neurons in V1 and V2 would encompass only a small portion of the visual display, whereas the larger RFs of neurons in V4, TEO, V3A, and MT would encompass all four stimuli. Therefore, suppressive interactions among the stimuli within RFs could take place most effectively in these more anterior extrastriate visual areas. In V1 and V2, it is likely that surround inhibition from regions outside the classical RF contributed to the small sensory suppressive effects observed (Knierim & Van Essen, 1992). Another possibility is that the complex, colorful stimuli we chose were more effective for activating areas V4 and TEO than areas V1 and V2, and therefore these stimuli were more likely to induce sensory suppression in the former areas.

To directly test the idea that sensory suppressive interactions are scaled to RF size, we undertook a second study in which the spatial separation between the four stimuli was increased (Kastner *et al.*, 2001). According to the RF hypothesis, the magnitude of sensory suppression should be inversely related to the degree

Table 4.1. *Receptive field sizes in monkey visual cortex and estimated receptive field sizes in human visual cortex at 5.5° eccentricity*

Area	Human	Monkey[a]
V1	<2	1.5
V2/VP	2–4	2.5
V4	4–6	4
TEO	>7[b]	8
V3A	>6[b]	?

[a] Gattass *et al.* (1981, 1988), Van Essen *et al.* (1984), and Boussaoud *et al.* (1991).

[b] Confined to a quadrant.

of spatial separation among the stimuli. In agreement with this idea, separating the stimuli by 4 degrees abolished sensory suppressive interactions in V2, reduced them in V4, but did not affect them in TEO. Separating the stimuli by 6 degrees led to a further reduction of sensory suppression in V4, but again had no effect in TEO. By systematically varying the spatial separation among the stimuli and measuring the magnitude of suppressive interactions, it was possible to get an estimate of average RF sizes across several areas in the human visual cortex. From these experiments, we estimated that, at an eccentricity of about 5 degrees, RF sizes were less than 2 degrees in V1, in the range of 2–4 degrees in V2, and about 6 degrees in V4. In TEO, the RFs were larger than in V4, but still confined to a single quadrant of the contralateral hemifield (Kastner *et al.*, 2001). It should be noted that these numbers may underestimate RF sizes due to additional suppressive influences from beyond the RF, which cannot be distinguished from interactions within RFs in our experimental paradigm. In monkeys, RF sizes have been defined at the level of single cells, whereas we have measured hemodynamic responses, that is, BOLD contrast, to determine RF sizes in the human visual cortex. Even though there are several important differences between these two methods, it was striking that these estimates of RF sizes in human visual cortex are similar to those measured in the homologous visual areas of monkeys (Table 4.1; Boussaoud *et al.*, 1991; Gattass *et al.*, 1981, 1988; Van Essen *et al.*, 1984). The results in humans need to be extended in future studies that will investigate RF sizes at different eccentricities.

In summary, these fMRI studies have begun to establish in the human visual cortex a neural basis for competition among multiple stimuli present at the same time in the visual field. Importantly, the degree to which this competition occurs appears to critically depend on the RF sizes of neurons across visual cortical areas. The role of additional factors in the competition, such as stimulus-driven bottom-up influences (e.g., stimulus contrast; Reynolds *et al.*, 2000) or the selectivity of neuronal populations to process certain stimulus features (e.g., color, motion), remains to be investigated.

4.3   Attentional response modulation in visual cortex

Converging evidence from single-cell recording studies in monkeys and functional brain imaging and event-related potential (ERP) studies in humans indicates that endogenous spatially directed attention can modulate neural processing in visual cortex. The first evidence of attentional modulation of visually evoked activity was provided by electrophysiological studies of selective attention in humans (Eason *et al.*, 1969; Van Voorhis & Hillyard, 1977). In single-cell recording studies in monkeys, neural responses to visual stimuli presented within a neuron's RF have been studied under conditions in which the animal covertly (i.e., without executing eye movements) directs its attention to a stimulus within the RF, or when the animal directs its attention away from the RF to another location in the visual field. Several studies have shown that neural responses to a single stimulus presented within the RF are enhanced when the animal directs its attention within the RF compared to when the animal attends outside the RF. This effect, which increases with task difficulty (Spitzer *et al.*, 1988; Spitzer & Richmond, 1991), has been demonstrated in V1 (Motter, 1993), in V2 (Luck *et al.*, 1997; Motter, 1993), in ventral extrastriate area V4 (Connor *et al.*, 1996, 1997; Haenny *et al.*, 1988; Luck *et al.*, 1997; McAdams & Maunsell, 1999; Motter, 1993; Reynolds *et al.*, 2000; Spitzer *et al.*, 1988), and in dorsal extrastriate areas MT/MST (Treue & Martinez, 1999; Treue & Maunsell, 1996) and LIP (Bushnell *et al.*, 1981; Colby *et al.*, 1996). This finding suggests that mechanisms of spatial attention operate by enhancing neural responses to stimuli at attended locations, thereby biasing information processing in favor of stimuli appearing at that location.

Similar results have been found in functional brain imaging and ERP studies in the human visual cortex. In these experiments, identical visual stimuli were presented simultaneously to corresponding peripheral field locations to the right and left of fixation, while subjects were instructed to direct attention covertly to the right or the left. Directing attention to the left hemifield led to increased stimulus-evoked activity in extrastriate visual areas of the right hemisphere, whereas directing attention to the right hemifield led to increased activity in extrastriate visual areas of the left hemisphere (Heinze *et al.*, 1994; Vandenberghe *et al.*, 1997). Thus, responses to the stimuli were enhanced on the side of extrastriate cortex containing the representations of the attended hemi-field. Response enhancement due to spatially directed attention that was found with ERP recordings from electrodes placed over extrastriate cortex occurred as early as 80–130 ms after stimulus onset (Heinze et al., 1994; Hillyard et al., 1998; Mangun, 1995; Mangun et al., 1998).

Thus far, we have considered that spatial attention enhances neural responses to a single stimulus at an attended location. However, a typical visual scene contains multiple stimuli that are often cluttered together in nearby locations, each competing for processing resources. As we have described above, competition among multiple stimuli in nearby locations for representation is evidenced by mutually suppressive sensory interactions that take place most effectively at the level of the RF; such interactions were demonstrated in both single-cell recording (Recanzone et al., 1997; Reynolds et al., 1999) and fMRI studies (Kastner et al., 1998, 2001). What is the role of spatially directed attention in this competition?

4.3.1   Filtering of unwanted information

Single-cell recording studies have demonstrated that spatially directed attention can bias the competition among multiple stimuli in favor of one of the stimuli by modulating sensory suppressive interactions. In particular, in extra-striate areas V2 and V4 it was shown that spatially directed attention to an effective stimulus within a neuron's RF eliminated the suppressive influence of a second ineffective stimulus presented within the same RF (Reynolds et al., 1999). This is illustrated in Figure 4.3B. When a monkey directed attention to one of two competing stimuli within a RF, the responses of V4 neurons were as large as those to that stimulus presented alone. The attentional effects were less pronounced when the second stimulus was presented outside the RF, suggesting that competition for processing resources within visual cortical areas takes place most strongly at the level of the RF. Similarly, in areas MT/MST, attentional response enhancement was found to be strongest when two stimuli rather than one stimulus moved through the RFs of neurons (Recanzone & Wurtz, 2000). These findings imply that attention may resolve the competition among multiple stimuli by counteracting the suppressive influences of nearby stimuli, thereby enhancing information processing at the attended location. This may be an important mechanism by which attention filters out unwanted information from cluttered visual scenes (Desimone, 1996; Desimone & Duncan, 1995).

Our fMRI studies suggest that a similar mechanism operates in the human visual cortex (Kastner et al., 1998). We studied the effects of spatially directed attention on multiple competing visual stimuli in a variation of the paradigm we used to examine sensory suppressive interactions among simultaneously presented stimuli, described above. In addition to the two different visual presentation conditions, sequential and simultaneous, two different attentional conditions were tested, where the peripheral stimuli were unattended or attended. During the unattended condition, attention was directed away from the peripheral visual display by having subjects count Ts or Ls at fixation, exactly as in our original study. In the attended condition, subjects were instructed to attend covertly to the peripheral stimulus location closest to fixation in the display and to count the occurrences of one of the four stimuli, which was indicated before the scan started. Based on the results from monkey physiology, we predicted that attention should reduce sensory suppression among stimuli. Thus, responses evoked by the competing, simultaneously presented stimuli should be enhanced more strongly than responses evoked by the noncompeting sequentially presented stimuli (Chelazzi *et al.*, 1993, 1998; Luck *et al.*, 1997; Moran & Desimone, 1985; Reynolds *et al.*, 1999; Treue & Maunsell, 1996).

The same areas in striate and extrastriate cortex were activated during both the unattended and attended condition, including V1, V2, V4, TEO, V3A, and MT. However, in the attended condition, activated volumes increased significantly in V4, TEO, V3A, and MT. The volume increase in V4 is illustrated for a single subject in Figure 4.4B. As illustrated in Figure 4.5B for area V4, directing attention to the location closest to fixation in the display enhanced responses to both the sequentially and the simultaneously presented stimuli. This finding confirmed the effects of attentional response enhancement shown in numerous previous studies in monkeys and humans, as cited above. More importantly, and in accordance with our prediction from monkey physiology, directed attention led to greater increases of fMRI signals to simultaneously presented stimuli than to sequentially presented stimuli. Additionally, the magnitude of the attentional effect scaled with the magnitude of the suppressive interactions among stimuli, with the strongest reduction of suppression occurring in ventral extrastriate areas V4 (Figure 4.5B) and TEO, suggesting that the effects scaled with RF size. These findings support the idea that directed attention enhances information processing of stimuli at the attended location by counteracting suppression induced by nearby stimuli, which compete for limited processing resources. In essence, unwanted distracting information is effectively filtered out.

In contrast to ventral extrastriate areas, in dorsal extrastriate areas V3A and MT, spatially directed attention led to comparable increases of activity to sequentially and simultaneously presented stimuli, indicating that the spatial filter mechanism did not operate within these areas. Because we used visual stimuli that activated ventral areas more effectively than dorsal areas, this finding suggests that the spatial filtering of unwanted information depends not only on RF size but also on the selectivity of neural populations to process preferred stimulus features.

It has been shown that attentional response enhancement in visual cortex occurs in the representations of the attended locations, that is, the attentional effects are retinotopically organized and spatially specific (Brefczynski & DeYoe, 1999; Tootell et al., 1998). In accordance with these findings, the attentional response modulation found with our paradigm was topographically organized, inasmuch as it was seen only in visual areas with a representation of the attended location (i.e., the upper right quadrant; see Figure 4.4B).

Importantly, the attentional response enhancement to both simultaneously and sequentially presented stimuli appeared to increase from early to later stages of visual processing. Attentional effects were absent or small in V1 and V2, respectively, and much stronger in more anterior extrastriate areas V4 and TEO, suggesting that the latter areas were the primary target of the attentional top-down biasing signals. Single-cell recording studies have shown that neural responses can be modulated by attention as early as in V1 (Motter, 1993; Roelfsema et al., 1998), and functional brain imaging studies have demonstrated attentional response modulation in V1 with moving (Ghandi et al., 1999; Somers et al., 1999; Watanabe et al., 1998a,b) and stationary stimuli (Martinez et al., 1999). Yet, in all of these studies, the magnitude of the attentional response modulation in V1 was smaller than that in more anterior extrastriate areas, suggesting that attentional effects in V1 may be caused by reactivation from higher order extrastriate areas (Martinez et al., 1999). This idea is supported by single-cell recording studies, which have shown that attentional effects in area TE of inferior temporal cortex have a latency of about 150 ms (Chelazzi et al., 1998), whereas attentional effects in V1 have a longer latency of about 230 ms (Roelfsema et al., 1998). However, experiments by Recanzone and Wurtz (2000) suggest that it takes several hundred milliseconds for the attentional effects found in areas MT/MST to be fully effective. Thus, an alternative view is that the latency differences found in these attention studies is not due to top-down feedback mechanisms but rather reflect local computations within areas. For example, facilitatory or suppressive effects of stimuli from beyond the classical RF on responses to stimuli shown in the RF occur with a delay (e.g., Knierim & Van Essen, 1992). This contextual response modulation has been attributed to local circuits within an area.

4.3.2   Increases of baseline activity

There is evidence that attentional biasing signals can be obtained not only for the modulation of visually driven activity, but also in the absence of any visual stimulation whatsoever. As illustrated in Figure 4.6, there was a moderate increase in spontaneous (baseline) firing rates in V2 neurons when the animal was cued to attend covertly to a location within the neuron's RF before the

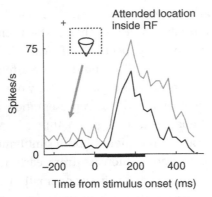

Figure 4.6 *Attention-related increases in spontaneous firing rates of neurons in area V4* (courtesy of J. Reynolds & R. Desimone, unpublished data). Single-cell recordings from a neuron in area V4. Spontaneous firing rates increased when the animal was cued to direct attention to the receptive field (RF) in anticipation of a stimulus onset compared to spontaneous firing rates when the animal attended elsewhere. These attention-related increases of baseline firing rates were interpreted as pure top-down signals, biasing neurons in favor of the attended location.

stimulus was presented there; that is, in the absence of visual stimulation. This increased baseline activity, termed the "baseline shift," has also been found in area V4 (Luck *et al.*, 1997) and in dorsal stream area LIP (Colby *et al.*, 1996). This attentional effect has been interpreted as a direct demonstration of a top-down signal that feeds back from higher order to lower order areas. In the latter areas, this feedback signal appears to bias neurons representing the attended location, thereby favoring stimuli that will appear there at the expense of those appearing at unattended locations. Thus, stimuli at attended locations are biased to "win" the competition for processing resources (Bundesen, 1990; Desimone, 1996; Desimone & Duncan, 1995; Duncan, 1996, 1998; Harter & Aine, 1984).

We studied attentional biasing signals in the human visual cortex in the absence of visual stimulation by adding a third experimental condition to the design used to investigate sensory suppressive interactions and their modulation by attention (Kastner *et al.*, 1999). In addition to the two visual presentation conditions, sequential and simultaneous, and the two attentional conditions, unattended and attended, an expectation period preceding the attended presentations was introduced. The expectation period, during which subjects were required to direct attention covertly to the target location and instructed to expect the occurrences of the stimulus presentations, was initiated by a marker presented briefly next to the fixation point 11 seconds before the onset of the stimuli. In this way, the effects of attention in the presence (ATT in Figure 4.7) and absence (EXP in Figure 4.7) of visual stimulation could be studied.

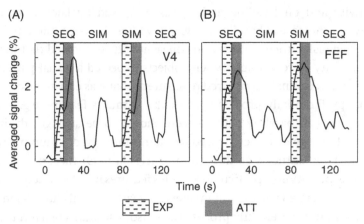

Figure 4.7 *Increases of baseline activity in the absence of visual stimulation* (adapted from Kastner *et al.*, 1999). (A) Time series of fMRI signals in V4. Directing attention to a peripheral target location in the absence of visual stimulation led to an increase of baseline activity (textured blocks), which was followed by a further increase after the onset of the stimuli (gray-shaded blocks). Baseline increases were found in both striate and extrastriate visual cortex. (B) Time series of fMRI signals in FEF. Directing attention to the peripheral target location in the absence of visual stimulation led to a stronger increase in baseline activity than in visual cortex; the further increase of activity after the onset of the stimuli was not significant. Sustained activity was seen in a distributed network of areas outside the visual cortex, including SPL, FEF, and SEF, suggesting that these areas may provide the source for the attentional top-down signals seen in visual cortex.

We found that, during the expectation period preceding the attended presentations, regions within visual areas with a representation of the attended location were activated. This activity was related to directing attention to the target location in the absence of visual stimulation (see activation of area V4 for a single subject in Figure 4.4C). Notably, the increase in activity during expectation was topographically specific, inasmuch as it was only seen in areas with a spatial representation of the attended location. As illustrated for area V4 in Figure 4.7A, the fMRI signals increased during the expectation period (textured epochs in the figure), before any stimuli were present on the screen. This increase of baseline activity was followed by a further increase of activity evoked by the onset of the stimulus presentations (gray shaded epochs in the figure). The baseline increase was found in all visual areas with a representation of the attended location. It was strongest in V4, but was also seen in early visual areas. It is noteworthy that baseline increases were found in V1, even though no significant attentional modulation of visually evoked activity was seen in this area. This dissociation suggests that different mechanisms underlie the effects of attention on visually evoked activity and on baseline activity, as suggested by Luck *et al.* (1997). Importantly, the increase in baseline activity in V1 has also been found to depend on the expected task difficulty. Ress and colleagues (2000) showed that increases in baseline activity were stronger when subjects expected a visual pattern that was difficult to discriminate compared to a pattern that was easy to discriminate. In areas that preferentially process a particular stimulus feature (e.g., color or motion), increases in baseline activity were shown to be stronger during the expectation of a preferred compared to a nonpreferred stimulus feature (Chawla *et al.*, 1999; Kastner *et al.*, 2000; Shulman *et al.*, 1999). Increases in activity caused by the expectation of particular stimulus features may be closely related to neural signals associated with visual imagery; the latter signals have been found in visual areas that preferentially process the sensory stimulus (Ishai *et al.*, 2000; Kosslyn *et al.*, 1995; O'Craven & Kanwisher, 2000).

The baseline increases found in human visual cortex (Chawla *et al.*, 1999; Kastner *et al.*, 1999, 2000; Shulman *et al.*, 1999) may be subserved by increases in spontaneous firing rate similar to those found in the single-cell recording studies (Colby *et al.*, 1996; Luck *et al.*, 1997), but summed over large populations of neurons. The increases evoked by directing attention to a target location in anticipation of a behaviorally relevant stimulus at that attended location are thus likely to reflect a top-down feedback bias in favor of the attended location in human visual cortex.

In summary, neural activity in visual cortex is modulated by spatially directed attention. Biasing signals due to spatial attention affect neural processing *in several ways*. These include: enhancement of neural responses to an attended stimulus; the filtering of unwanted information by counteracting the suppression induced by nearby distracters; and the biasing of signals in favor of an attended location by increases of baseline activity in the absence of visual stimulation.

4.4   The role of areas V4 and TEO in filtering irrelevant information

In the imaging study described earlier, it was found that spatially directed attention reduced the sensory suppressive effects of multiple competing stimuli (Kastner *et al.*, 1998). Further, attentional response enhancement increased from early to later stages of visual processing, with the strongest effects found in areas V4 and TEO. These findings suggest that these extrastriate visual areas are important sites where attentional top-down signals can bias competition among stimuli and effectively filter out irrelevant information. If so, then damage to areas V4 and TEO should impair the ability to use attention to ignore distracting stimuli when they are presented close to a behaviorally relevant target stimulus in a visual array. We tested this hypothesis by

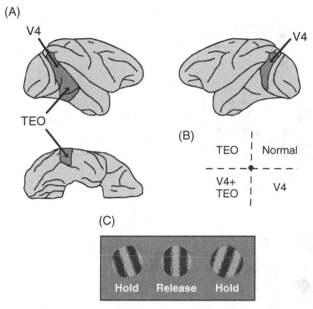

Figure 4.8 *Extent of V4 and TEO lesions in monkeys* (adapted from De Weerd *et al.*, 1999). (A) Lateral view of the left hemisphere showing a lesion (in dark shading) in the dorsal part of V4 and lateral and ventral views of the right hemisphere showing a lesion in the dorsal part of V4 and in TEO. (B) Distribution of lesion effects in the four quadrants of the visual field, derived from retinotopy in areas V4 and TEO. (C) Task and stimuli used in the experiments. Monkeys were rewarded for releasing a bar when the stimulus was vertical, and holding the bar for any other orientation.

examining the ability of monkeys with lesions of areas V4 and TEO to ignore distracters while performing a visual discrimination task (De Weerd *et al.*, 1999).

We prepared two monkeys with retinotopic "mosaic" lesions of areas V4 and TEO, such that the dorsal portion of V4 was removed bilaterally, thereby affecting the lower quadrant of both hemifields, and all of TEO was removed unilaterally, thereby affecting the upper and lower quadrants of the contralateral hemifield. As shown in Figure 4.8, this resulted in a V4-affected quadrant, a TEO-affected quadrant, a combined V4 + TEO-affected quadrant, and a normal intact quadrant. By having the monkeys fixate a central fixation spot, we could then compare their visual discrimination performance in each lesion-affected quadrant to their performance in the normal quadrant, both in the absence and in the presence of irrelevant distracters.

Monkeys were first trained to discriminate the orientation of gratings contained within a circular disk. They were rewarded for releasing a bar for a

(A)

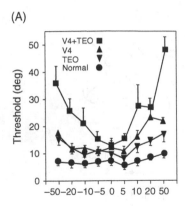

(B)

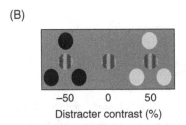

Distracter contrast (%)

Figure 4.9 *Effects of distracter contrast on grating orientation discrimination* (adapted from De Weerd *et al.*, 1999). (A) Grating orientation thresholds as a function of distracter contrast in each visual field quadrant for the two monkeys averaged. Grating contrast, the contrast between dark and light stripes, was 50%. Distracter contrast was defined as the contrast between distracter and background luminances (Michelson index), which were in the mesopic range. There were nine distracter conditions, ranging from −50% to +50%. Vertical bars indicate standard deviations. (B) Example of conditions with dark distracters (−50% contrast), bright distracters (50% contrast), and without distracters (0% contrast). Distracter positions were varied, but the grating's position was constant. Typical V4 and TEO cells contain the target and much of the distracters in their RF (see Table 4.1).

vertically oriented grating and holding the bar for any orientation other than vertical. In this way, we could measure their orientation thresholds, the smallest detectable difference they could discriminate. The thresholds were measured with a staircase procedure (Wetherill & Levitt, 1965) which estimated the 84% correct point of the psychometric distribution. Distracters, three luminance disks surrounding the target grating, were then added to the display and we manipulated their contrast by increasing or decreasing their brightness relative to the background.

The effect of distracter contrast on grating orientation in the three lesion-affected quadrants and the normal quadrant is shown, averaged over the two monkeys, in Figure 4.9. As predicted, in the three lesion-affected quadrants, orientation thresholds for target gratings (of 50% contrast) were larger with surrounding distracters than without. Further, the severity of the deficit increased as a function of the contrast of the distracters, with the brightest and darkest luminance distracters having the greatest effect. In contrast to the lesion-affected quadrants, in the normal quadrant, orientation thresholds were unaffected by the distracters, indicating that in the intact quadrant the animals could use attention to filter out the irrelevant distracters. Threshold increases were more pronounced in the visual field quadrant affected by lesions in both areas V4 and TEO (V4 + TEO-affected quadrant) than in quadrants affected by a lesion in V4 or TEO alone. This suggests that the loss of one of these extrastriate areas can be partially compensated for by the other.

The distracter-induced impairment on grating discrimination found in our study is remarkably similar to the impairment recently demonstrated in a patient with a putative V4 lesion (Gallant et al., 2000). Our data are also in agreement with two previous studies, which reported impairments in detecting a target less salient (dimmer or smaller) than surrounding elements in monkeys with V4 lesions (Schiller, 1993; Schiller & Lee, 1991). Together, these studies point to an inability to filter out distracting information after removal of V4 and/or TEO.

If impairments caused by distracters in the lesion-affected quadrants reflected competition between stimuli no longer biased by attention (or biased to a lesser extent), then impairments should be observed for any combination in which target grating contrast is much lower than distracter contrast. Likewise, performance should be restored by increasing target grating contrast above that of the distracters. In addition, without distracters, there should be no competition and hence performance should be stable in lesion-affected quadrants when grating contrast is decreased. These predictions were tested by varying both grating and distracter contrast simultaneously (De Weerd et al., 1999).

Figure 4.10 illustrates the results of this experiment for the quadrant affected by the combined V4 and TEO lesion. Orientation thresholds in this quadrant increased by about 40 degrees above baseline when distracters of 50% contrast were placed around a grating of similar contrast, in agreement with the results of the previous experiment. When the contrast of the grating was reduced below that of the distracters, further threshold increases were observed and, ultimately, thresholds were raised beyond a measurable range. Thus, the monkeys were severely impaired in discriminating a grating surrounded by distracters of equal or higher contrast. When weak distracters (10% contrast) surrounded the grating, however, and when the contrast of the grating exceeded that of the distracters, orientation thresholds were only slightly elevated compared to thresholds obtained with the grating presented alone. Thus, increasing the contrast of the target grating relative to that of the distracters enabled the monkeys to perform the task quite well. Indeed, under those conditions, they

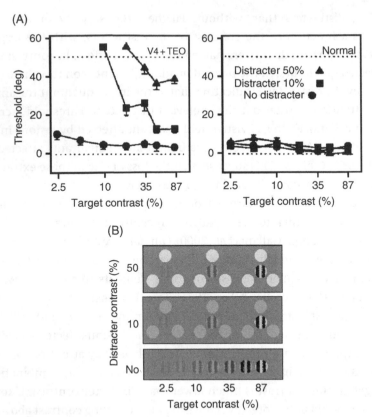

Figure 4.10 *Effects of grating and distracter contrast on grating orientation discrimination* (adapted from De Weerd *et al.*, 1999). (A) Orientation grating thresholds as a function of target grating contrast (log scale) in the presence and absence of distracters in the V4 + TEO-affected and normal quadrants for the two monkeys averaged. Threshold increases were calculated by subtracting the average baseline threshold in a given quadrant, obtained from separate measurements without distracters at 50–87% grating contrast, from each individual threshold collected within that quadrant in each monkey, after which the data were pooled over monkeys. Symbols above upper dotted lines indicate conditions in which no threshold could be determined in at least half of the measurements. Data for different distracter conditions were obtained in separate experiments, during which grating contrast was decreased from session to session. (B) Examples of stimuli used in the experiment, with three distracter conditions (no distracters, 10%, and 50% distracter contrast) and seven grating contrasts, ranging from 2.5 to 87% contrast.

could see, "attend to," and discriminate the grating almost as well as a normal monkey. In sum, the data suggest that the activity in visual areas that process stimuli placed in the combined V4 + TEO-affected quadrant was dominated by the higher contrast stimulus, regardless of whether it was the target or the distracter. This implies that the ability of the animals to use attention to selectively process one stimulus over another in the V4 + TEO lesion-affected quadrant was lost. Similar but less pronounced effects were observed in the two quadrants affected by the V4 and TEO lesions alone (data not illustrated). These behavioral data are in accord with recent physiological results, demonstrating that when attention is absent (i.e., directed away from the RF) neuronal responses in V4 to a pair of stimuli within the RF are dominated by the stimulus that has the higher contrast (Reynolds et al., 2000).

The results in the three lesion-affected quadrants were strikingly different from the results in the normal quadrant, in which the monkeys could easily attend to the grating's orientation at all contrast levels, in spite of strong distracters (Figure 4.10). This shows that, under normal conditions, attention can put a physically weak stimulus at a competitive advantage against strong distracters. It is important to note that, in the absence of distracters, decreases in the contrast of the target grating induced threshold increases in the three lesion-affected quadrants that were comparable to those in the normal quadrant. The data thus indicate that contrast sensitivity in these monkeys can be considered normal. Together with the findings that grating acuity was virtually unimpaired and that there was good-to-excellent discriminative ability in the absence of distracters, the data suggest that the distracter-induced threshold increases are unlikely to be sensory in nature. Furthermore, because the discrimination of a low-contrast grating is an attention-demanding task, it does not appear that the lesions caused a general, nonspecific loss of attentional capacity. Instead, the lesions specifically impaired the use of attention to resolve competition among multiple stimuli.

In both neurophysiological and imaging studies, both competitive interactions among stimuli and the resolution of competition by attention have been shown to take place at the level of the RF (Kastner et al., 1998; Reynolds et al., 1999). Accordingly, one would predict that, in monkeys with V4 and TEO lesions, if the distracters were moved a sufficient distance from the target, such that the target and distracters would not be contained within a typical RF in V4 or TEO, then the distracters should not influence target discriminations. We tested this prediction by systematically varying the distance between target and distracters using stimulus arrays of different sizes in the V4-affected and TEO-affected quadrants (De Weerd et al., 1999).

The results of this experiment showed that for a 5.6 by 5.6 degree array size, threshold increases were similar in the V4-affected and in the TEO-affected quadrants, presumably because the array was small enough to be contained within typical RFs in both V4 and TEO. Compared to the 5.6 degree array size, the effect of distracters for array sizes of 7.5 and 9 degrees was strongly reduced in the V4-affected quadrant, but not in the TEO-affected quadrant. In the TEO-affected quadrant, a significant reduction of the distracter effect was observed only when the distracters were placed outside that quadrant. In the normal quadrant, no effect of the distracters was found. Thus, distracter-induced deficits caused by V4 and TEO lesions were maximal for stimulus arrays contained within their respective typical RFs (see Table 4.1), and then decreased as stimulus arrays significantly exceeded those typical RF sizes. These data, like those from neuroimaging (Kastner *et al.*, 2001), indicate that the RF size in a given visual area sets an upper limit for the spatial extent over which competitive interactions among stimuli can occur.

In summary, fine perceptual analysis of a stimulus requires selective attention when distracters are present. After lesions of extrastriate areas V4 and TEO, top-down biasing signals are no longer operational to filter irrelevant distracters so that relevant, albeit less salient, visual targets can be processed. Instead, processing resources are devoted to whichever stimulus, be it the target or the distracter, is more salient. Thus, in the absence of attention, performance is governed by bottom-up sensory-driven inputs. Although the data point to the crucial importance of areas V4 and TEO as a substrate for the interaction between top-down and bottom-up signals, as we discuss in the next section, the source of the top-down biasing signals is likely to be a network of fronto-parietal areas that modulates competition among stimuli in these extrastriate visual areas (for review, see Kastner & Ungerleider, 2000). Friedman-Hill *et al.* (2000) recently provided support for this idea by demonstrating that patient RM, who has a bilateral parietal lesion, is impaired in target-distracter tasks similar to the ones used in our monkeys.

4.5   Source areas generating attentional top-down bias

Thus far, we have argued that there is competition among objects within visual cortical areas for neural representation. Further, we have proposed that this competition can be biased in favor of a particular object by mechanisms of selective attention; that is, through top-down inputs. Although extrastriate areas appear to be critical sites where the competition among multiple stimuli is resolved, there is evidence that the top-down biasing signals derive from areas outside visual cortex and are transmitted via feedback projections to visual cortex (Buchel & Friston, 2000; Hopfinger *et al.*, 2000; Kastner *et al.*, 1999; Kastner & Ungerleider, 2000; Martinez *et al.*, 1999; Mesulam, 1999; Miller & Cohen, 2001). What areas might be the source of these top-down signals?

Both studies in patients suffering from attentional deficits due to brain damage and functional brain imaging studies in healthy subjects performing attention tasks have given insights into a distributed network of higher order areas in frontal and parietal cortex. This network appears to be involved in the generation and control of attentional top-down feedback signals.

4.5.1   Lesion studies

There is a long history demonstrating that unilateral brain lesions in humans often cause an impairment in spatially directing attention to the contralateral hemifield, a syndrome known as "visuospatial neglect." In severe cases, patients suffering from neglect will completely disregard the visual hemifield contralateral to the side of the lesion (Bisiach & Vallar, 1988; Heilman et al., 1993; Rafal, 1994). For example, they will read from only one side of a book, apply make-up to only one half of their face, or eat from only one side of a plate. In less severe cases, the deficit is more subtle and becomes apparent only if the patient is confronted with competing stimuli, as in the case of visual extinction. In visual extinction, patients are able to orient attention to a single visual object presented to their impaired visual hemifield; but, if two stimuli are presented simultaneously, one in the impaired and the other in the intact hemifield, the patients will only detect the one presented to the intact side, denying that any other object had been presented. These findings suggest that visual extinction reflects an attentional bias toward the intact hemifield in the presence of competing objects (Duncan, 1998; Kinsbourne, 1993; but see Cocchini et al., 1999).

Visuospatial neglect may follow unilateral lesions at very different sites, including the parietal lobe, especially its inferior part and the temporo-parietal junction (Vallar & Perani, 1986), regions of the frontal lobe (Damasio et al., 1980; Heilman & Valenstein, 1972), the anterior cingulate cortex (Janer & Pardo, 1991), the basal ganglia (Damasio et al., 1980), and the thalamus, in particular the pulvinar (Watson & Heilman, 1979). Studies in monkeys have implicated the same brain regions (Gaffan & Hornak, 1997; Latto & Cowey, 1971; Lynch & McLaren, 1989; Petersen et al., 1987; Watson et al., 1973, 1974; Welch & Stuteville, 1958). The finding that lesions of many different areas may cause visuospatial neglect has led to the notion that these areas form a distributed network for directed attention (Mesulam, 1981; Posner & Petersen, 1990).

Neglect occurs more often with right-sided parietal lesions than with left-sided parietal lesions, suggesting a specialized role for the right hemisphere in directed attention (Vallar, 1993). Based on this hemispheric asymmetry, it has been proposed that the right hemisphere mediates directed attention to both sides of visual space, whereas the left hemisphere mediates directed attention only to the contralateral, right side of visual space (Heilman & Van Den Abell, 1980; Mesulam, 1981). According to this view, in the case of a left-hemisphere lesion, the intact right hemisphere would take over the attentional function of the damaged left hemisphere, whereas a right hemisphere lesion would result in a left-sided hemispatial neglect because of the bias of the intact left hemisphere for the right hemifield. This right hemispheric dominance of parietal cortex has been demonstrated only in cases of severe neglect; visual extinction appears to result as frequently from left as from right-sided lesions (Rafal, 1994).

Importantly, stimulus-driven bottom-up mechanisms within visual cortex, such as figure-ground segmentation or perceptual grouping, which determine the salience of a stimulus, are preserved in the neglected hemifield and may influence the patients' behavior (Driver, 1995; Driver & Mattingley, 1998; Driver *et al.*, 1992; Grabowecky *et al.*, 1993; Marshall & Halligan, 1994; Mattingley *et al.*, 1997). For example, Mattingley *et al.* (1997) reported a patient with parietal damage whose extinction was less severe when bilateral stimuli were arranged to form an illusory Kanisza-square, a percept based on automatic filling-in of illusory boundaries. This result shows that the patient could use the information from his neglected left hemifield to form the percept of a common surface. It therefore appears that, following parietal damage, the competition among multiple stimuli can be biased equally well across the entire visual field by bottom-up processes, whereas mechanisms under top-down control, such as directing attention to a particular location, are biased toward the intact hemifield.

4.5.2   Functional brain imaging studies

Results from our and other functional brain imaging studies support the idea that top-down signals related to spatially directed attention may be generated by a distributed network of areas in frontal and parietal cortex. In addition to activations within visual cortex, we were able to examine activations of parietal and frontal cortex with the experimental design used to study competitive interactions and their modulation by spatial attention, as described above (Kastner *et al.*, 1998). Results for a single subject are shown in Figure 4.11B. In this subject, the frontal eye fields (FEF) were activated bilaterally, together with the supplementary eye field (SEF) and the superior parietal lobule (SPL). Remarkably, none of these areas were activated to a significant degree when subjects were processing visual information in an unattended condition (Figure 4.11A). A network consisting of areas in the SPL, FEF, and the SEF was consistently activated across subjects. A similar network has been found to be activated in a variety of visuospatial tasks (Corbetta *et al.*, 1993, 1998; Culham *et al.*, 1998; Fink *et al.*, 1997; Gitelman *et al.*, 1999; Kim *et al.*, 1999; Nobre *et al.*, 1997; Rosen *et al.*, 1999; Vandenberghe *et al.*, 1997). In addition, but less consistently, activations in the inferior parietal lobule (IPL), the lateral prefrontal

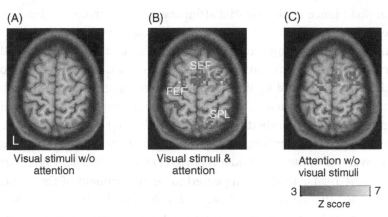

Figure 4.11 *A fronto-parietal network mediating biased competition and spatially directed attention.* Axial slice through frontal and parietal cortex; same subject and experimental conditions as in Figure 4.4. (A) Visual stimulation did not activate frontal or parietal cortex reliably when attention was directed elsewhere in the visual field. (B) When the subject directed attention to a peripheral target location and performed an object discrimination task, a distributed fronto-parietal network was activated including the SEF, the FEF, and the SPL. (C) The same network of frontal and parietal areas was activated when the subject directed attention to the peripheral target location in the expectation of the stimulus onset, that is, in the absence of any visual input whatsoever. This activity therefore does not reflect attentional modulation of visually evoked responses, but rather attentional control operations themselves. L indicates left hemisphere (for color image please see www.cambridge.org/9780521143400).

cortex in the region of the middle frontal gyrus (MFG), and the anterior cingulate cortex have been reported. A common feature among these visuospatial tasks is that subjects were asked to maintain fixation at a central fixation point and to direct attention covertly to peripheral target locations in order to detect a stimulus (Corbetta *et al.*, 1993, 1998; Gitelman *et al.*, 1999; Kim *et al.*, 1999; Nobre *et al.*, 1997; Rosen *et al.*, 1999), to discriminate it (Fink *et al.*, 1997; Kastner *et al.*, 1999; Vandenberghe *et al.*, 1997), or to track its movement (Culham *et al.*, 1998). Thus, there appears to be a general spatial attention network that operates independent of the specific requirements of the visuospatial task (for a meta-analysis, see Kastner & Ungerleider, 2000). Interestingly, the same areas of parietal cortex have been shown to be activated to a similar extent during different spatial and non-spatial attention tasks including peripheral shifts of attention, object matching, and nonspatial conjunction search (Wojciulik & Kanwisher, 1999). Hence, in parietal cortex, spatially and nonspatially based attentional selections may be mediated by a common neural substrate.

There are two notable differences in the results from patient and from functional brain imaging studies. First, the patient studies suggest a right parietal dominance in visuospatial attention; that is, directing attention to the left hemifield is presumed to be exclusively subserved by the right parietal cortex, whereas directing attention to the right hemifield is presumed to be subserved by both the left and the right parietal cortex. This notion has not been unequivocally supported by functional brain imaging studies. Although some investigators have found a stronger or an even exclusive activation of areas in the right parietal lobe (Corbetta *et al.*, 1993; Gitelman *et al.*, 1999; Kim *et al.*, 1999; Nobre *et al.*, 1997; Vandenberghe *et al.*, 1997), others have found largely symmetrical activations in the right and left parietal lobes (Fink *et al.*, 1997). Moreover, these symmetrical activations appeared to be independent of the visual hemifield attended (Vandenberghe *et al.*, 1997). A second difference between the results from patient and from functional brain imaging studies concerns which portion of the parietal lobe plays a key role in attention. The patient literature has consistently identified the IPL, including the temporo-parietal junction, as the critical lesion site in neglect patients (Vallar, 1993). By contrast, the majority of functional brain imaging studies points to the SPL rather than the IPL as the part of the parietal lobe that is involved in visuospatial attention. One possible explanation for this discrepancy is that many tasks used in the imaging studies involved a cue to indicate the location at which the visual stimulus would appear; these tasks thus had an expectancy component. Results from lesion studies suggest that the ability to maintain expectancy depends on the SPL rather than the IPL (Friedrich *et al.*, 1998; Posner *et al.*, 1984).

Evidence from fMRI studies suggests that the attention-related activity in parietal and frontal areas may not reflect attentional modulation of visual responses; instead, the activity is largely due to the attentional operations themselves. In a study conducted by Rees *et al.* (1997), attentional modulation of visually evoked activity was found to be rate-dependent in the inferior temporal cortex, but rate-independent in prefrontal cortex. This result thus suggests two distinct effects of attention: one, in the frontal lobe, which may generate modulatory influences; and another, in the temporal lobe, in which the visually evoked responses themselves are modulated. In a more recent study, we investigated activations in frontal and parietal cortex during directed attention in the presence and in the absence of visual stimulation in the paradigm described above (Kastner *et al.*, 1999). During directed attention in the absence of visual stimulation, the same distributed network for spatial attention as during directed attention in the presence of visual stimulation was activated, consisting of the FEF, the SEF, and the SPL (Figure 4.11C). A time course analysis of the fMRI signals revealed that, as in visual cortical areas, there was an increase in activity in these frontal and parietal areas due to directed attention in the absence of visual input. However, first, this increase in activity was stronger in SPL, FEF, and SEF than the increase in activity seen in visual cortex (as exemplified for FEF in Figure 4.7B), and second, there was no further increase in activity evoked by the attended stimulus presentations in these parietal and frontal areas. Rather, there was sustained activity throughout the expectation period and the attended presentations (Figure 4.7B). Taken together, these findings suggest that the activity reflected the attentional operations of the task and not visual processing. These and other studies (Hopfinger et al., 2000) have provided evidence that the distributed fronto-parietal attention network may be the source of feedback that generated the top-down biasing signals seen in visual cortex. Because the magnitude of the activity in the parietal and frontal areas was the same during directed attention in the absence and in the presence of visual stimulation, it appears that this activity may be independent of the particular visual task, be it detection or discrimination. This would explain the finding that functional brain imaging studies using different visuospatial attention tasks have described very similar attentional networks.

The anatomical connections of SPL, FEF, and SEF put them in a position to serve as sources of top-down biasing signals within visual cortex. In the monkey, FEF and SEF are reciprocally connected with ventral stream areas (Ungerleider et al., 1989; Webster et al., 1994) and posterior parietal cortex (Cavada & Goldman-Rakic, 1989), and the posterior parietal cortex is connected with ventral stream areas via the lateral intraparietal area (area LIP) (Webster et al., 1994).

The functional roles of these frontal and parietal areas in attentional selection and control are not well understood. In regions of parietal cortex, it has been shown that neural responses are enhanced during covert shifts of attention to peripheral visual stimuli (Bushnell et al., 1981; Colby et al., 1996; Robinson et al., 1978). The strongest determinant of neural responsiveness in parietal cortex turned out to be the salience of the stimulus (Colby & Goldberg, 1998). Therefore, it may be speculated that parietal cortex provides a "saliency map" for exogeneous stimuli that will capture attention rapidly. Recent functional brain imaging studies suggest that distinct parietal regions subserve different attentional processes. It was found that regions within the intraparietal sulcus were activated when subjects voluntarily directed attention to a pre-cued location before the presentation of a visual target stimulus. In contrast, regions of the right temporo-parietal junction were activated when target stimuli were detected at unattended locations (Corbetta et al., 2000). In the FEF and SEF, attentional response enhancement was originally shown in the context of activity related to the preparation of saccadic eye movements (Goldberg & Bushnell, 1981; Wurtz & Mohler, 1976), supporting the notion that covert shifts of attention precede overt shifts of gaze. More recent recording studies suggest, however, that the response enhancement in these frontal areas during covert shifts of attention to peripheral visual stimuli does not depend on the subsequent execution of saccades (Bon & Lucchetti, 1997; Kodaka *et al.*, 1997). The intimate functional relationship between covert shifts of attention and eye movements in frontal cortical areas has also been demonstrated in functional brain imaging studies. Areas including the FEF and SEF that were engaged by covert shifts of attention and by executing saccadic eye movements were shown to greatly overlap (Corbetta *et al.*, 1998; Nobre *et al.*, 2000; Perry & Zeki, 2000). Taken together, these studies have begun to define functional roles for distinct areas within frontal and parietal cortex in attentional control, which need further refinement in future research.

Thus far, results from single-cell recording and functional brain imaging studies clearly converge to support the idea that areas in parietal and frontal cortex are potential sources for generating and controlling attentional top-down bias. However, because results from functional brain imaging studies demonstrate only correlated activity of distributed brain areas and cannot establish the functional significance of a particular brain area in a given task, future studies using reversible lesion techniques such as cooling of brain tissue or transcranial magnetic stimulation are needed to test these ideas further.

4.6   Summary and conclusions

In this review, we have considered the mechanisms of selective attention in human visual cortex in the context of a biased competition account of attention. Evidence from functional brain imaging studies in humans, supported by results from single-cell recording studies in monkeys, indicates that, first, there is competition among multiple stimuli for representation in visual cortex. Thus, multiple stimuli presented at the same time are not processed independently, but rather interact with each other in a mutually suppressive way. Such sensory suppressive interactions are scaled to the RF size of neurons within visual cortical areas. Second, competition among multiple stimuli can be biased by top-down feedback mechanisms. Top-down influences on visual cortex, as in the case of selective attention, can affect neural processing in several ways, which include: (1) the enhancement of neural responses to attended stimuli; (2) the filtering of unwanted information by counteracting the suppression induced by nearby distracters; and (3) the biasing of signals in favor of an attended location by increases of baseline activity in expectation of a visual stimulus. Thus, attentional modulation of activity in visual cortex can occur not only in the presence, but also in the absence, of visual stimulation. Third, as suggested by lesion studies in monkeys, extrastriate visual areas V4 and TEO appear to be important sites where attention acts to resolve the competition among multiple stimuli for neural representation. Fourth, although competition is resolved in visual cortex, the source of top-down biasing signals may derive from a network of areas outside visual cortex. For spatially directed visual attention, these areas include the superior parietal lobule, the frontal eye field, the supplementary eye field, and, less consistently, areas in the inferior parietal lobule, the mid-lateral prefrontal cortex, and the anterior cingulate cortex. Attention-related activity in frontal and parietal areas may not reflect attentional modulation of visually evoked responses, but rather attentional control operations. Future studies will be needed to elucidate the functional nature of these operations and to determine the functional significance of these higher order areas in spatially directed attention. Finally, the stimulus that wins the competition for representation in visual cortex will gain further access to memory systems for mnemonic encoding and retrieval, and to motor systems for guiding action and behavior.

References

Andersen, R. A., Snowden, R. J., Treue, S., and Graziano, M. (1990). Hierarchical processing of motion in the visual cortex of moneky. *Cold Spring Harbor Symposia Quantitative Biology*, **55**, 741–8.

Bandettini, P. A., Wong, E. C., Hinks, R. S., Tikofsky, R. S., and Hyde, J. S. (1992). Time course EPI of human brain function during task activation. *Magnetic Resonance in Medicine*, **25**, 390–7.

Bashinski, H. S. and Bacharach, V. R. (1980). Enhancement of perceptual sensitivity as the result of selectively attending to spatial locations. *Perception & Psychophysics*, **28**, 241–8.

Beauchamp, M. S., Haxby, J. V., Jennings, J. E., and DeYoe, E. A. (1999). An fMRI version of the Farnsworth Munsell 100-Hue Test reveals multiple color-selective areas in human ventral occipitotemporal cortex. *Cerebral Cortex*, **9**, 257–63.

Bisiach, E. and Vallar, G. (1988). Hemineglect in humans. In F. Boller and J. Grafman, eds., *Handbook of Neuropsychology*, Vol. 1. Amsterdam: Elsevier, pp. 195–222.

Bon, L. and Lucchetti, C. (1997). Attention-related neurons in the supplementary eye field of the macaque monkey. *Experimental Brain Research*, **113**, 180–5.

Boussaoud, D., Desimone, R., and Ungerleider, L. G. (1991). Visual topography of area TEO in the macaque. *Journal of Computational Neurology*, **306**, 554–75.

Brefczynski, J. A. and DeYoe, E. A. (1999). A physiological correlate of the 'spotlight' of visual attention. *Nature Neuroscience*, **2**, 370–4.

Broadbent, D. E. (1958). *Perception and Communication*. London: Pergamon Press.

Buchel, C. and Friston, K. J. (2000). Assessing interactions among neuronal systems using functional neuroimaging. *Neural Networks*, **13**, 871–82.

Bundesen, C. (1990). A theory of visual attention. *Psychology Review*, **97**, 523–47.

Bushnell, M. C., Goldberg, M. E., and Robinson, D. L. (1981). Behavioral enhancement of visual responses in monkey cerebral cortex. *Journal of Neurophysiology*, **46**, 755–72.

Carrasco, M. and Yeshurun, Y. (1998). The contribution of covert attention to the set-size and eccentricity effects in visual search. *Journal of Experimental Psychology: Human Perception Performance*, **24**, 673–92.

Cavada, C. and Goldman-Rakic, P. S. (1989). Posterior parietal cortex in rhesus monkey: II. Evidence for segregated cortico-cortical networks linking sensory and limbic areas with the frontal lobe. *Journal of Computational Neurology*, **287**, 422–45.

Chawla, D., Rees, G., and Friston, K. J. (1999). The physiological basis of attentional modulation in extrastriate visual areas. *Nature Neuroscience*, **2**, 671–6.

Chelazzi, L., Duncan, J., Miller, E. K., and Desimone, R. (1998). Responses of neurons in inferior temporal cortex during memory-guided visual search. *Journal of Neurophysiology*, **80**, 2918–40.

Chelazzi, L., Miller, E. K., Duncan, J., and Desimone, R. (1993). A neural basis for visual search in inferior temporal cortex. *Nature*, **363**, 345–7.

Cocchini, G., Cubelli, R., Della Sala, S., and Beschin, N. (1999). Neglect without extinction. *Cortex*, **35**, 285–313.

Colby, C. L., Duhamel, J. R., and Goldberg, M. E. (1996). Visual, presaccadic, and cognitive activation of single neurons in monkey lateral intraparietal area. *Journal of Neurophysiology*, **76**, 2841–52.

Colby, C. L. and Goldberg, M. E. (1998). Space and attention in parietal cortex. *Annual Review of Neuroscience*, **22**, 319–49.

Connor, C. E., Gallant, J. L., Preddie, D. C., and Van Essen, D. C. (1996). Responses in area V4 depend on the spatial relationship between stimulus and attention. *Journal of Neurophysiology*, **75**, 1306–8.

Connor, C. E., Preddie, D. C., Gallant, J. L., and Van Essen, D. C. (1997). Spatial attention effects in macaque area V4. *Journal of Neuroscience*, **17**, 3201–14.

Corbetta, M., Akbudak, E., Conturo, T. E., *et al.* (1998). A common network of functional areas for attention and eye movements. *Neuron*, **21**, 761–73.

Corbetta, M., Kincade, J. M., Ollinger, J. M., McAvoy, M. P., and Shulman, G. L. (2000). Voluntary orienting is dissociated from target detection in human posterior parietal cortex. *Nature Neuroscience*, **3**, 292–7.

Corbetta, M., Miezin, F. M., Shulman, G. L., and Petersen, S. E. (1993). A PET study of visuospatial attention. *Journal of Neuroscience*, **13**, 1202–26.

Culham, J. C., Brandt, S. A., Cavanagh, P., *et al.* (1998). Cortical fMRI activation produced by attentive tracking of moving targets. *Journal of Neurophysiology*, **80**, 2657–70.

Damasio, A. R., Damasio, H., and Chang, C. H. (1980). Neglect following damage to frontal lobe or basal ganglia. *Neuropsychologia*, **18**, 123–32.

Desimone, R. (1991). Face-selective cells in the temporal cortex of monkeys. *Journal of Cognitive Neuroscience*, **3**, 1–8.

Desimone, R. (1996). Neural mechanisms for visual memory and their role in attention. *Proceedings of the National Academy of Sciences USA*, **26**, 13494–9.

Desimone, R. (1998). Visual attention mediated by biased competition in extrastriate visual cortex. *Philosophical Transactions of the Royal Society of London*, **353**, 1245–55.

Desimone, R. and Duncan, J. (1995). Neural mechanisms of selective visual attention. *Annual Review of Neuroscience*, **18**, 193–222.

Desimone, R. and Ungerleider, L. G. (1986). Multiple visual areas in the caudal superior temporal sulcus of the macaque. *Journal of Computational Neurology*, **248**, 164–89.

Desimone, R. and Ungerleider, L. G. (1989). Neural mechanisms of visual processing in monkeys. In F. Boller and J. Grafman, eds., *Handbook of Neuropsychology*, Vol. 2. Amsterdam: Elsevier, pp. 267–99.

DeYoe, E. A., Carman, G. J., Bandettini, P., *et al.* (1996). Mapping striate and extrastriate visual areas in human cerebral cortex. *Proceedings of the National Academy of Sciences USA*, **93**, 2382–6.

De Weerd, P., Peralta III, M. R., Desimone, R., and Ungerleider, L. (1999). Loss of attentional selection after extrastriate cortical lesions in macaques. *Nature Neuroscience*, **2**, 753–7.

Driver, J. (1995). Object segmentation and visual neglect. *Behavior Brain Research*, **71**, 135–46.

Driver, J. and Baylis, G. C. (1989). Movement and visual attention: the spotlight metaphor breaks down. *Journal of Experimental Psychology: Human Perception Performance*, **15**, 448–56.

Driver, J., Baylis, G. C., and Rafal, R. D. (1992). Preserved figure-ground segmentation and symmetry perception in visual neglect. *Nature*, **360**, 73–5.

Driver, J. and Mattingley, J. B. (1998). Parietal neglect and visual awareness. *Nature Neuroscience*, **1**, 17–22.

Duffy, C. J. and Wurtz, R. H. (1991). Sensitivity of MST neurons to optic flow stimuli. II. Mechanisms of response selectivity revealed by small-field stimuli. *Journal of Neurophysiology*, **65**, 1346–59.

Duncan, J. (1980). The locus of interference in the perception of simultaneous stimuli. *Psychology Review*, **87**, 272–300.

Duncan, J. (1984). Selective attention and the organization of visual information. *Journal of Experimental Psychology*, **113**, 501–17.

Duncan, J. (1996). Cooperating brain systems in selective perception and action. In T. Inui and J. L. McClelland, eds., *Attention and Performance XVI*. Cambridge: MIT Press, pp. 549–78.

Duncan, J. (1998). Converging levels of analysis in the cognitive neuroscience of visual attention. *Philosophical Transactions of the Royal Society of London B*, **353**, 1307–17.

Duncan, J. and Humphreys, G. W. (1989). Visual search and stimulus similarity. *Psychology Review*, **96**, 433–58.

Duncan, J. and Humphreys, G. W. (1992). Beyond the search surface: visual search and attentional engagement. *Journal of Experimental Psychology: Human Perception Performance*, **18**, 578–88.

Eason, R. G., Harter, M. R., and White, C. T. (1969). Effects of attention and arousal on visually evoked cortical potentials and reaction time in man. *Physiology and Behavior*, **4**, 283–9.

Engel, S. A., Glover, G. H., and Wandell, B. A. (1997). Retinotopic organization in human visual cortex and the spatial precision of functional MRI. *Cerebral Cortex*, **7**, 181–92.

Felleman, D. J. and Van Essen, D. C. (1991). Distributed hierarchical processing in the primate cerebral cortex. *Cerebral Cortex*, **1**, 1–47.

Fink, G. R., Dolan, R. J., Halligan, P. W., Marshall, J. C., and Frith, C. D. (1997). Space-based and object-based visual attention: shared and specific neural domains. *Brain*, **120**, 2013–28.

Fox, P. T. and Raichle, M. E. (1986). Focal physiological uncoupling of cerebral blood flow and oxidative metabolism during somatosensory stimulation in human subjects. *Proceedings of the National Academy of Sciences USA*, **83**, 1140–4.

Friedman-Hill, S. R., Robertson, L. C., Ungerleider, L. G., and Desimone, R. (2000). Impaired attentional filtering in a patient with bilateral parietal lesions. *Society of Neuroscience Abstracts*, 106.11.

Friedrich, F. J., Egly, R., Rafal, R. D., and Beck, D. (1998). Spatial attention deficits in humans: a comparison of superior parietal and temporal-parietal junction lesions. *Neuropsychology*, **12**, 193–207.

Gaffan, D. and Hornak, J. (1997). Visual neglect in the monkey: representation and disconnection. *Brain*, **120**, 1647–57.

Gallant, J. L., Shoup, R. E., and Mazer, J. A. (2000). A human extrastriate area functionally homologous to macaque V4. *Neuron*, **27**, 227–35.

Gattass, R., Gross, C. G., and Sandell, J. H. (1981). Visual topography of V2 in the macaque. *Journal of Computational Neurology*, **201**, 519–39.

Gattass, R., Sousa, A. P. B., and Gross, C. G. (1988). Visuotopic organization and extent of V3 and V4 of the macaque. *Journal of Neuroscience*, **8**, 1831–45.

Ghandi, S. P., Heeger, D. J., and Boynton, G. M. (1999). Spatial attention affects brain activity in human primary visual cortex. *Proceedings of the National Academy of Sciences USA*, **96**, 3314–19.

Gitelman, D. R., Nobre, A. C., Parrish, T. B., *et al.* (1999). A large-scale distributed network for covert spatial attention. *Brain*, **122**, 1093–106.

Goldberg, M. E. and Bushnell, M. C. (1981). Behavioral enhancement of visual responses in monkey cerbral cortex. *Journal of Neurophysiology*, **46**, 773–87.

Goldberg, M. E. and Colby, C. L. (1989). The neurophysiology of spatial vision. In F. Boller and J. Grafman, eds., *Handbook of Neuropsychology*, Vol. 2. Amsterdam: Elsevier, pp. 301–15.

Goodale, M. A. and Milner, A. D. (1992). Separate visual pathways for perception and action. *Trends Neuroscience*, **15**, 20–5.

Grabowecky, M., Robertson, L. C., and Treisman, A. (1993). Preattentive processes guide visual search: evidence from patients with unilateral visual neglect. *Journal of Cognitive Neuroscience*, **5**, 288–302.

Grill-Spector, K., Kushnir, T., Hendler, T., *et al.* (1998). A sequence of object-processing stages revealed by fMRI in the human occipital lobe. *Human Brain Mapping*, **6**, 316–28.

Hadjikhani, N. K., Liu, A. K., Dale, A. M., Cavanagh, P., and Tootell, R. B. H. (1998). Retinotopy and color sensitivity in human visual cortical area V8. *Nature Neuroscience*, **1**, 235–41.

Haenny, P. E., Maunsell, J. H. R., and Schiller, P. H. (1988). State dependent activity in monkey visual cortex. *Experimental Brain Research*, **69**, 245–59.

Halgren, E., Dale, A. M., Sereno, M. I., *et al.* (1999). Location of human face-selective cortex with respect to retinotopic areas. *Human Brain Mapping*, **7**, 29-37.

Harter, M. R. and Aine, C. J. (1984). Brain mechanisms of visual selective attention. In R. Parasuraman and D. R. Davies, eds., *Varieties of Attention*. Orlando, FL: Academic, pp. 293–321.

Haxby, J. V., Horwitz, B., Ungerleider, L. G., *et al.* (1994). The functional organization of human extrastriate cortex: a PET-rCBF study of selective attention to faces and locations. *Journal of Neuroscience*, **14**, 6336-53.

Heilman, K. M. and Valenstein, E. (1972). Frontal lobe neglect in man. *Neurology*, **22**, 660-4.

Heilman, K. M. and Van Den Abell, T. (1980). Right hemisphere dominance for attention: the mechanism underlying hemispheric asymmetries of inattention (neglect). *Neurology*, **30**, 327-30.

Heilman, K. M., Watson, R. T., and Valenstein, E. (1993). Neglect and related disorders. In K. M. Heilman and E. Valenstein, eds., *Clinical Neuropsychology*, pp. 279–336.

Heinze, H. J., Mangun, G. R., Burchert, W., *et al.* (1994). Combined spatial and temporal imaging of brain activity during visual selective attention in humans. *Nature*, **372**, 543-6.

Hillyard, S. A., Vogel, E. K., and Luck, S. J. (1998). Sensory gain control (amplification) as a mechanism of selective attention: electrophysiological and neuroimaging evidence. *Philosophical Transactions of the Royal Society of London*, **353**, 1257-70.

Hopfinger, J. B., Buonocore, M. H., and Mangun, G. R. (2000). The neural mechanisms of top-down attentional control. *Nature Neuroscience*, **3**, 284-91.

Ishai, A., Ungerleider, L. G., and Haxby, J. V. (2000). Distributed neural systems for the generation of visual images. *Neuron*, **28**, 979-90.

Janer, K. W. and Pardo, J. V. (1991). Deficits in selective attention following bilateral anterior cingulotomy. *Journal of Cognitive Neuroscience*, **3**, 231-41.

Kanwisher, N., McDermott, J., and Chun, M. M. (1997). The fusiform face area: a module in human extrastriate cortex specialized for face perception. *Journal of Neuroscience*, **17**, 4302-11.

Kastner, S., De Weerd, P., Desimone, R., and Ungerleider, L. G. (1998). Mechanisms of directed attention in the human extrastriate cortex as revealed by functional MRI. *Science*, **282**, 108-11.

Kastner, S., De Weerd, P., Pinsk, M. A., *et al.* (2001). Modulation of sensory suppression: implications for receptive field sizes in the human visual cortex. *Journal of Neurophysiology*, **86**, 1398-411.

Kastner, S., De Weerd, P., and Ungerleider, L. G. (2000). Texture segregation in the human visual cortex: a functional MRI study. *Journal of Neurophysiology*, **83**, 2453-7.

Kastner, S., Pinsk, M. A., De Weerd, P., Desimone, R., and Ungerleider, L. G. (1999). Increased activity in human visual cortex during directed attention in the absence of visual stimulation. *Neuron*, **22**, 751–61.

Kastner, S. and Ungerleider, L. G. (2000). Mechanisms of visual attention in the human cortex. *Annual Review of Neuroscience*, **23**, 315–41.

Kim, Y. H., Gitelman, D. R., Nobre, A. C., *et al.* (1999). The large-scale neural network for spatial attention displays multifunctional overlap but differential asymmetry. *NeuroImage*, **9**, 269–77.

Kinsbourne, M. (1993). Orientational bias model of unilateral neglect: evidence from attentional gradients within hemispace. In I. H. Robertson and J. C. Marshall, eds., *Unilateral Neglect: Clinical and Experimental Studies*. Hillsdale, NJ: Lawrence Erlbaum, pp. 63–86.

Kleinschmidt, A., Lee, B. B., Requardt, M., and Frahm, J. (1996). Functional mapping of color processing by magnetic resonance imaging of responses to selective P- and M-pathway stimulation. *Experimental Brain Research*, **110**, 279–88.

Knierim, J. J. and Van Essen, D. C. (1992). Neuronal responses to static texture patterns in area V1 of the alert macaque monkey. *Journal of Neurophysiology*, **67**, 961–80.

Kodaka, Y., Mikami, A., and Kubota, K. (1997). Neuronal activity in the frontal eye field of the monkey is modulated while attention is focused on to a stimulus in the peripheral visual field, irrespective of eye movement. *Neuroscience Research*, **28**, 291–8.

Kosslyn, S. M., Thompson, W. L., Kim, I. J., and Alpert, N. M. (1995). Topographical representations of mental images in primary visual cortex. *Nature*, **378**, 496–8.

Kwong, K. K., Belliveau, J. W., Chesler, D. A., *et al.* (1992). Dynamic magnetic resonance imaging of human brain activity during primary sensory stimulation. *Proceedings of the National Academy of Sciences USA*, **89**, 5675–9.

Latto, R. and Cowey, A. (1971). Visual field defects after frontal eye-field lesions in monkeys. *Brain Research*, **30**, 1–24.

Lavie, N. and Driver, J. (1996). On the spatial extent of attention in object-based visual selection. *Perception & Psychophysics*, **58**, 1238–51.

Lu, Z. L. and Dosher, B. A. (1998). External noise distinguishes attention mechanisms. *Vision Research*, **38**, 1183–98.

Luck, S. J., Chelazzi, L., Hillyard, S. A., and Desimone, R. (1997). Neural mechanisms of spatial selective attention in areas V1, V2, and V4 of macaque visual cortex. *Journal of Neurophysiology*, **77**, 24–42.

Lynch, J. C. and McLaren, J. W. (1989). Deficits of visual attention and saccadic eye movements after lesions of parietooccipital cortex in monkeys. *Journal of Neurophysiology*, **61**, 74–90.

Mangun, G. R. (1995). Neural mechanisms of visual selective attention. *Psychophysiology*, **32**, 4–18.

Mangun, G. R., Buonocore, M. H., Girelli, M., and Jha, A. P. (1998). ERP and fMRI measures of visual spatial selective attention. *Human Brain Mapping*, **6**, 383–9.

Marshall, J. C. and Halligan, P. W. (1994). The yin and the yang of visuo-spatial neglect: a case study. *Neuropsychologia*, **32**, 1037–57.

Martinez, A., Vento, L. A., Sereno, M. I., *et al.*, (1999). Involvement of striate and extrastriate visual cortical areas in spatial attention. *Nature Neuroscience*, **2**, 364–9.

Mattingley, J. B., Davis, G., and Driver, J. (1997). Preattentive filling-in of visual surfaces in parietal extinction. *Science*, **275**, 671–4.

Maunsell, J. H. R. and Van Essen, D. C. (1983). Functional properties of neurons in middle temporal visual area of the macaque monkey. *Journal of Neurophysiology*, **49**, 1127–47.

McAdams, C. J. and Maunsell, J. H. R. (1999). Effects of attention on orientation-tuning functions of single neurons in macaque cortical area V4. *Journal of Neuroscience*, **19**, 431–41.

McCarthy, G., Puce, A., Gore, J. C., and Allison, T. (1997). Face-specific processing in the human fusiform gyrus. *Journal of Cognitive Neuroscience*, **9**, 605–10.

McKeefry, D. J. and Zeki, S. (1997). The position and topography of the human colour centre as revealed by functional magnetic resonance imaging. *Brain*, **120**, 2229–42.

Mesulam, M. M. (1981). A cortical network for directed attention and unilateral neglect. *Annals of Neurology*, **10**, 309–25.

Mesulam, M. M. (1999). Spatial attention and neglect: parietal, frontal and cingulate contributions to the mental representation and attentional targeting of salient extrapersonal events. *Philosophical Transactions of the Royal Society of London B Biology Science*, **354**, 1325–46.

Miller, E. K. and Cohen, J. D. (2001). An integrative theory of prefrontal cortex function. *Annual Review of Neuroscience*, **24**, 167–202.

Miller, E. K., Li, L., and Desimone, R. (1993). Activity of neurons in anterior inferior temporal cortex during a short-term memory task. *Journal of Neuroscience*, **13**, 1460–78.

Moran, J. and Desimone, R. (1985). Selective attention gates visual processing in the extrastriate cortex. *Science*, **229**, 782–4.

Motter, B. C. (1993). Focal attention produces spatially selective processing in visual cortical areas V1, V2, and V4 in the presence of competing stimuli. *Journal of Neurophysiology*, **70**, 909–19.

Neisser, U. (1967). *Cognitive Psychology*. New York: Appleton.

Newsome, W. T. and Salzman, C. D. (1990). Neuronal mechanisms of motion perception. *Cold Spring Harbor Symposia Quantitative Biology*, **55**, 697–705.

Nobre, A. C., Gitelman, D. R., Dias, E. C., and Mesulam, M. M. (2000). Covert visual spatial orienting and saccades: overlapping neural systems. *NeuroImage*, **11**, 210–16.

Nobre, A. C., Sebestyen, G. N., Gitelman, D. R., *et al.* (1997). Functional localization of the system for visuospatial attention using positron emission tomography. *Brain*, **120**, 515–33.

Nothdurft, H. C. (1993). The role of features in preattentive vision: comparison of orientation, motion and colour cues. *Vision Research*, **33**, 1937–58.

O'Craven, K. M. and Kanwisher, N. (2000). Mental imagery of faces and places activates corresponding stimulus-specific brain regions. *Journal of Cognitive Neuroscience*, **12**, 1013–23.

Ogawa, S., Tank, D. W., Menon, R., *et al.* (1992). Intrinsic signal changes accompanying sensory stimulation: functional brain mapping with magnetic resonance imaging. *Proceedings of the National Academy of Sciences USA*, **89**, 5951–5.

Perry, R. J. and Zeki, S. (2000). The neurology of saccades and covert shifts in spatial attention. *Brain*, **123**, 2273–88.

Petersen, S. E., Robinson, D. L., and Morris, J. D. (1987). Contributions of the pulvinar to visual spatial attention. *Neuropsychologia*, **25**, 97–105.

Posner, M. (1980). Orienting of attention. *Quarterly Journal of Experimental Psychology*, **32**, 3–25.

Posner, M. I. and Petersen, S. E. (1990). The attention system of the human brain. *Annual Review of Neuroscience*, **13**, 25–42.

Posner, M. I., Walker, J. A., Friedrich, F. J., and Rafal, R. D. (1984). Effects of parietal injury on covert orienting of attention. *Journal of Neuroscience*, **4**, 1863–74.

Prinzmetal, W. (1981). Principles of feature integration in visual perception. *Perception & Psychophysics*, **30**, 330–40.

Puce, A., Allison, T., Asgari, M., Gore, J. C., and McCarthy, G. (1996). Differential sensitivity of human visual cortex to faces, letterstrings, and textures: a functional magnetic resonance imaging study. *Journal of Neuroscience*, **16**, 5205–15.

Rafal, R. D. (1994). Neglect. *Current Opinion in Neurobiology*, **4**, 231–6.

Recanzone, G. H. and Wurtz, R. H. (2000). Effects of attention on MT and MST neuronal activity during pursuit initiation. *Journal of Neurophysiology*, **83**, 777–90.

Recanzone, G. H., Wurtz, R. H., and Schwarz, U. (1997). Responses of MT and MST neurons to one and two moving objects in the receptive field. *Journal of Neurophysiology*, **78**, 2904–15.

Ress, D., Backus, B. T., and Heeger, D. J. (2000). Activity in primary visual cortex predicts performance in a visual detection task. *Nature Neuroscience*, **3**, 940–5.

Rees, G., Frackowiak, R. S. J., and Frith, C. D. (1997). Two modulatory effects of attention that mediate object categorization in human cortex. *Science*, **275**, 835–8.

Reynolds, J. H., Chelazzi, L., and Desimone, R. (1999). Competitive mechanisms subserve attention in macaque areas V2 and V4. *Journal of Neuroscience*, **19**, 1736–53.

Reynolds, J. H., Pasternak, T., and Desimone, R. (2000). Attention increases sensitivity of V4 neurons. *Neuron*, **26**, 703–14.

Robinson, D. L., Goldberg, M. E., and Stanton, G. B. (1978). Parietal association cortex in the primate: sensory mechanisms and behavioral modulations. *Journal of Neurophysiology*, **91**, 910–32.

Roelfsema, P. R., Lamme, V. A. F., and Spekreijse, H. (1998). Object-based attention in the primary visual cortex of the macaque monkey. *Nature*, **395**, 376–81.

Rolls, E. T. and Tovee, M. J. (1995). Sparseness of the neuronal representation of stimuli in the primate temporal visual cortex. *Journal of Neurophysiology*, **73**, 713–26.

Rosen, A. C., Rao, S. M., Caffarra, P., *et al.* (1999). Neural basis of endogenous and exogenous spatial orienting: a functional MRI study. *Journal of Cognitive Neuroscience*, **11**, 135–52.

Sakai, K., Watanabe, E., Onodera, Y., *et al.* (1995). Functional mapping of the human colour centre with echo-planar magnetic resonance imaging. *Proceedings of the Royal Society of London B*, **261**, 89–98.

Sato, T. (1989). Interactions of visual stimuli in the receptive fields of inferior temporal neurons in awake monkeys. *Experimental Brain Research*, **77**, 23–30.

Schein, S. J. and Desimone, R. (1990). Spectral properties of V4 neurons in the macaque. *Journal of Neuroscience*, **10**, 3369–89.

Schiller, P. H. (1993). The effects of V4 and middle temporal (MT) area lesions on visual performance in rhesus monkey. *Visual Neuroscience*, **10**, 717–46.

Schiller, P. H. and Lee, K. (1991). The role of the primate extrastriate area V4 in vision. *Science*, **251**, 1251–3.

Schneider, W., Noll, D. C., and Cohen, J. D. (1993). Functional topographic mapping of the cortical ribbon in human vision with conventional MRI scanners. *Nature*, **365**, 150–3.

Schneider, W. and Shiffrin, R. M. (1977). Controlled and automatic human information processing: I. detection, search, and attention. *Psychology Review*, **84**, 1–66.

Sereno, M. I., Dale, A. M., Reppas, J. B., *et al.* (1995). Borders of multiple visual areas in humans revealed by functional magnetic resonance imaging. *Science*, **268**, 889–93.

Shiu, L. P. and Pashler, H. (1995). Spatial attention and vernier acuity. *Vision Research*, **35**, 337–43.

Shulman, G. L., Ollinger, J. M., Akbudak, E., *et al.* (1999). Areas involved in encoding and applying directional expectations to moving objects. *Journal of Neuroscience*, **21**, 9480–96.

Somers, D. C., Dale, A. M., Seiffert, A. E., and Tootell, R. B. H. (1999). Functional MRI reveals spatially specific attentional modulation in human primary visual cortex. *Proceedings of the National Academy of Sciences USA*, **96**, 1663–8.

Spitzer, H., Desimone, R., and Moran, J. (1988). Increased attention enhances both behavioral and neuronal performance. *Science*, **240**, 338–40.

Spitzer, H. and Richmond, B. J. (1991). Task difficulty: ignoring, attending to, and discriminating a visual stimulus yield progressively more activity in inferior temporal neurons. *Experimental Brain Research*, **83**, 340–8.

Tanaka, K. and Saito, H. (1989). Analysis of motion of the visual field by direction, expansion/contraction, and rotation cells clustered in the dorsal part of the medial superior temporal area of the macaque monkey. *Journal of Neurophysiology*, **62**, 626–41.

Tootell, R. B. H., Hadjikhani, N., Hall, E. K., *et al.* (1998). The retinotopy of visual spatial attention. *Neuron*, **21**, 1409–22.

Tootell, R. B., Mendola, J. D., Hadjikhani, N. K., *et al.* (1997). Functional analysis of V3A and related areas in human visual cortex. *Journal of Neuroscience*, **17**, 7060–78.

Tootell, R. B. H, Reppas, J. B., Kwong, K. K., *et al.* (1995). Functional analysis of human MT and related visual cortical areas using magnetic resonance imaging. *Journal of Neuroscience*, **15**, 3215–30.

Treisman, A. M. (1969). Strategies and models of selective attention. *Psychology Review*, **76**, 282–99.

Treisman, A. M. and Gelade, G. (1980). A feature-integration theory of attention. *Cognitive Psychology*, **12**, 97–136.

Treisman, A. and Gormican, S. (1988). Feature analysis in early vision: evidence from search asymmetries. *Psychology Review*, **95**, 15–48.

Treue, S. and Martinez, J. C. (1999). Feature-based attention influences motion processing gain in macaque visual cortex. *Nature*, **399**, 575–9.

Treue, S. and Maunsell, J. H. R. (1996). Attentional modulation of visual motion processing in cortical areas MT and MST. *Nature*, **382**, 539–41.

Tsotsos, J. K. (1990). Analyzing vision at the complexity level. *Behavioral Brain Science*, **13**, 423–69.

Ungerleider, L. G. (1995). Functional brain imaging studies of cortical mechanisms for memory. *Science*, **270**, 769–75.

Ungerleider, L. G., Gaffan, D., and Pelak, V. S. (1989). Projections from inferior temporal cortex to prefrontal cortex via the uncinate fascicle in rhesus monkeys. *Experimental Brain Research*, **76**, 473–84.

Ungerleider, L. G. and Haxby, J. V. (1994). What and where in the human brain. *Current Opinion Neurobiology*, **4**, 157–65.

Ungerleider, L. G. and Mishkin, M. (1982). Two cortical visual systems. In D. J. Ingle, M. A. Goodale, and R. J. W. Mansfield, eds., *Analysis of Visual Behavior*. Cambridge: MIT Press, pp. S49–86.

Vallar, G. (1993). The anatomical basis of spatial neglect in humans. In I. H. Robertson and J. C. Marshall, eds., *Unilateral Neglect: Clinical and Experimental Studies*. Hillsdale, NJ: Lawrence Erlbaum, pp. 27–62.

Vallar, G. and Perani, D. (1986). The anatomy of unilateral neglect after right-hemisphere stroke lesions: a clinical/CT-scan correlation study in man. *Neuropsychologia*, **24**, 609–22.

Vandenberghe, R., Duncan, J., Dupont, P., *et al.* (1997). Attention to one or two features in left or right visual field: a positron emission tomography study. *Journal of Neuroscience*, **17**, 3739–50.

Van Essen, D. C., Newsome, W. T., and Maunsell, J. H. (1984). The visual field representation in striate cortex of the macaque monkey: asymmetries, anisotropies, and individual variability. *Vision Research*, **24**, 429–48.

Van Voorhis, S. and Hillyard, S. A. (1977). Visual evoked potentials and selective attention to points in space. *Perception & Psychophysics*, **22**, 54–62.

Watanabe, T., Harner, A. M., Miyauchi, S., *et al.* (1998a). Task-dependent influences of attention on the activation of human primary visual cortex. *Proceedings of the National Academy of Sciences USA*, **95**, 11489–92.

Watanabe, T., Sasaki, Y., Miyauchi, S., *et al.* (1998b). Attention-regulated activity in human primary visual cortex. *Journal of Neurophysiology*, **79**, 2218–21.

Watson, R. T. and Heilman, K. M. (1979). Thalamic neglect. *Neurology*, **29**, 690–4.

Watson, R. T., Heilman, K. M., Cauthen, J. C., and Frederick, A. K. (1973). Neglect after cingulectomy. *Neurology*, **23**, 1003–7.

Watson, R. T., Heilman, K. M., Miller, B. D., and King, F. A. (1974). Neglect after mesencephalic reticular formation lesions. *Neurology*, **24**, 294–8.

Watson, J. D. G., Myers, R., Frackowiak, R. S. J., *et al.* (1993). Area V5 of the human brain: evidence from combined study using positron emission tomography and magnetic resonance imaging. *Cerebral Cortex*, **3**, 79–94.

Webster, M. J., Bachevalier, J., and Ungerleider, L. G. (1994). Connections of inferior temporal areas TEO and TE with parietal and frontal cortex in macaque monkeys. *Cerebral Cortex*, **4**, 470–83.

Welch, K. and Stuteville, P. (1958). Experimental production of unilateral neglect in monkeys. *Brain*, **81**, 341–7.

Wetherhill, G. B. and Levitt, R. (1965). Sequential estimation of points on a psychometrical function. *The British Journal of Mathematical and Statistical Psychology*, **18**, 1–10.

Wojciulik, E. and Kanwisher, N. (1999). The generality of parietal involvement in visual attention. *Neuron*, **23**, 747–64.

Wolfe, J. M. (1994). Guided search 2.0: a revised model of visual search. *Psychonomic Bulletin & Review*, **1**, 202–38.

Wolfe, J. M., Cave, K. R., and Franzel, S. L. (1989). Guided search: an alternative to the feature integration model for visual search. *Journal of Experimental Psychology: Human Perception and Performance*, **15**, 419–33.

Wurtz, R. H. and Mohler, C. W. (1976). Enhancement of visual responses in monkey striate cortex and frontal eye fields. *Journal of Neurophysiology*, **39**, 766–72.

Zeki, S. M. (1974). Functional organization of a visual area in the posterior bank of the superior temporal sulcus of the rhesus monkey. *Journal of Physiology (London)*, **236**, 549–73.

Zeki, S. M. (1978). Uniformity and diversity of structure and function in rhesus monkey prestriate visual cortex. *Journal of Physiology (London)*, **277**, 273–90.

Zeki, S., Watson, J. D. G., Lueck, C. J., *et al.* (1991). A direct demonstration of functional specialization in human visual cortex. *Journal of Neuroscience*, **11**, 641–9.

PART II LANGUAGE

Introduction to Language Section

HELEN J. NEVILLE

The last decade of the twentieth century was unprecedented in its progress toward discoveries linking the anatomical structures and physiological systems of the brain to the human mind. This enterprise is possible now, both because of a large body of behavioral data characterizing the operations and subsystems within different domains of cognitive processing and because of great advances in the methods and techniques available to noninvasively image the structure and the physiology of the functioning human brain. The focus of this part is to consider different perspectives and approaches to the study of the brain systems important in language processing and in the development and differentiation of the language systems of the brain.

The study of language is particularly well poised to benefit from knowledge about underlying neural mechanisms. It has been recognized since the 1950s that the study of language is a model case for understanding the species-specific capacities of human learners and the brain mechanisms in human adults and infants that permit them. Language in humans is an extraordinary ability, showing many properties without parallel in other species; understanding the mechanisms underlying human language will therefore shed special light on human cognition. At the same time the lack of animal models that have made such powerful contributions to the characterization of nonlinguistic cognitive systems underscores the importance of the new noninvasive techniques for imaging the language systems of the human brain.

Additionally, the study of language acquisition in relation to human brain development can be particularly powerful because of the well-developed state of the theoretical and descriptive fields studying the structure of human languages. Indeed formal descriptions of language may be the most highly developed theories we have of a specific cognitive capacity. There is enormous

Topics in Integrative Neuroscience: From Cells to Cognition, ed. James R. Pomerantz. Published by Cambridge University Press. © Cambridge University Press 2008.

societal import for understanding the neural mechanisms underlying human language development and the behavioral and neural routes to remediating its disorders. Overall level of language still has a profound impact on the ability of children and adults to form relationships with others and to succeed on a wide range of cognitive tasks. Improvement in our understanding of how to optimize normal language development and treat and rehabilitate disorders of language development will have profound consequences for both a basic understanding of human development and for human society.

In this section are included chapters representative of very different empirical approaches to the study of the neurobiology of language. Ultimately it will be the convergence of evidence from such multiple perspectives that will indicate we are closer to a veridical characterization of the architecture, neurobiology, and ontogeny of human language. The chapter by Poeppel and Hackl addresses the neural and functional architecture of speech perception. They describe the many sources of complexity and variability in natural speech and the structural and sequencing constraints that demand high level linguistic competence in order to achieve speech perception. Their analysis and description make it clear why phonemes are not elemental, but are instead composites of distinctive features. Indeed, they make the provocative suggestion that the phoneme may be an epiphenomenon that alphabetic writing systems incorrectly imply as the most basic, smallest unit of sound structure. They demonstrate the predictive power of the framework that takes distinctive feature complexes, rather than phonemes, as the fundamental unit of speech, and moreover show that distinctive features themselves can be understood as articulatory constraints and instructions. Poeppel and Hackl take the distinctive feature complex as central in their rigorous description of the cortical systems active during speech perception. Drawing on an elegant series of studies, Poeppel and Hackl propose a specific and testable functional anatomy of the speech processing system including a new proposal to account for the different contributions of cortical fields in the left and right temporal lobes. Specifically, they provide evidence that the sampling rates of the two hemispheres are different (left higher), rendering the left hemisphere biased to process rapid acoustic changes (including formant transitions) and the right hemisphere favored in the analysis of slow acoustic changes (as are important in intonation contours). Their proposal is powerful in accounting for diverse findings within the literature on speech processing of normal adults, and also for profiles of aphasia.

The next chapter (Patterson *et al.*) is a forceful reminder that the study of the impact of neurodegenerative diseases is uniquely powerful in revealing fundamental facts about the neural representation and organization of language and demonstrates how the power of this approach has been amplified when used in conjunction with new neuroimaging techniques. These studies highlight the highly local and specific effects on language of degenerative diseases, leading to both fluent and nonfluent aphasia. The atrophy of anterior, inferior lateral temporal lobe structures leaves phonological and syntactic processing intact but leads to an inexorable loss of semantic (conceptual) knowledge. Moreover, this damage leads to an effective, "functional" lesion of more posterior inferior temporal lobe structures important in conceptual representations – these are rendered virtually inactive. In sharp contrast is the profile of non-fluent aphasia associated with atrophy of the left perisylvian and frontal lobe structures. These patients retain good vocabulary but display severe phonological disruptions. The production of connected speech is very effortful. This series of studies highlight the power of this approach in characterizing the boundaries between different subsystems of language, and their neural substrates. In addition, this type of approach, unlike other neural-based methodologies, can identify brain systems that are necessary for particular language functions, by virtue of the observations that specific abilities are deficient when they are damaged.

Mehler and Nespor's chapter addresses the fundamental question of how the language systems are acquired by the young infant. They describe the theoretical differences that have dominated the study of language acquisition and propose a new framework in which the analysis of how speech signals are initially processed and represented can lead to a deep understanding of the complexities and uniqueness of the syntactic structure of language.

Whereas many psycholinguistic studies of language acquisition eschew the first year of life – since syntax does not develop until later – Mehler and Nespor propose and provide considerable data in support of the hypothesis that the sound pattern of language (prosody) which is available to the infant even before birth contains information that is central in constraining and triggering the acquisition of even the most abstract properties of language, that is syntax. They argue that it is important to study specific cortical areas before language is acquired in order to assess the direction of the relationship between language acquisition and left hemisphere specialization for language. They report an initial study of the left and right hemispheres of neonates using the technique of optical topography, recently derived from near-infrared technology. This method permits an estimate, from optic fibers placed on the scalp, of the relative shifts of oxy- and deoxy-hemoglobin that occur in response to different types of stimulation. They report that even in the neonate there is evidence for specialized processing of speech by the left hemisphere. Overall, this chapter illustrates the advantages of combining behavioral and imaging levels of analysis within the context of development. This multi-faceted approach will be powerful in future studies of language acquisition.

The chapter of Sanders, Weber-Fox, and Neville provides another developmental perspective on the relative roles of intrinsic constraints and the role of experience in the differentiation of the language systems of the brain. They report behavioral and neuroimaging studies of adults who had different kinds of language experience in development, including congenitally deaf adults and bilinguals who learned their second language at different ages. Their studies of semantic, syntactic, and phonological processing in these different groups show that there is tremendous variability in the extent and timing of experience-dependent plasticity of different subsystems within language. Just as the case within sensory and perceptual development, some linguistic subsystems change very little, even when experience is very different; others are dependant on and modified by early experience but only during particular time periods ("sensitive periods") – for example, aspects of phonology and syntax; and there are many different such time periods. Still other systems, for example aspects of lexical semantics, retain the ability to change in response to experience throughout life. These differences in experience-dependent plasticity can help define and draw boundaries between different linguistic subsystems and in the long run this type of information will contribute to the design of educational and rehabilitative programs.

Taken together, these chapters illustrate the rapid growth of knowledge of the neurobiology of language over the past decade, and highlight the unique advantages that a characterization based on multiple perspectives and methodologies can provide.

5

Varying degrees of plasticity in different subsystems within language

LISA D. SANDERS, CHRISTINE M. WEBER-FOX, AND HELEN J. NEVILLE

There are periods in development during which experience plays its largest role in shaping the eventual structure and function of mature language-processing systems. These spans of peak cortical plasticity have been called "sensitive periods." Here, we describe a series of studies investigating the effects of delays in second language (L2) acquisition on different subsystems within language. First, we review the effects of the altered language experience of congenitally deaf subjects on cerebral systems important for processing written English and American Sign Language (ASL). Second, we present behavioral and electrophysiological studies of L2 semantic and syntactic processing in Chinese-English bilinguals who acquired their second language over a wide range of ages. Third, we review semantic, syntactic, and prosodic processing in native Spanish and native Japanese late-learners of English. These approaches have provided converging evidence, indicating that delays in language acquisition have minimal effects on some aspects of semantic processing. In contrast, delays of even a few years result in deficits in some types of syntactic processing and differences in the organization of cortical systems used to process syntactic information. The different subsystems of language which rely on different cortical areas, including semantic, syntactic, phonological, and prosodic processing, may have different developmental time courses that in part determine the different sensitive period effects observed.

Humans, in comparison to other animals, go through a protracted period of post-natal development that lasts at least 15 years (Chugani & Phelps, 1986; Huttenlocher, 1990). During this extended time period, there is opportunity for experience to interact with neural development such that neurocognitive systems are eventually established to optimally process the types of information these systems are exposed to during development. The developmental time

Topics in Integrative Neuroscience: From Cells to Cognition, ed. James R. Pomerantz. Published by Cambridge University Press. © Cambridge University Press 2008.

span during which experience has its greatest effects on how the mature system will eventually function has been called a "sensitive or critical period." A full characterization of sensitive periods is important for basic understanding of the role of experience in neural and cognitive development and can contribute to the design of educational and rehabilitative programs by identifying which systems are most influenced by environmental input and when they are most affected.

Much of our current knowledge about plasticity during neural development has come from studies of sensory systems (Rauschecker & Marler, 1987). Different neural systems and associated behavioral capabilities are affected by environmental input at highly variable time periods, supporting the idea that they develop along distinct time courses (Harwerth *et al.*, 1986; Maurer & Lewis, 1998; Mitchell, 1981; Neville & Bavelier, 1999). Importantly, the sensitive periods and developmental time courses for subsystems within major sensory systems can differ dramatically. For example, visual processes thought to arise within the retina (e.g., the sensitivity of the scotopic visual system) display relatively short sensitive periods. By contrast, binocular functions that rely on later developing cortical neurons display considerably longer sensitive periods (Harwerth *et al.*, 1986). Cross-modal plasticity also shows considerable variability within a single domain. For example, congenitally deaf and hearing individuals have very similar brain responses to stimuli presented to the center of the visual field and to color information. By contrast, congenitally deaf individuals display enhanced behavioral responses, electrophysiological responses, and cerebral blood flow to peripheral visual stimuli (Bavelier *et al.*, 2000; Neville & Bavelier, 1999, 2001).

The concept of sensitive periods has been central in the study of language processing and language acquisition. Penfield and Roberts (1959) were among the first to discuss the idea that children might be better language learners than adults. Lenneberg (1967) suggested that just as maturational constraints define a period of time during which visual experience is necessary for setting up a normal visual processing system, there may be a period of time in development during which language experience is critical for setting up normal linguistic processing systems. He presented evidence from patients with left-hemisphere lesions that occurred early or late in development and showed that children (younger than 9 years of age) inevitably recovered language function after a unilateral lesion, whereas adults with the same types of lesions failed to fully recover. These data suggest that children, unlike adults, retain the cortical plasticity in both hemispheres necessary to acquire language. Additionally, evidence from a few children not exposed to normal language input until later in life due to either extreme abuse (Curtiss, 1977) or deafness (Curtiss, 1989;

Emmorey & Corina, 1990; Mayberry & Fischer, 1989; Newport, 1990) indicates that exposure to a first language early in life is necessary for full language attainment.

Similarly, studies focusing on second language acquisition have shown that children are more likely to attain native-like proficiency in a second language than are adults (Flege *et al.*, 1999; Lamendella, 1977; Long, 1990; Patkowski, 1994; Scovel, 1988; Singleton, 1989). The study of second language acquisition offers an opportunity to determine the boundaries of the sensitive period for language since individuals who learn second languages at a wide range of ages are readily available. However, the results of some studies have suggested that native-like language processing cannot be attained by second language learners no matter how early they began learning the second language (Cutler *et al.*, 1983, 1989, 1992; Pallier *et al.*, 1997; Sebastian-Galles & Soto-Faraco, 1999), while other studies find that at least some adult second language learners are able to perform some language tasks in a native-like manner (Birdsong, 1999; Bongaerts, 1995). From these studies, it is not clear whether the offset of the sensitive period for language is extremely early in life (less than 1 year of age), very late in life (continuing into adulthood), or does not exist at all. The lack of a single age after which native-like language processing cannot be achieved has been used to argue that there is no sensitive period for language. However, this argument fails to address two issues: first, the fact that some individuals of any age fail to attain a specific aspect of language does not disprove the hypothesis that there is a peak in plasticity during development in which native-like attainment of a language is more likely; second, the argument ignores the possibility that the time window for a sensitive period for language may differ for different subsystems within language as is the case for the development of the visual system (as noted above). To address this hypothesis, we review here research that has assessed the effects of age of acquisition on different subsystems within language, including semantic, syntactic, and phonological processing.

The literature on phonetic and prosodic processing suggests that experience with a language very early in life is necessary for native-like performance. For example, studies of pronunciation have shown that delays of as little as 4 years in exposure to a second language can result in an accent in that second language even after decades of use (Flege *et al.*, 1999; Yeni-Komshian *et al.*, 1997). Furthermore, there is evidence that perception of the sounds of a second language is not native-like even for those who are exposed to the second language as early as 3 or 4 years of age (Pallier *et al.*, 1997; Sebastian-Galles & Soto-Faraco, 1999). Studies of young infants listening to sounds in their native language and a nonnative language indicate that, by the end of the first year of life, infants show categorical perception that is specific to the language to which they have been exposed (Best, 1993; Kuhl, 1993; Kuhl *et al.*, 1992; Werker & Tees, 1992, 1999). Since phonological perception is already influenced by language experience within the first year of life, it is possible (although not necessary) that this defines the sensitive period for phonological processing. Although more research will be necessary to determine the exact offset of a phonological processing sensitive period, it is clear that this offset occurs early in life, perhaps before the age of 4.

The few studies that specifically address the effects of age of acquisition on syntactic processing suggest that the sensitive period for this subsystem of language may also be within the first decade of life. In several of the case studies in which first language acquisition was delayed, deficits specific to syntactic processing were reported (Curtiss, 1977, 1989; Newport, 1990). In these studies, children who did not acquire a first language until they were 4 to 6 years old showed deficits in some types of grammatical processing in their first language as adults. Studies of second language acquisition provide corroborating evidence: children who began learning a second language at 8 to 10 years of age scored lower on tests of grammar in that second language (Johnson & Newport, 1989). In fact, deficits in making grammaticality judgements on some types of sentences have been found in adults who acquired their second language as early as 3 years of age (Weber-Fox & Neville, 1996). As with phonological processing, more research will be necessary to precisely characterize the sensitive period for syntactic processing, as well as the types of syntactic processing that are most affected by a lack of experience with a given language during the sensitive period. However, the evidence to date clearly suggests that at least some types of grammatical processing require early experience.

In contrast, semantic processing does not seem to depend on early exposure to a language. Research has shown that people who learn either a first or second language later in life are able to learn new lexical items in that language (Curtiss, 1977, 1989; Newport, 1990) and are able to judge whether or not sentences in that language make sense (Weber-Fox & Neville, 1996). These data suggest that there may not be a sensitive period for semantic and lexical processing, or that the sensitive period for this type of language skill may extend well into adulthood.

While behavioral testing can be used to determine if delays in language learning affect the ability to process language, neuroimaging studies can be used to investigate whether or not first and second language processing makes use of the same neural systems. For example, cortical stimulation studies have found that stimulation of at least some cortical areas affects only one of a bilingual's two languages (Ojemann, 1983; Ojemann & Whitaker, 1978).

However, for the most part, these studies have not compared the different types of linguistic processing (semantic, syntactic, and phonological) necessary to perform the tasks used. As with behavioral studies, this lack of task specificity has created a contradictory picture, with some studies finding no differences in processing native and nonnative languages (Chee et al., 1999; Illes, et al., 1999; Klein et al., 1995, 1999) and others suggesting that different cortical areas are used for languages learned early and late in life (Kim et al., 1997; Klein et al., 1994; Perani et al., 1996).

This evidence suggests that the sensitive periods for subsystems within language are nonidentical and that characterizing the development of language processing will require characterizing each of these subsystems separately. Taking such an approach may help to clarify the currently contradictory results from neuroimaging studies of first and second language processing. In addition, it may be that even within specific subsystems different aspects of language processing are differentially affected by delays in learning. For example, within the syntactic subsystem, delays in language learning seem to have less of an effect on the ability to process word order than other types of syntactic information (Weber-Fox & Neville, 1996). Therefore, it will be important to use a variety of tasks that tap into different types of lexical, syntactic, and phonological processing to determine which aspects of language processing are most affected by delays in language learning.

Below we present evidence on these issues, first from a comparison of semantic and syntactic processing and related neural organization in English and ASL by deaf and hearing individuals who acquired these languages at different ages. Next we describe a series of studies concerning the effects of age of acquisition on grammaticality and meaningfulness judgments and on the event-related brain potentials (ERPs) to different word classes, violations of grammar, and violations of meaning within sentences. Finally, we present a series of behavioral and ERP studies in which we assess the ability of native and nonnative speakers to use stress-pattern, syntax, and lexical information to segment speech.

5.1   Studies of congenitally deaf individuals

The comparison of the processing of English in deaf and hearing subjects provides an important opportunity to study sensitive periods during development. While hearing subjects learn English from birth, deaf individuals are introduced to English much later. ERPs recorded while deaf and hearing subjects read English sentences suggest that semantic and grammatical processing are differentially vulnerable to altered early language experience (Neville et al.,

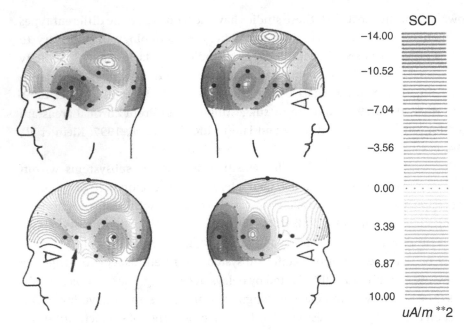

Figure 5.1 Distribution of current flow for the N280 peak elicited by closed-class words in English. Maps in the top row show the prominent response in the left hemisphere of hearing subjects (marked by arrow). Bottom row maps display results from congenitally deaf individuals who lack the response (arrow) (Figure 5.9 from Neville *et al.*, 1992; with permission from *Cerebral Cortex*) (for color image please see www.cambridge.org/9780521143400).

1992). Deaf subjects displayed ERPs to open-class words and other semantic information in English that were similar to those observed when normal hearing subjects processed English. These results suggest that aspects of semantic processing are robust following deaf subjects' altered early language experience. In contrast, deaf subjects' ERPs to closed-class words that carry grammatical information were markedly different from those of hearing subjects reading the same sentences. Deaf subjects' ERPs lacked the negative (N280) potential over anterior regions of the left hemisphere and did not display any evidence of left hemisphere advantage (Figure 5.1). These results are in accord with the idea that language experience has different effects on the development of the several different brain systems that mediate language. Brain systems that mediate grammatical aspects of language processing appear to be more sensitive to altered language experience. This idea is supported by our observation that deaf subjects whose grammar skills were excellent displayed an N280 response that was prominent and asymmetrical just as in normal hearing subjects (Neville, 1991).

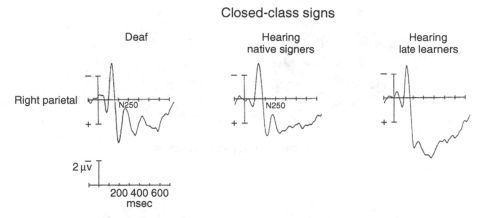

Figure 5.2   ERPs to closed-class signs in ASL sentences from 10 deaf, 10 hearing native signers, and 10 late-learners of ASL. Recordings from parietal areas of the right hemisphere (Figure 7.6 from Neville & Bavelier, 1999; with permission from MIT Press).

Recently, we have employed ERPs to pursue this hypothesis further and to obtain evidence on the question of whether the strongly biased role of the left hemisphere in language occurs independently of the structure and modality of the language first acquired (Neville et al., 1997, 1998). ERPs recorded in response to open- and closed-class signs in ASL sentences displayed similar timing and anterior/posterior distributions to those observed in previous studies of English. But, whereas in native speakers of English responses to closed-class English words were largest over anterior regions of the left hemisphere, in native signers closed-class ASL signs elicited activity that extended posteriorly over both the left and right hemispheres. These results imply that the acquisition of a language that relies on spatial contrasts and the perception of motion may result in the inclusion of right-hemisphere regions. As seen in Figure 5.2, both hearing and deaf native signers displayed this effect. However, hearing people who acquired ASL in the late teens did not show this effect, suggesting there may be a limited time (sensitive) period when this type of organization for grammatical processing can develop.

In fMRI studies comparing sentence processing in English and ASL we also observed evidence for biological constraints and effects of experience on the mature organization of the language systems of the brain. As seen at the top of Figure 5.3, when hearing adults read English (L1), there is robust activation within the left but not the right hemisphere and in particular within the left inferior frontal (Broca's) region. When deaf people read English (L2), we do not observe activation of these regions within the left hemisphere (Figure 5.3, middle). Is the absence of left-hemisphere activation in the deaf linked to lack of

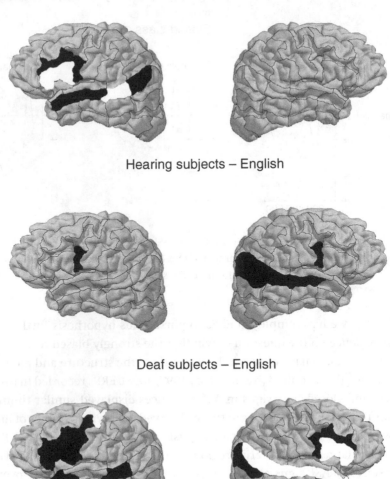

Hearing subjects – English

Deaf subjects – English

Deaf subjects – ASL

$P < 0.0005$ 0.005

Figure 5.3 Cortical areas showing increases in blood oxygenation on fMRI when normal hearing adults read English sentences (top), when congenitally deaf native signers read English sentences (middle), and when congenitally deaf native signers view sentences in their native sign language (American Sign Language) (bottom) (Figure 7.7 from Neville & Bavelier, 1999; with permission from MIT Press) (for color image please see www.cambridge.org/9780521143400).

auditory experience with language or to incomplete acquisition of the grammar of the language? ASL is not sound-based, but displays each of the characteristics of all formal languages including a complex grammar that makes extensive use of spatial location and hand motion (Klima & Bellugi, 1979). Studies of the same deaf subjects when viewing sentences in their native ASL clearly show activation within the same inferior frontal regions of the left hemisphere that are active when native speakers of English process English (Figure 5.3, bottom). These data suggest a strong biological bias for these neural systems to mediate grammatical language regardless of the structure and modality of the language acquired. However, if the language is not acquired within the appropriate time window, this strong bias is not expressed. Biological constraints and language experience interact epigenetically, as has been described for many other systems in developmental biology.

The fMRI data also indicate a robust role for the right hemisphere in processing ASL. These results suggest that the nature of the language input, in this case the co-occurrence of location and motion information with language, shapes the organization of the language systems of the brain. The right-hemisphere activation observed in deaf native signers viewing ASL sentences was also observed in hearing individuals who acquired ASL as a native language from their deaf parents (Neville et al., 1998). However, hearing signers who acquired ASL after the age of 15 did not show the same extent of right-hemisphere activation as did native signers (Newman et al., 2001). These results imply that like other oral–aural, natural languages the acquisition of aspects of ASL display sensitive period effects.

5.2   Syntactic and semantic processing in hearing bilinguals

As reviewed above, converging evidence points to specialized subsystems for language processing that are differentially sensitive to delays in second language learning. Based on the behavioral findings of linguistic proficiency in second language learners (Johnson & Newport, 1989; Newport, 1988) as well as the neurophysiological evidence for language processing in hearing and deaf individuals (Neville et al., 1992), we hypothesized that the neural subsystems for syntactic processing would be more vulnerable to delays in language learning compared to those associated with semantic processing. This hypothesis was tested in two ways. One approach was to measure the differential effects of processing violations in syntactic structure and in semantic expectation. In another experiment, the effects of delays in second language immersion were examined for processing two different word classes that were used appropriately in sentences.

Both of these paradigms examined the ERP responses obtained from Chinese–English bilingual speakers and monolingual English speakers (Weber-Fox &

Neville, 1996, 2001). The bilingual participants were grouped according to the age at which they were initially immersed in English: 1–3, 4–6, 7–10, 11–13, and after 15 years of age. Age of immersion corresponded, for the most part, to the time that these individuals arrived in the US. All of the bilingual participants had been immersed in English for a minimum of 5 years at the time of testing. The years of English experience naturally ranged from the highest for the bilinguals who were immersed in English at the youngest age (1–3 group – mean of 17.9 years) to progressively shorter durations. However, it should be noted that the two latest learning groups (11–13 and >15) had comparable years of experience with English (means of 7.8 and 7.6 years, respectively).

5.2.1   Linguistic proficiency

Consistent with previous behavioral studies (Johnson & Newport, 1989; Newport, 1988), the English proficiency demonstrated by these bilingual participants was related to their age of English immersion (Weber-Fox & Neville, 1996, 2001). This relationship was reflected in both the participants' self-rated proficiency scores as well as their performance on tests of knowledge of English syntax and grammar. The self-rated proficiency scores were virtually identical for comprehension and speaking abilities (Weber-Fox & Neville, 1996, 2001). Specifically, the bilingual speakers who were immersed in English prior to the age of 11 years rated themselves more proficient and nearly perfect in English as compared to Chinese. The bilingual speakers who arrived in the US around the age of puberty (11–13 years) rated themselves equally proficient in English and Chinese, and interestingly did not consider themselves perfect in either of their languages. The latest learning bilinguals, who were immersed in English after the age of 15 years, rated their proficiency in Chinese as perfect and higher than their abilities in English. The results of standardized testing in English also revealed that longer delays in second language learning were associated with reduced English proficiency. Performance scores on the CELF Sentence Structure Subtest (Semel-Mintz & Wiig, 1982) revealed reduced proficiency for bilingual speakers who were immersed in English as early as 7–10 years of age (Weber-Fox & Neville, 1996, 2001). Figure 5.4 illustrates the syntactic proficiency of the bilingual groups compared to monolingual English speakers.

5.2.2   Semantic and syntactic anomalies

Sentence stimuli that had previously revealed distinct neural subsystems for syntactic and semantic processing in monolinguals were utilized (Neville *et al.*, 1991). This paradigm allowed the comparison of ERPs that were elicited by violations in syntactic structure, specifically a phrase structure violation (e.g., "The boys heard Joe's <u>about</u> stories Africa"), and violations in semantic

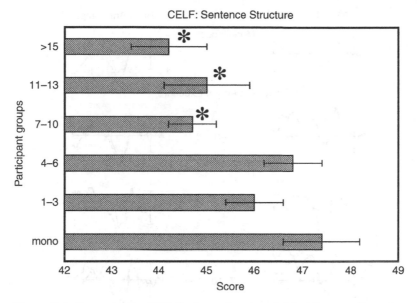

Figure 5.4   Scores for the CELF: Sentence Structure Subtest for monolinguals and each of the bilingual groups. Asterisks indicate decreased syntactic proficiency in English for bilinguals who were immersed in English after 7 years of age.

expectation (e.g., "The boys heard Joe's <u>orange</u> about Africa"). Participants were also presented with control sentences that contained no violations of English syntax or semantics (e.g., "The boys heard Joe's *stories about* Africa"). The randomized sentences were displayed one word at a time (2 words/second) on a monitor while the participants' electroencephalographic (EEG) signals were recorded. The underlined words in the examples of the phrase structure violations and semantic anomalies indicate the comparison points for ERPs elicited by those violation conditions and their control sentences.

After reading each sentence, participants were asked to judge whether or not the sentence was a "good English sentence." The accuracies in detecting syntactic and semantic violations were differentiated among the bilingual groups (Weber-Fox & Neville, 1996). Consistent with our predictions, the judgment accuracy for phrase structure violations was affected by shorter delays in second language exposure compared to the detection of semantic anomalies. While only the latest learning bilingual group (>15) performed less accurately than the monolinguals in detecting semantic anomalies, the detection of phrase structure violations was reduced in bilinguals who were immersed in English as young as 7–10 years old (Weber-Fox & Neville, 1996).

Consistent with these behavioral findings, the ERP responses elicited by phrase structure violations and semantic anomalies displayed differential sensitivity to delays in second language learning. The electrophysiological

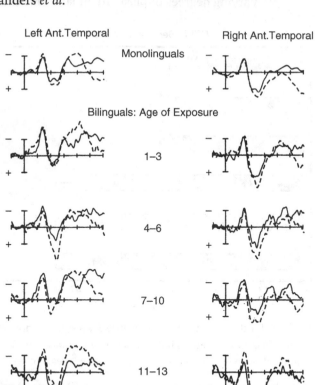

Figure 5.5   ERPs elicited by phrase structure violations for monolinguals and each of the bilingual groups. Responses over the left and right anterior temporal electrode sites are illustrated. Negative potentials are plotted upward (from Weber-Fox & Neville, 1999; with permission from Lawrence Erlbaum).

responses to phrase structure violations showed marked changes in the distribution, amplitude, and actual presence of ERP components (Weber-Fox & Neville, 1996). For example, the asymmetry in the left anterior negativity (LAN) between 300 and 500 ms elicited by phrase structure violations in monolinguals was decreased with longer delays in English immersion, and a more bilateral response emerged in the late-learners (Figure 5.5). As Figure 5.5 illustrates, longer delays in second language learning were associated with increased involvement of the right hemisphere between 300 and 500 ms. This result suggests that less specialized and more broadly distributed language systems are used by later learning bilinguals for this task.

Another aspect of the ERP responses elicited by phrase structure violations was sensitive to delays in second language learning as well: the syntactic positive shift (SPS). The SPS, measured in the 500–700 ms latency window, was absent in the ERPs of bilinguals immersed in English after 11 years of age (also depicted in Figure 5.5). Further analysis revealed that the ERPs from bilinguals immersed in English at around the time of puberty (11–13 years) displayed an SPS in a later latency range (700–900 ms). However, no evidence of an SPS was found in the ERPs of the latest learning group (>15 years), despite a similar number of years of experience with English. These results suggest that later learners of English might have been processing and interpreting these syntactic violations in an atypical manner.

In contrast, semantic anomalies elicited characteristic N400 responses for each of the bilingual groups, regardless of age of second language immersion (Figure 5.6). No differences in the distribution or amplitude of the N400 across the bilingual groups were found. However, the peak latency of the N400 was longer for the bilinguals immersed in English after 11 years of age, suggesting a slight slowing in processing (approximately 20 ms) for the latest learning bilingual groups.

Thus, both the behavioral and neurophysiological results for detecting linguistic violations indicate that the subsystems for processing syntactic and semantic information are differentially impacted by delays in second language immersion. Further, both the behavioral and electrophysiological results indicate that the subsystems for syntactic processing are more sensitive and impacted to a greater extent by delayed immersion compared to the subsystems utilized for semantic interpretation.

5.2.3   Closed- and open-class words

In a complementary study, the effects of delays in second language learning were examined for closed- and open-class words that were used appropriately in sentences (Weber-Fox & Neville, 2001). These two word classes were selected because they have different functions during sentence processing. Open-class words primarily provide referential meaning and are more closely related to semantic processing. In contrast, closed-class words provide information regarding the relationships between open-class words and are primarily related to syntactical processing (Hagoort et al., 1999; Neville et al., 1992). As in the study described above, effects of delayed language immersion could thus be observed separately for the functional neural subsystems associated with

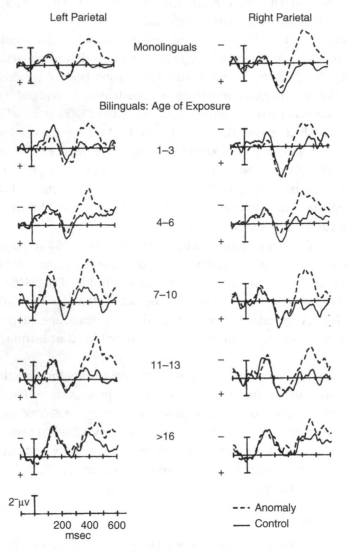

SEMANTIC ANOMALY

Left Parietal   Right Parietal

Monolinguals

Bilinguals: Age of Exposure

1–3

4–6

7–10

11–13

>16

2⁻µv

200 400 600
msec

- - - Anomaly
— Control

Figure 5.6 ERPs elicited by violations in semantic expectations for monolinguals and each of the bilingual groups. Responses over the left and right parietal electrode sites are illustrated. Negative potentials are plotted upward (from Weber-Fox & Neville, 1999; with permission from Lawrence Erlbaum).

syntactic and semantic processing. Therefore, this study extended the observations of our previous findings to include processing of words used appropriately in sentences. Given the differential functions of open- and closed-class words in sentence processing and electrophysiological evidence (Neville *et al.*, 1992, 1993), we hypothesized that the neural subsystems associated with these two word classes would be differentially affected by delays in second language immersion. Evidence from deaf individuals (Neville *et al.*, 1992) and children with language impairment (Neville *et al.*, 1993) predicted that the neural subsystems associated with processing closed-class words would be impacted to a greater extent by delays in second language immersion than the neural systems associated with processing open-class words.

Parallel to the previous study (Weber-Fox & Neville, 1996), participants were grouped according to the age at which they were initially immersed in English. Monolingual and bilingual speakers read 120 sentences previously used in a study of hearing and deaf individuals (Neville *et al.*, 1992). The sentences were presented one word at a time on a monitor. Half of them ended in a semantic anomaly and participants indicated whether the sentences made sense or not. With the exception of the first and last words in the sentences, each of the words was categorized as open- or closed-class. The ERPs were then averaged separately for each word class (Weber-Fox & Neville, 2001).

Similar to previous findings (Neville *et al.*, 1992), the ERPs elicited by closed- and open-class words displayed distinctions in functional neural subsystems in monolingual and bilingual speakers; that is, the responses to open-class words were characterized by a bilateral negativity, peaking around 350 ms after word onset that was largest over posterior regions. In contrast, the ERPs elicited by closed-class words displayed an earlier negative peak (280 ms after word onset) that was lateralized over anterior and temporal regions of the left hemisphere (Weber-Fox & Neville, 2001).

The effects of delays in second language immersion were evidences by the peak latencies of the N280 over the left hemisphere. Peak latencies of the N280 were later (approximately 35 ms) with delays in second language learning as short as 7 years (Weber-Fox & Neville, 2001) (Figure 5.7). Further analyses revealed that these latencies were significantly correlated with English syntactic proficiency as measured by the CELF Sentence Structure Subtest (Semel-Mintz & Wiig, 1982; see Weber-Fox & Neville, 2001, for further details). In contrast, the latencies and distribution of the ERPs elicited by open-class words (N350) were similar across monolinguals and each of the bilingual groups. No age of immersion effects were observed for open-class words (Weber-Fox & Neville, 2001).

Consistent with our findings for processing syntactic and semantic violations, the findings for closed- and open-class words support the hypothesis that delays in second language immersion do not uniformly affect neural subsystems for language. Furthermore, whether participants were processing linguistic violations or different word classes used appropriately in sentences, the neural subsystems for syntactic/grammatical functions were more sensitive to shorter delays in second language learning. Thus, these studies support the

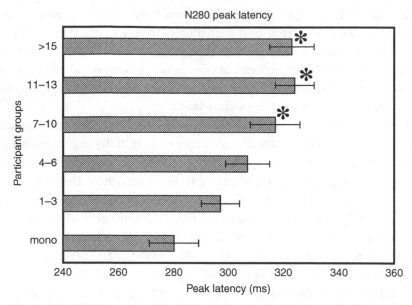

Figure 5.7   Peak latencies of the N280 elicited by closed-class words for monolinguals and each of the bilingual groups. Measures are illustrated for the left anterior temporal electrode site. Asterisks indicate longer latencies for bilinguals who were immersed in English after 7 years of age.

hypothesis that the timing of second language experience has differential degrees of impact in the development of specialized neural subsystems for language.

5.3   Speech segmentation in bilinguals

Unlike with written English, people do not usually leave spaces or pauses between words in spoken English. However, listeners must somehow determine where boundaries occur in continuous speech in order to map the sounds onto familiar lexical items. Many different types of information in speech have been hypothesized to be useful in this process of speech segmentation, including lexical information (Norris *et al.*, 1995), syntactic information (Cole *et al.*, 1980), and, in at least some languages, stress pattern information (Cutler & Butterfield, 1992). In a recent study, we showed that all of these types of information are not only available in English speech, but also that native speakers use each of these cues to determine where word onsets occur in continuous speech (Sanders & Neville, 2000). Since native speakers used lexical, syntactic, and stress-pattern cues to perform the segmentation task, we employed the same task as a measure of nonnative speakers' abilities to use each of these aspects of language as well. Thus, the segmentation task provided an opportunity to measure the effects of delays in second language acquisition on an additional subsystem of language – prosody.

Based on the literature reviewed above, we hypothesized that nonnative speakers would be able to use lexical information to segment English speech, even if they did not learn the language until late in life. In contrast, we expected that nonnative speakers who learned English late in life would not be able to use syntactic information to the same extent as native speakers. Based on the research of phonological processing and the finding that nonnative speakers fail to learn to use syllabification as a segmentation cue (Cutler *et al.*, 1983, 1989, 1992), we hypothesized that nonnative speakers would not be able to use stress pattern to the same extent as native speakers. We were also interested in the ways in which the stress-pattern characteristics of the native language might affect nonnative speakers' ability to use English stress-pattern as a segmentation cue.

5.3.1   *Behavioral study*

Five groups of participants were included in this study: monolingual English speakers (ME), native Japanese late-learners of English (JLE), native Spanish late-learners of English (SLE), native Japanese speakers who had little experience with English and were tested in Japan (JJ), and monolingual Spanish speakers (MS). Both groups of late-learners began learning English after the age of 12 but had lived in an English-speaking country for an average of 6 years. The two groups of nonnative speakers were selected such that one native language (Japanese) would provide no experience with lexical stress as it is used in English, and the other native language (Spanish) would provide experience with lexical stress, but with a different stress pattern than is typical in English.

All subjects were asked to perform the same task. For each sentence that they heard, they were first given a target phoneme or phoneme combination. They were asked to press one button if they heard the target at the beginning of a word or nonword in the subsequent sentence. They were asked to press a different button if they heard the target in the middle of a word or nonword. The amount of lexical information available in the sentences was varied by taking normal English sentences (semantic sentence type) and replacing all of the content words with pronounceable nonwords (syntactic sentence type). The amount of syntactic information available in the sentences was varied by taking the syntactic sentences and replacing all of the remaining words and mor-phemes with nonwords (acoustic sentence type). Prosody was maintained across all three sentence types, but stress pattern was manipulated by including target phonemes in words with normal English stress pattern (strong stress on the

Table 5.1. *Examples of semantic, syntactic, and acoustic sentences*

Condition	Type	Sentence
Target present		
SI	Semantic	In order to recycle *b*ottles you have to separate them.
	Syntactic	In order to lefatal *b*okkers you have to thagamate them.
	Acoustic	Ah ilgen di lefatal *b*okkerth ha maz di thagamate fon.
SM	Semantic	If the only thing in it were to*b*acco it wouldn't cause so much harm.
	Syntactic	If the ilmy shord in it were do*b*atty it wouldn't gaff so much hilm.
	Acoustic	Os fa ilmy shord el ok hon do*b*atty ag hapsel gaff sha nes hilm.
WI	Semantic	The child stopped crying when a *b*alloon was given to her.
	Syntactic	The ferp trepped plawing when a *b*arreal was kaffen to her.
	Acoustic	Sa ferp trepp plawel ron i *b*arreal hof kaffem gi wem.
WM	Semantic	I saved money since lowgrade tim*b*er worked for this project.
	Syntactic	I cheft rono since miltrok del*b*er meld for this plassig.
	Acoustic	O cheft rono zalf miltrok del*b*er meld sith foch plassig.
Target absent		
	Semantic	Try looking under the afghan for the toy you lost.
	Syntactic	Qui medding under the ithdon for the kay you moft.
	Acoustic	Qui medden amkel fa ithdon sal cha kay wa moft.

Note: All example sentences use /b/ as the target phoneme which is indicated by italics in the sentences. SI = Strong stress, Initial position; SM = Strong stress, Medial position; WI = Weak stress, Initial position; WM = Weak stress, Medial position.
Source: From Sanders and Neville (2000)

initial syllable and weak stress on the medial syllables) and words with an infrequent English stress pattern (weak stress on the initial syllable and strong stress on the medial syllable). Examples of each sentence type and stress patterns are shown in Table 5.1. The groups' abilities to use lexical information were measured by comparing performance on the semantic sentences, which contained complete lexical information, and the syntactic sentences, which had degraded lexical information. Use of syntactic information was measured by comparing performance on the syntactic sentences with performance on the acoustic sentences, which had less syntactic information available. The use of stress pattern to segment speech was measured by comparing performance on targets that occurred in words with normal English stress pattern to performance on those that occurred in words with infrequent English stress pattern.

As reported previously (Sanders & Neville, 2000; Sanders, *et al.*, 2002), the comparison of performance on the semantic and syntactic sentence types (shown in Figure 5.8) revealed that both groups of late-learners of English (JLE, SLE) used lexical information to the same extent as native English speakers, as

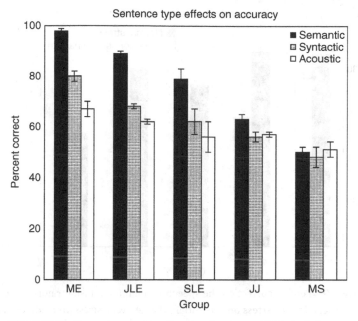

Figure 5.8   Percent correct on the speech segmentation task for semantic, syntactic, and acoustic sentence types. ME = Monolingual English speakers; JLE = Native Japanese late-learners of English; SLE = Native Spanish late-learners of English; JJ = Native Japanese speakers tested in Japan (native Japanese speakers with little English experience); MS = Monolingual Spanish speakers. Both groups of late-learners of English used lexical information to the same extent as native English speakers (difference in performance on semantic and syntactic sentence types). However, the late-learners of English did not use syntactic information to the same extent (difference in performance on syntactic and acoustic sentence types).

hypothesized. The fact that both groups who did not know English (JJ, MS) did not use the lexical information to as great an extent as the native English speakers confirms that lexical information, and not acoustic factors that could be processed regardless of language experience, was the key difference between the two sentence types.

In contrast to the lexical information, a comparison of the syntactic and acoustic sentence types (also shown in Figure 5.8) revealed that none of the nonnative speakers (JLE, SLE, JJ, and MS) used syntactic information to the same extent as native English speakers. These findings support the hypothesis that delays in second language acquisition affect syntactic processing to a greater extent than lexical or semantic processing.

The comparison of normal and infrequent stress pattern (Figure 5.9) revealed that both the acquisition of English and the specific native language acquired affected the ability to use this segmentation cue. First, both groups of

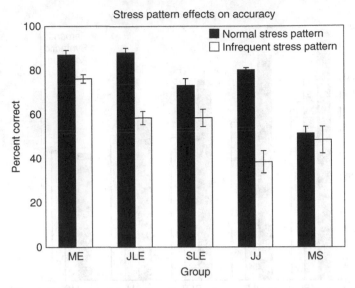

Figure 5.9 Percent correct on the speech segmentation task for normal English stress pattern (strong stress on the initial syllable, weak stress on medial syllables) and an infrequent English stress pattern (weak stress on the initial syllable, strong stress on a medial syllable). ME = Monolingual English speakers; JLE = Native Japanese late-learners of English; SLE = Native Spanish late-learners of English; JJ = Native Japanese speakers tested in Japan (native Japanese speakers with little English experience); MS = Monolingual Spanish speakers. All groups with any experience with English (ME, JLE, SLE, and JJ) were more accurate with normal English stress than infrequent English stress. However, the extent to which stress pattern was used as a segmentation cue depended on the stress pattern characteristics of the native language.

late-learners (JLE, SLE) were able to use stress-pattern to at least the same extent as native English speakers. Second, both groups of native Japanese speakers (JLE, JJ) relied on normal English stress pattern to an even greater extent than the native English speakers did. Third, neither group of native Spanish speakers (SLE, MS) relied on stress pattern to the same extent as either group of native Japanese speakers (JLE, JJ). This pattern of results was interpreted as evidence that stress pattern, and perhaps other prosodic information, can be learned even if exposure to a language that uses lexical stress occurs after the age of 12 and even without many years of experience. Furthermore, the results suggest that the specific type of experience gained with a native language (here, the stress rules) can affect the degree to which similar aspects of a second language are learned and used.

Overall, the results of this behavioral study are consistent with the hypothesis that delays in learning a second language affect syntactic processing to a greater extent than semantic processing. Additionally, they indicate that at least some types of prosodic processing, specifically stress pattern, can be learned later in life. Although the behavioral study indicates that nonnative speakers used lexical and stress-pattern segmentation cues in ways similar to native speakers, this study does not address the issue of whether or not native and nonnative speakers process these types of information at the same rate or using the same neural systems. To answer this question, the same stimuli were presented to subjects while ERPs were recorded.

5.3.2   Event-related potential study

Two groups of subjects were included in this experiment: monolingual English speakers (ME) and native Japanese late-learners of English (JLE). As with the previous study, the native Japanese late-learners of English all began learning English in school in Japan at the age of 12. They continued learning English in school until they moved to the United States and used English as their primary language for an average of 5 years. Both groups of subjects were asked to listen to sentences of the three types described above (semantic, syntactic, and acoustic). They were not given any target phonemes and the only task they completed was to answer "yes" or "no" to the question "Was the word ____ in the previous sentence?" after a randomly selected 5% of the sentences.

Based on the behavioral data described above, we hypothesized that native and nonnative speakers would process semantic information similarly. To test this hypothesis, we compared the ERPs elicited by words in the normal English sentences (semantic) to those evoked by the equivalent nonwords in the syntactic sentences. As reported previously (Sanders & Neville, 2003), in monolingual English speakers, words elicited a greater negativity than nonwords starting by 150 ms after onset in continuous speech (Figure 5.10). This negativity was broadly distributed, but largest at posterior electrode sites over the right hemisphere. The evoked responses to words in comparison to nonwords were equivalent in the native Japanese late-learners of English; that is, a negativity with similar latency and distribution was also evident in this group (Sanders & Neville, 2003). The only differences found in the response to lexical information in the two groups was that the evoked response was of greater amplitude in the native English speakers.

The behavioral data for syntactic processing, unlike lexical processing, indicated that native speakers and late-learners of a language do not process grammatical information in the same way. To further assess this hypothesis, we compared the ERPs to nonwords in the sentences which retained syntactic structure (syntactic sentences) to the same nonwords in the sentences which contained less syntactic structure (acoustic sentences). In the native English speakers,

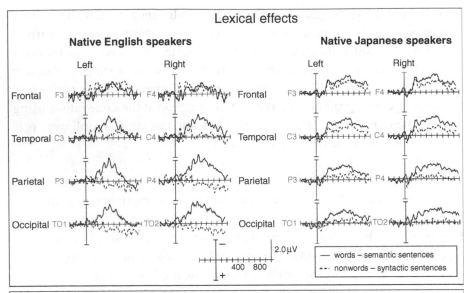

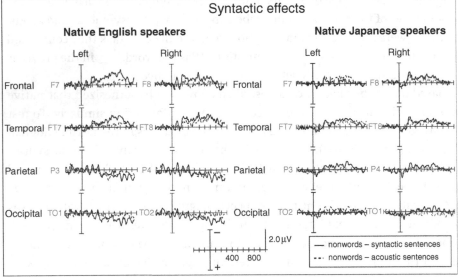

Figure 5.10   ERPs from selected electrode sites for monolingual English speakers and native Japanese late-learners of English. For both groups, words, in comparison to nonwords, elicited a negativity that was largest at posterior areas over the right hemisphere. In contrast, nonwords in the syntactic sentences as compared to nonwords in the acoustic sentences elicited different potentials only in the native English speakers. These differences were found over anterior regions of the left hemisphere.

nonwords in the syntactically intact sentences elicited a negativity that was focally distributed over anterior regions of the left hemisphere (also shown in Figure 5.10). In contrast, no differences in the responses evoked by nonwords in the two types of sentences were found for the native Japanese speakers.

Consistent with the results of the behavioral study, the results of these comparisons indicated that delays in second language learning as long as 12 years had little effect on the ability to use lexical information to segment speech or the cortical organization of processing lexical information. In contrast, these same second language learning delays affected both the ability to use syntactic information in a segmentation task and the cortical organization of syntactic processing.

Lexical stress in English is associated with physical differences in speech such that strongly stressed syllables are both louder and longer than weakly stressed syllables. Since hearing differences in loudness and length do not require specific language experience, it seemed likely that both native and nonnative speakers would show differences in the evoked responses to strongly and weakly stressed syllables. Furthermore, the behavioral evidence indicated that monolingual English speakers and native Japanese late-learners of English are both able to use lexical stress as a cue for speech segmentation. Therefore, we hypothesized that there would be no differences evident in the cortical responses to the two types of stress.

The monolingual English speakers showed a larger negative peak around 100 ms to strong stresses in comparison to weak stresses (shown in Figure 5.11). This difference was predictable in light of research showing that the N100 is larger to louder sounds in comparison to softer sounds. However, the native Japanese late-learners of English showed no differences in the response to strong and weak stresses until after 200 ms. Both groups showed a larger negativity to strong stresses in this later time range. This suggests that, in continuous speech, the early-evoked responses to stress differences may be dependent on language experience. Furthermore, it suggests that delays in learning a language that makes use of lexical stress can affect which neural populations are responsible for processing this type of information.

Additionally, we assessed whether these were differences in the ERPs elicited by word-initial syllable onsets and word-medial syllable onsets (Sanders & Neville, 2003). A comparison of the responses to syllables of equivalent loudness and length in word-initial and word-medial positions, revealed that the word-initial syllables elicited a larger N100, similar to that found for strong stresses, in native English speakers (also shown in Figure 5.11). If the nonnative speakers were segmenting speech in the same way as native speakers, we would expect the same results for the native Japanese speakers. However, for this group, no differences in the responses evoked by word-initial and word-medial syllables were found in the first 300 ms after presentation (Sanders & Neville, 2003). Along with the results for strong and weak stresses, these findings suggest that although both native English speakers and native Japanese late-learners of English were able to perform the speech segmentation task and made use of

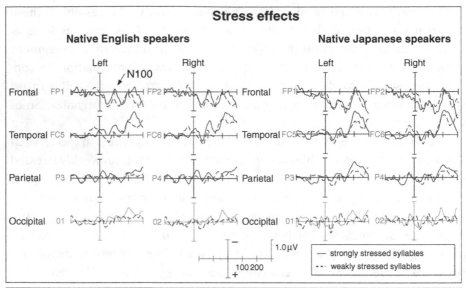

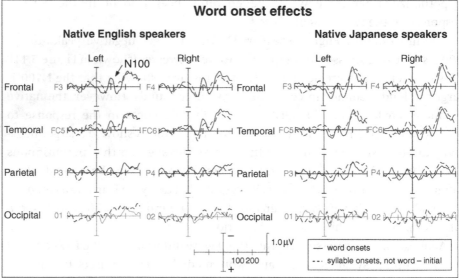

Figure 5.11 ERPs from selected electrode sites for monolingual English speakers and native Japanese late-learners of English. Although strongly stressed syllables elicited a larger negativity than weakly stressed syllables in both groups, this difference was earlier in the monolingual English speakers (100 ms) than in the native Japanese speakers (200 ms). Additionally, a word-onset effect was only found for the native English speakers.

stress-pattern information to do so, processing stress information and segmenting speech take place over different time courses and involve different neural populations for the two groups.

In summary, these studies suggest that delays in second language acquisition affect semantic, syntactic, and prosodic processing in different ways. Results from both behavioral and electrophysiological measures indicate that delays of up to 12 years do not affect at least certain aspects of semantic/lexical processing. In contrast, the same delays in second language acquisition affect the extent to which syntactic information can be used and the way in which syntactic information is processed. Further, the behavioral data indicate that late-learners of English are able to learn to use stress-pattern information; however, the electrophysiological measures indicate that stress information is processed along different time-courses and using nonidentical neural systems by native and nonnative speakers. The differential effects of delays in second language acquisition on lexical, syntactic, and prosodic processing clearly indicate that, as is the case for the sensory systems of the brain, there is considerable variability in the degree to which and the time periods during which different subsystems depend upon and can be modified by input from the environment: some systems retain the ability to change throughout life while others display multiple, different sensitive periods of peak plasticity.

Acknowledgments

This research was supported by NIH, NIDCD grant R01 DC00128.

References

Bavelier, D., Tomann, A., Hutton, C., *et al.* (2000). Visual attention to the periphery is enhanced in congenitally deaf individuals. *Journal of Neuroscience*, **20**, RC93, 1–6.

Best, C. T. (1993). Emergence of language-specific constraints in perception of non-native speech: a window on early phonological development. In B. de Boysson-Bardies, S. de Schonen, P. Jusczyk, P. MacNeilage, and J. Morton, eds., *Developmental Neurocognition: Speech and Face Processing in the First Year of Life.* Dordrecht, Netherlands: Kluwer, pp. 289–304.

Birdsong, D. (1999). Introduction: whys and why nots of the critical period hypothesis for second language acquisition. In D. Birdsong, ed., *Second Language Acquisition and the Critical Period Hypothesis.* Mahwah, NJ: Lawrence Erlbaum, pp. 1–22.

Bongaerts, T. (1995). Can late starters attain a native accent in a foreign language? A test of the critical period hypothesis. In D. Singleton and Z. Lengyel, eds., *The Age Factor in Second Language Acquisition: A Critical Look at the Critical Period Hypothesis.* Clevedon, UK: Multilingual Matters, pp. 30–50.

Chee, M. W. L., Tan, E. W. L., and Thiel, T. (1999). Mandarin and English single word processing studied with functional magnetic resonance imaging. *The Journal of Neuroscience*, **19**, 3050–6.

Chugani, H. T. and Phelps, M. E. (1986). Maturational changes in cerebral function in infants determined by FDG positron emission tomography. *Science*, **23**, 840–3.

Cole, R. A., Jakimik, J., and Cooper, W. E. (1980). Segmenting speech into words. *Journal of the Acoustical Society of America*, **67**, 1323–32.

Curtiss, S. (1977). *Genie: A Psycholinguistic Study of a Modern-day "Wild Child."* New York: Academic Press.

Curtiss, S. (1989). The case of Chelsea: a new test case of the critical period for language acquisition. Unpublished manuscript, University of California, Los Angeles.

Cutler, A. and Butterfield, S. (1992). Rhythmic cues to speech segmentation: evidence from juncture misperception. *Journal of Memory and Language*, **31**, 218–36.

Cutler, A., Mehler, J., Norris, D., and Segui, J. (1983). A language-specific comprehension strategy. *Nature*, **304**, 159–60.

Cutler, A., Mehler, J., Norris, D., and Segui, J. (1989). Limits on bilingualism. *Nature*, **340**, 229–30.

Cutler, A., Mehler, J., Norris, D., and Segui, J. (1992). The monolingual nature of speech segmentation by bilinguals. *Cognitive Psychology*, **24**, 381–410.

Emmorey, K. and Corina, D. (1990). Lexical recognition in sign language: effects of phonetic structure and morphology. *Perceptual and Motor skills*, **71**, 1227–52.

Flege, J. E., Yeni-Komshian, G. H., and Liu, S. (1999). Age constraints on second-language acquisition. *Journal of Memory and Language*, **41**, 78–104.

Hagoort, P., Brown, C. M., and Osterhout, L. (1999). The neurocognition of syntactic processing. In C. M. Brown and P. Hagoort, eds., *The Neurocognition of Language*. New York: Oxford University Press, pp. 273–316.

Harwerth, R., Smith, E., Duncan, G., Crawford, M., and von Noorden, G. (1986). Multiple sensitive periods in the development of the primate visual system. *Science*, **232**, 235–8.

Huttenlocher, P. R. (1990). Morphometric study of human cerebral cortex development. *Neuropsychologia*, **28**, 517–27.

Illes, J., Francis, W. S., Desmond, J. E., *et al.* (1999). Convergent cortical representation of semantic processing in bilinguals. *Brain and Language*, **70**, 347–63.

Johnson, J. and Newport, E. (1989). Critical period effects in second language learning: the influence of maturational state on the acquisition of English as a second language. *Cognitive Psychology*, **21**, 60–99.

Kim, K. H. S., Relkin, N. R., Lee, K.-M., and Hirsch, J. (1997). Distinct cortical areas associated with native and second languages. *Nature*, **388**, 171–4.

Klein, D., Milner, B., Zatorre, R. J., Meyer, E., and Evans, A. C. (1995). The neural substrates underlying word generation: a bilingual functional-imaging study. *Proceedings of the National Academy of Sciences USA*, **92**, 2899–903.

Klein, D., Milner, B., Zatorre, R. J., Zhao, V., and Nikelski, J. (1999). Cerebral organization in bilinguals: a PET study of Chinese-English verb generation. *NeuroReport*, **10**, 2841–6.

Klein, D., Zatorre, R. J., Milner, B., Meyer, E., and Evans, A. C. (1994). Left putaminal activation when speaking a second language: evidence from PET. *NeuroReport*, **5**, 2295–7.

Klima, E. S. and Bellugi, U. (1979). *The Signs of Language*. Cambridge, MA: Harvard University Press.

Kuhl, P. A. (1993). Innate predispositions and the effects of experience in speech perception: the native language magnet theory. In B. de Boysson-Bardies, S. de Schonen, P. Jusczyk, P. MacNeilage, and J. Morton, eds., *Developmental Neurocognition: Speech and Face Processing in the First Year of Life*. Dordrecht, Netherlands: Kluwer, pp. 259–74.

Kuhl, P. K., Williams, K. A., Lacerda, F., Stevens, K. N., and Lindblom, B. (1992). Linguistic experience alters phonetic perception in infants by 6 months of age. *Science*, **255**, 606–8.

Lamendella, J. T. (1977). General principles of neurofunctional organization and their manifestation in primary and nonprimary language acquisition. *Language Learning*, **27**, 155–96.

Lenneberg, E. H. (1967). *Biological Foundations of Language*. New York: Wiley.

Long, M. (1990). Maturational constraints on language development. *Studies in Second Language Acquisition*, **12**, 251–85.

Maurer, D. and Lewis, T. L. (1998). Overt orienting toward peripheral stimuli: normal development and underlying mechanisms. In J. E. Richards, ed., *Cognitive Neuroscience of Attention: A Developmental Perspective*. Hillsdale, NJ: Erlbaum, pp. 51–102.

Mayberry, R. and Fischer, S. D. (1989). Looking through phonological shape to lexical meaning: the bottleneck of non-native sign language processing. *Memory and Cognition*, **17**, 740–54.

Mitchell, D. (1981). Sensitive periods in visual development. In R. Aslin, J. Alberts, and M. Petersen, eds., *Development of Perception*. New York: Academic Press, pp. 3–43.

Neville, H. and Bavelier, D. (1999). Specificity and plasticity in neurocognitive development in humans. In M. Gazzaniga, ed., *The New Cognitive Neurosciences*, 2nd edn. Cambridge, MA: MIT Press, pp. 83–98.

Neville, H. J. (1991). Neurobiology of cognitive and language processing: effects of early experience. In K. R. Gibson and A. C. Petersen, eds., *Brain Maturation and Cognitive Development: Comparative and Cross-cultural Perspectives*. Hawthorne, NY: Aldine de Gruyter Press, pp. 355–80.

Neville, H. J. and Bavelier, D. (2001). Effects of auditory and visual deprivation on human brain development. *Clinical Neuroscience Research*, **1**, 248–57.

Neville, H. J., Bavelier, D., Corina, D., *et al.* (1998). Cerebral organization for language in deaf and hearing subjects: biological constraints and effects of experience. *Proceedings of the National Academy of Sciences USA*, **95**, 922–9.

Neville, H. J., Coffey, S. A., Holcomb, P. J., and Tallal, P. (1993). The neurobiology of sensory and language processing in language impaired children. *Journal of Cognitive Neuroscience*, **5**(2), 235–53.

Neville, H. J., Coffey, S. A., Lawson, D. S., *et al.* (1997). Neural systems mediating American Sign Language: effects of sensory experience and age of acquisition. *Brain and Language*, **57**, 285–308.

Neville, H. J., Mills, D. L., and Lawson, D. S. (1992). Fractionating language: different neural subsystems with different sensitive periods. *Cerebral Cortex*, **2**(3), 244–58.

Neville, H. J., Nicol, J., Barss, A., Forster, K., and Garrett, M. (1991). Syntactically based sentence processing classes: evidence from event related brain potentials. *Journal of Cognitive Neuroscience*, **3**, 155–70.

Newman, A. J., Bavilier, D., Corina, D., Jezzard, P., and Neville, H. J. (2001). A critical period for right hemisphere recruitment in American Sign Language processing. *Nature Neuroscience*, **5**, 76–80.

Newport, E. L. (1988). Constraints on learning and their role in language acquisition: studies of the acquisition of American Sign Language. *Language Sciences*, **10**, 147–72.

Newport, E. L. (1990). Maturational constraints on language learning. *Cognitive Science*, **14**, 11–28.

Norris, D., McQueen, J. M., and Cutler, A. (1995). Competition and segmentation in spoken-word recognition. *Journal of Experimental Psychology: Learning, Memory, and Cognition*, **21**, 1209–28.

Ojemann, G. A. (1983). Brain organization for language from the perspective of electrical stimulation mapping. *Behavioral Brain Science*, **6**, 189–230.

Ojemann, G. A. and Whitaker, H. A. (1978). The bilingual brain. *Archives of Neurology*, **35**, 409–12.

Pallier, C., Bosch, L., and Sebastian-Galles, N. (1997). A limit on behavioral plasticity in speech perception. *Cognition*, **64**, B9–17.

Patkowski, M. S. (1994). The critical age hypothesis and interlanguage phonology. In M. Yavas, ed., *First and Second Language Phonology*, San Diego: Singular, pp. 205–21.

Penfield, W. and Roberts, L. (1959). *Speech and Brain Mechanisms*. New York: Atheneum.

Perani, D., Dehaene, S., Grassi, F., *et al.* (1996). Brain processing of native and foreign languages. *NeuroReport*, **7**, 2439–44.

Rauschecker, J. P. and Marler, P. (1987). *Imprinting and Cortical Plasticity*. New York: Wiley.

Sanders, L. D. and Neville, H. J. (2000). Lexical, syntactic, and stress-pattern cues for speech segmentation. *Journal of Speech, Language, and Hearing, Research*, **43**, 1301–21.

Sanders, L. D. and Neville, H. J. (2003). An ERP study of continuous speech processing: I. Segmentation, semantics, and syntax in native English speakers. *Cognitive Brain Research*, **15**, 228–40.

Sanders, L. D. and Neville, H. J. (2003). An ERP study of continuous speech processing: II. Segmentation, semantics, and syntax in non-native speakers. *Cognitive Brain Research*, **15**, 214–27.

Sanders, L. D., Neville, H. J., and Woldorff, M. G. (2002). Speech segmentation by native and non-native speakers: the use of lexical, syntactic, and stress-pattern cues. *Journal of Speech, Language, and Hearing Research*, **45**, 519–30.

Scovel, T. (1988). *A Time to Speak: A Psycholinguistic Inquiry into the Critical Period for Human Speech*. USA: Newbury House.

Sebastian-Galles, N. and Soto-Faraco, S. (1999). Online processing of native and non-native phonemic contrasts in early bilinguals. *Cognition*, **72**, 111–23.

Semel-Mintz, E. and Wiig, E. H. (1982). *Clinical Evaluation of Language Functions (CELF)*. Columbus, OH: Charles E. Merrill.

Singleton, D. (1989). *Language Acquisition: The Age Factor*. Clevedon, UK: Multilingual Matters.

Weber-Fox, C. M. and Neville, H. J. (1996). Maturational constraints on functional specializations for language processing: ERP and behavioral evidence in bilingual speakers. *Journal of Cognitive Neuroscience*, **8**, 231–56.

Weber-Fox, C. M. and Neville, H. J. (1999). Functional neural subsystems are differentially affected by delays in second language immersion: ERP and behavioral evidence in bilinguals. In: D. Birdsong, ed., *Second Language Acquisition and the Critical Period Hypothesis*. Mahwah, NJ: Lawrence Erlbaum, pp. 23–38.

Weber-Fox, C. and Neville, H. J. (2001). Sensitive periods differentiate processing of open- and closed-class words: an ERP study of bilinguals. *Journal of Speech, Language, and Hearing Research*, **44**, 1338–53.

Werker, J. F. and Tees, R. C. (1992). The organization and reorganization of human speech perception. *Annual Review of Neuroscience*, **15**, 377–402.

Werker, J. F. and Tees, R. C. (1999). Influences on infant speech processing: toward a new synthesis. *Annual Review of Psychology*, **50**, 509–35.

Yeni-Komshian, G., Flege, J. E., and Liu, H. (1997). Pronunciation proficiency in L1 and L2 among Korean-English bilinguals: the effect of age of arrival in the US. *Journal of the Acoustical Society of America*, **102**, 3138.

6

The functional architecture of speech perception

DAVID POEPPEL AND MARTIN HACKL

6.1   Introduction

The language system is that aspect of mind/brain function that forms the basis for phonological, morphological, syntactic, and semantic computation. The "currencies" (or the ontology) of this central and abstract computational system are representations that are amodal, for example the concepts "feature" (phonology) or "affix" (morphology) or "phrase" (syntax) or "generalized quantifier" (semantics). Representation and computation with such concepts is typically considered independent of sensory modalities. Of course, the linguistic computational system is not isolated but interacts with other cognitive systems and with sensory–motor interface systems.

With regard to the input and output, the system has at least three modality-specific interfaces: an acoustic-articulatory system (speech perception and production), a visuo-motor system (reading/writing and sign), and a somato-sensory interface (Braille). Speech and sign are the canonical interfaces and develop naturally; written language and Braille are explicitly taught: barring gross pathology, every child learns to speak or sign (rapidly, early, without explicit instruction, to a high level of proficiency), whereas learning to read/write Braille requires explicit instruction, is not universal, and occurs later in development.

In this chapter we focus on speech perception, specifically with regard to linguistic constraints and cortical organization. We first outline the key linguistic assumptions, including the concept of "distinctive feature," and then discuss a functional-anatomic model that captures a range of empirical findings.

Topics in Integrative Neuroscience: From Cells to Cognition, ed. James R. Pomerantz. Published by Cambridge University Press. © Cambridge University Press, 2008.

6.2   The linguistic basis of speech perception

6.2.1   *The central importance of words for language use and understanding*

An essential part of the cognitive ability underlying the linguistic behavior of a competent speaker of a language consists of knowing the words of the language or their constituents (roots). Words cast the two fundamental aspects of language – form and meaning – into single, elementary units. These units are the basic building blocks that are combined in various ways to form larger expressions (pairs of form and meaning) such as phrases, sentences, or texts that are used for communicating information. Models of linguistic competence therefore typically assume two core components: an inventory of building blocks (the set of words stored in the mental lexicon) and a generative engine that manipulates these building blocks to form larger expressions (Figure 6.1).

A central property of this architecture that accounts for the versatility and unparalleled expressive power of natural language is that it is compositional; that is, while at the word level the particular combination of form and meaning is entirely arbitrary, the form and meaning of combinations of words is to a large extent determined by the form and meaning of the words they contain and the particular way these words are put together. To give an example: the English word *cow* is a combination of the phonological form [kau] and the meaning [fully grown female of domestic cattle]. This particular combination of phonological form and meaning into one expression ⟨[kau],[fully grown female of domestic cattle]⟩ is entirely arbitrary. Nothing in the meaning of the word *cow* dictates that its phonological form is [kau]. In fact, the same concept can be described for instance in German with the word *Kuh*, whose phonological form is [ku:]. Vice versa: nothing in the phonological form of *cow* dictates that its (dominant) meaning exponent is [fully grown female of domestic cattle]. In German the meaning associated with the same phonological form [kau] is the root as well as the imperative form of the verb *chew*. Since the particular combination of form and meaning cast into a word is unpredictable, speakers have to learn words one by one and store them in a repository called the mental lexicon. Once words are combined with other words, the resulting expression has predictable form and meaning exponents. For instance, if *cow* is combined with the determiner

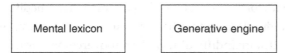

Figure 6.1   The two main components of the language system in the context of contemporary generative linguistic theories include the repository of lexical knowledge as well as the set of elementary operations that generate expressions.

quantifier *every*, the result is the phrase *every cow* whose form is [every cow] and whose meaning is the generalized quantifier [{A: {x: x is a cow} ⊆ A}] – both of which are determined by the properties of the components and the particular way English syntax and semantics demands them to be combined.[1]

A simple illustration of the importance of the compositionality of natural language is provided by the fact that competent speakers understand sentences that they have never encountered before with (roughly) the same ease with which they understand sentences they have encountered many times. To give an example, consider the sentence in (1a), which even though you most likely have never seen before you understand easily to mean the same as the sentence in (1b).

(1) a.   John read more books than there are prime numbers smaller than 5.
     b.   John read more than three books.

This is a remarkable feat that every competent speaker of English is able to accomplish with astonishing ease because she knows all the words in the sentence (1a) and the particular rules that determine how these words are combined to form that sentence. In general, then, understanding an utterance requires of a listener to analyze the signal so that the words that make up the utterance can be identified. The primary cues to achieve this are given by the phonological form of the words. Once the phonological form of a word is recognized it can be used to access the meaning of the word, which in turn is used to build up a representation of the information conveyed by the utterance.

6.2.2   Identifying words in written language is easy

The specifics of the task of identifying the words in an utterance depend, of course, on the modality in which the utterance is presented to the recipient. If the utterance is in English and presented in written form, the task is relatively easy because the writing system used to transcribe English typically indicates word boundaries with blank spaces.[2] If that were not the case, understanding written language would be a lot harder. For instance, even a skilled reader will find it much more difficult to read the paragraph below (although it says exactly the same thing as the following paragraph) simply because word boundaries are omitted.

(2) sincetherearenowordboundarysignsinspokenlanguagethedifficulty
     wefeelinreadingandunderstandingtheaboveparagraphprovidesasimple
     illustrationofoneofthemaindifficultieswehavetoovercomeinorderto
     understandspeechratherthananeatlyseparatedsequenceofletterstrings
     correspondingtothephonologicalformofwordsthespeechsignalisa
     continuousstreamofsoundsthatrepresentthephonologicalformsof

wordsinadditionthesoundsofneighboringwordsoftenoverlapwhich
makestheproblemofidentifyingwordboundariesevenharder

6.2.3   Identifying words in spoken language should be much harder

Since there are no word boundary signs in spoken language, the difficulty we feel in reading and understanding the above paragraph provides a simple illustration of one of the main difficulties we have to overcome when we try to understand speech. Rather than a neatly separated sequence of letter strings corresponding to the phonological form of words, the speech signal is a continuous stream of sounds that represent the phonological forms of words. Worse, not only are the sounds that correspond to the words in an utterance not neatly separated by pauses, they often overlap with sounds of neighboring words (the problem of "linearity"). Additional difficulties arise because actual speech sounds are highly variable across speakers, speech rate and acoustics of the environment (the invariance problem), making the task of speech perception – even if we simplify it in a first approximation as a process of mapping a continuous acoustic signal to a sequence of discrete phonological forms of words – seemingly impossible to master. It is therefore prima facie astonishing how effortless and robust speech perception is for competent speakers of a language.

6.2.4   Speech sounds that correspond to words are highly structured acoustic events

The robustness of speech perception across adverse conditions such as speaker variability, rate of speech, environmental conditions, etc. makes it highly unlikely that all there is to speech perception is a simple, analogue one-to-one mapping between speech sound and the phonological form of a word. (The violation of linearity in the signal is due to factors such as coarticulation.) Instead, it suggests that the speech signal is broken down into more abstract and invariant, linguistically significant components, while many acoustic properties of the signal are filtered out for the purpose of understanding a spoken utterance.[3] But, what are the linguistically relevant components of a speech sound and how is the phonological form of a word represented in an acoustic signal?

We can approach these questions from the other end, so to speak. Minimally, identifying a specific word requires the listener to distinguish it from all other words – in particular from those words that are very similar and differ only minimally from the target. The difference between minimal word pairs can typically be localized to segments of the word. For instance, the difference between the minimal pair *cup* and *cop* is localized in the quality of the vowel. The consonants flanking the vowel are identical. On the other hand, the differences between the minimal pairs *but* and *cut* and *cup* and *cut* are located at the beginning and end of the words, in the identity of the initial and final consonants,

respectively. Observations of this kind lead naturally to the view that the components of the phonological form of a word are segments with distinct melodic
identity and the task that speech perception has to accomplish is to identify the
segments of the words in the acoustic signal.[4] Segments whose particular melodic
identity is exploited by the language to code different words are called *phonemes*
and a competent speaker needs to have a representation of the phonemes of her
language; that is, she needs to know the ways in which phonological forms of
words can minimally differ in her language. On the other hand, the inventory or
distinctive segments provide a rough characterization of the space of possible
words of a language.[5] Knowing what the possible word forms in your language are
is rather useful to solve the problem of speech perception because it constrains
the search for the target word given an input signal.

6.2.5   *Sequencing constraints*

Of course, it is not the case that any old combination of phonemes results
in a legitimate word. In fact, there are severe restrictions as to what kinds of
phoneme sequences are possible. For instance, there are no words in English that
contain the phoneme sequence [pf], even though both sounds are phonemes of
English. German, on the other hand, allows this sequence. Similarly, certain
phoneme sequences are highly restricted in their distribution within a word.
For instance, there are no words in English that start with the sequence [rt]
although the sequence itself is allowed, as illustrated by the final phoneme
sequence of the word *cart*. Constraints of this sort – known as "sonority sequencing constraints" – typically make reference to prosodic units such as syllables,
feet, etc. within a word. For instance, the distribution of the sequence [rt] in
English is restricted to follow the nucleus of a syllable that is occupied by a
vowel while the sequence [tr] is restricted to precede the nucleus as in *track*.
Constraints of this sort are highly significant for speech perception because
they suggest that the signal is broken down into linguistically significant chunks
like syllables and feet[6] within which sequencing constraints provide a powerful
filter that constrains the mapping between acoustic signal and phoneme.
Although there are a number of universal constraints on syllable structure and
sequencing, it is worth pointing out that languages differ as to what kinds of
syllables and what kinds of sequencing constraints they employ. If syllable structure and sequencing constraints indeed matter for speech perception, it goes to
show that the linguistic competence of speakers – which is thought to be a rather
abstract knowledge base of one's language – affects speech perception, often
thought to be a lower-level cognitive ability. Compelling results pointing to the
relevance of native phonology (syllabic constraints) to perception are shown by,
among others, Dupoux *et al.* (1999) and Dehaene-Lambertz *et al.* (2000).

6.2.6 Allophonic variability

While this simplifies the perceptual task considerably by temporally narrowing down the problem of identifying which portion of the acoustic signal corresponds to which phoneme, the difficulties mentioned above (variability across conditions, coarticulation) still have to be dealt with. As a simple illustration of the difficulties speakers of English encounter, consider the well-known variation in the realization of the phoneme [t] in American English exemplified in the words listed below (examples from Kenstowicz, 1994).

(3) a. stem   [t]
    b. ten   [tʰ]   "aspirated t"
    c. strip   [ʈ]   "retroflexed t"
    d. atom   [D]   "flapped"
    e. panty   [N]   "nasal flap"
    f. hit   [tʔ]   "glottalized t"
    g. bottle   [ʔ]   "glottal stop"
    h. pants   zero

The examples in (3) show that there are at least eight rather different acoustic-phonetic realizations of the same phoneme. Interestingly, speakers of American English report to "hear" the same sound in all these contexts despite the large range of phonetic variability. This suggests that there is a common core to all of these sounds, namely the phoneme /t/, while the various sounds described in (4) are allophonic variations of it.[7] Of course, knowing that English does not make phonemic distinctions between the various realizations listed above simplifies the task of identifying the phoneme in the signal considerably. This suggests once more that linguistic competence matters a great deal for speech perception. Even more, it suggests that the problem of speech perception should be stated in terms of linguistically significant units – especially if they are rather abstract entities such as phonemes that are related to the signal by a many-to-one mapping.

6.2.7 Phonological processes

In addition to allophonic variation, there are numerous systematic alternations that phonemes undergo when the words they appear in are combined with other morphemes to form a larger unit. A simple example is given by the alternation the English indefinite article *a* undergoes, depending on whether the following word starts with a vowel or consonant.

(4) a. a book
    b. a dog

c.   a cat

d.   an apple

e.   an egg

f.   an island

Processes of this kind are very common across languages. Modern Arabic, for instance, displays a slightly more radical version of this phenomenon involving the definite article *al*. Specifically, as the examples listed in (5) and (6) show, the final phoneme of the definite article *al* mimics the melodic identity of the first phoneme of the word following the article (data from Kaye, 1989).

(5) a.   al bab   "the father"

     b.   al firaash   "the bed"

     c.   al ɣurfa   "the bedroom"

     d.   al miftaah   "the key"

     e.   al baab   "the door"

     f.   al qamar   "the moon"

     g.   al kitaab   "the book"

     h.   al yasaar   "the left"

(6) a.   ad dars   "the lesson"

     b.   ar ruzz   "the rice"

     c.   az zuba   "the butter"

     d.   al turb   "the land"

     e.   as sayyaara   "the car"

     f.   al luɣa   "the language"

     g.   an naas   "the people"

     h.   ash shams   "the sun"

An inspection of these examples suggests that the particular phonemic make-up of the word-beginning determines whether the preceding definite article changes its appearance or not. In (5), the article keeps its basic form if it combines with words like the ones listed. The data listed in (6) illustrate a robust generalization in Modern Arabic: words that begin with one of the phonemes [d], [r], [z], [t], [s], [l], [n], or [sh] *always* assimilate the preceding determiner, while words that do not begin with one of these phonemes do not (cf. 5). Interestingly, this grouping of phonemes into ones that do and do not affect the preceding article is not random. All of the phonemes listed in the second group that trigger assimilation share an articulatory gesture. Specifically, all of them are produced with the front of the tongue raised toward the top of the mouth, while none of the phonemes listed in the first set of examples (that do not affect the shape of the preceding definite determiner) employs this gesture. The gesture is called *coronal*.

Observations of this kind are abundant across languages and have been taken by linguists to show that phonemes are not atomic units. Instead, they are composites of more elementary entities, so called *distinctive features*. The idea that phonemes are complexes of distinctive features provides a natural and elegant explanation for the fact that phonemes can be grouped into natural classes with respect to phonological processes. In the Arabic example above, the phonemes that trigger regressive assimilation are those that contain the feature [+coronal].[8] A well-known example from the plural morphology of English provides a nice illustration of the explanatory power of the hypothesis that phonological processes are defined over the features that make phonemes rather than the phonemes themselves. Regular English plural formation of nouns employs three distinct suffixes, as the examples in (7) demonstrate (examples from Halle, 1990).

(7) [ɪz]   places, mazes, porches, cabbages, ambushes, camouflages
    [s]   lips, lists, maniacs, telegraphs, hundredths
    [z]   clubs, herds, colleagues, phonemes, terns, fangs, holes, gears, pies, apostrophes, avenues, cellos, violas

Inspection of these examples shows – quite similar to the assimilation process of Modern Arabic – that the choice of the particular plural suffix is governed by the last phoneme of the word that is pluralized. Specifically, the pattern can be described by the rule in (8):

(8) [ɪz]   if the word ends with [s],[z],[č],[š], or [ž], otherwise
    [s]   if the word ends with [p], [t], [k], [f], or [θ], otherwise
    [z]

Even though the rule in (8) is descriptively adequate, it is intrinsically unsatisfactory because it does not explain why the phonemes are grouped in exactly those ways rather than any other combination. The hypothesis that phonemes are feature complexes provides the means to identify the various groups in a principled way: phonemes form a natural class with respect to phonological processes if they share a distinctive feature relevant for the process in question. In the case of regular plural morphology of English nouns, the features in question are [+coronal], [+strident], and [−voice]. The rule that describes the generalization therefore takes on the form in (9).

(9) [ɪz]   if the word ends with [+coronal, +strident], otherwise
    [s]   if the word ends with [−voice], otherwise
    [z]

Even though both rules are equally successful in describing the pattern listed in (7), they make different predictions for words that end in phonemes that are not native to English. One such example is provided by the German name *Bach*. Since the last phoneme of this word is the velar fricative [χ] which contains as one of its components the feature [−voice], the rule schema in (9) predicts correctly that its plural form is realized by [s] and that speakers of English will say [baχs]. The rule schema in (8), on the other hand, incorrectly predicts that the plural of *Bach* is marked by [z] because the phoneme [χ] is not listed in the set that requires the [s]-plural. Clearly, the rule schema that makes reference to the distinctive feature [−voice] offers the better explanation of these facts. Generalizations stated in terms of distinctive features are more powerful in that they do not depend on the specific inventory of phonemes. Instead, they depend on the presence or absence of features, which allows words that employ nonnative phonemes to behave regularly as long as their feature make-up subjects the item to phonological processes native to the language.

Phenomena of this sort are far from being isolated cases. On the contrary, they have been documented in language after language in numerous morphological environments, supporting the same conclusion: phonological processes are defined over units that are smaller than phonemes, that is distinctive features.

The theoretical framework that incorporates these results rejects the significance of the concept phoneme. Rather than being the elementary unit of phonological processes, the phoneme appears to be a mere epiphenomenon that alphabetic writing systems misleadingly present as the fundamental and atomic unit of sound structure. Current phonological theories assume a universal feature inventory of up to 20 distinct features that are used in various combinations by various languages to generate the phoneme inventories of these languages. By the same token, words are no longer viewed as sequences of phonemes. Instead they are sequences of feature complexes. Furthermore, to explain, among other things, the fact that not any combination of features makes a good phoneme, it is typically assumed that the set of features that make up a phoneme is partially hierarchically organized. To illustrate these ideas, consider how the word *cat*, traditionally represented as the phoneme sequence [cæt], is represented in Figure 6.2 in an abbreviated and simplified way as a sequence of feature complexes each associated to a distinct timing slot "x."

6.2.8   *Distinctive features have an articulatory interpretation*

The set of distinctive features is not only motivated by phonological processes; distinctive features have – as pointed out in the example from Modern Arabic – articulatory significance. Recall that the distinctive feature [+coronal] that unifies the phonemes that trigger regressive assimilation of the definite determiner has an interpretation in terms of articulatory gestures. Specifically,

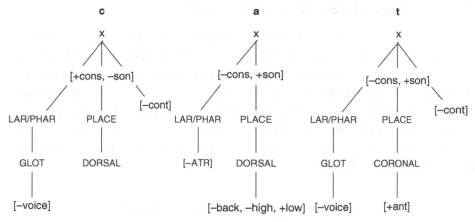

Figure 6.2   The specification of the word "cat" using distinctive features. Each timing slot "x" contains a bundle of features which specify a particular speech sound. This abstract characterization of how words are represented makes explicit the articulatory basis of lexical representation.

[±coronal] represents instructions that the corona of the tongue has to execute in the production of the sounds that are classified as [±coronal]. Similarly, the feature [±voice] represents instructions that the vocal cords execute in the production of sounds that are voiced or voiceless. Quite generally and rather surprisingly, distinctive features, which are the basic units of phonological organization, can be seen as (abstract) instructions of articulatory movements. These articulatory movements have very specific acoustic effects. For instance, the feature [±voice] determines whether the acoustic signal is periodic while the feature [±coronal] has a distinct pattern of formant transitions as an acoustic correlate. In general, the feature complex that constitutes a particular phoneme can be seen as a set of instructions of articulatory movements (quite similar to a ballet score) that the vocal tract has to execute in order to pronounce that phoneme.

6.2.9   The role of distinctive features in perception

Given the central importance of distinctive features for the organization of linguistically significant sounds and the fact that their articulatory interpretation results in specific acoustic correlates, it is natural to assume that one of the central aspects of speech perception is the extraction of distinctive features from the signal. In other words, the fact that the basic units of phonological organization can be interpreted as articulatory gestures with distinct acoustic consequences suggests a rather tight and efficient architectural organization of the language system in which speech production and speech perception are intimately connected through the unifying concept of distinctive features.

6.3   The neural basis of speech perception

In the first section we motivated the critical roles that words, syllables, and distinctive features play for the representation of speech. Specifically, we argued that distinctive features play a unifying role in the characterization and explanation of the mental lexicon, speech production, and speech perception. We now turn to a model of the functional anatomy of speech perception. The model builds on the concept of distinctive feature and illustrates how a model for the cortical organization of speech sound processing is natural in the context of the assumptions detailed above.

6.3.1   *The auditory cortex (bilaterally) builds spectro-temporal representations*

The basic challenge for the perceptual system is to transform the incoming signal, a continuously time-varying waveform, into a format that allows the information in the signal to interface with words in the mental lexicon. If words are stored in a format that uses features (Figure 6.2), the goal is thus to extract features (or feature complexes) from the input waveform. The auditory word recognition process thus must minimally include the analysis of the acoustic signal in the ascending auditory pathway and the construction of a spectro-temporal representation of the signal, the extraction of featural information from that representation, and the interface with stored lexical forms. Figure 6.3 illustrates the implicated processes. There is debate about the extent to which these processes are entirely bottom-up or top-down modulated; this debate is not critical to our considerations, although based on present evidence one might favor an "analysis-by-synthesis" view, by which a significant proportion of perceptual analysis involves the (internal) synthesis of potential candidate representations based on sparse data. Recent physiological evidence (van Wassenhove *et al.*, 2005) suggests that such a model is viable.

What brain areas are implicated in this set of processes? Ignoring the (large) contribution of the ascending auditory pathway up to and including the medial geniculate body, the present evidence suggests that primary (core) auditory cortex and adjacent cortical fields (i.e., Brodmann areas 42 and 22) construct

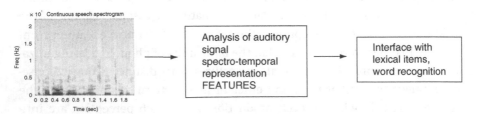

Figure 6.3   The processes implicated in the transformation of the input signal.

spectrotemporal representations of the signal. Neurophysiological data show that there are multi-scale representations that reflect frequency, amplitude, phase, and timing information of acoustic signals. Furthermore, speech perception, when occurring in an ecologically valid way (i.e., "passive" listening without executing laboratory tasks), typically is associated with *bilateral* activity in the auditory cortices, notwithstanding the "left hemisphere imperialism" typical of neurolinguistic research. A variety of findings suggest that the construction of auditory representations of speech is mediated by both hemispheres. *First*, hemodynamic imaging studies show that the activation pattern obtained when subjects listen to speech is always bilateral, including nonprimary areas along Brodmann area 22/STS (Binder *et al.*, 1996, 2000; Mazoyer *et al.*, 1993; Norris & Wise, 2000; Poeppel *et al.*, 1996, 2004; Scott *et al.*, 2000; Zatorre *et al.*, 1992). *Second*, deficit-lesion data suggest that the most selective speech perception deficit, pure word deafness, is a consequence of a lesion pattern that implicates both hemispheres, either directly or by virtue of deafferenting the relevant areas from one another (Buchman *et al.*, 1986; Griffiths *et al.*, 1999; Poeppel, 2001). *Third*, patients in which the dominant (typically left) hemisphere is anaesthetized as part of a presurgical evaluation perform quite well at speech discrimination tasks (Boatman *et al.*, 1998). Overall, the data suggest that (at least one aspect of) speech perception is mediated by the superior temporal lobes of both hemispheres. This general point has been discussed and reviewed in detail by Norris and Wise (2000), Binder *et al.* (2000), and Hickok and Poeppel (2000, 2004).

The hypothesis that the auditory cortex is not just analyzing acoustic structure but is actually sensitive to *featural* information has recently been tested in several MEG studies. Phillips *et al.* (2000) used a mismatch negativity design and manipulated the standard/deviant distributions in a manner such that the analysis of featural information could yield the canonical mismatch responses. These investigators showed that an auditory mismatch field was generated when the only available cue was the featural mismatch, that is the acoustic variation in the test and control conditions could not predict the response. This response localized to auditory cortex. Further experiments by Phillips suggested that the sensitivity to the featural composition is probably left lateralized. To what extent left and right auditory cortices are involved and what their respective contributions might be is discussed below.

6.3.2   *The interface of auditory representations of speech with lexical information*

By conceptual necessity, there must be an interface between sound-based representations of speech and lexical-semantic representations. Where are words represented – or where is the interface? Several kinds of evidence speak to this question. *First*, neuropsychological and neuroimaging data have implicated left posterior temporo-parietal cortex (but also middle and inferior anterior temporal lobe) in conditions such as semantic dementia, in which the lexical-semantic system appears to be compromised (Damasio, 1992; Price, 2000). *Second*, neuroimaging data often show activation in left posterior temporal cortex for words, including the middle and inferior temporal gyri. *Third*, MEG studies show that the typical "lexical" response (N400/M350) is generated in left posterior temporal cortex, consistent with the position that this part of cortex plays a privileged role in lexical processing (Helenius *et al.*, 1998; Pylkkanen *et al.*, 2002). *Finally*, the large literature on Wernicke's aphasia has as its main generalization that posterior temporal cortex is the neural substrate for the processing of word meaning. Based on such data we hypothesize that the output of the analysis executed in the (bilateral) temporal lobes interfaces with left posterior temporal lobe areas to jointly mediate lexical access.

6.3.3   *Frontal areas are involved in production – but also segmentation*

So far we have been concerned with comprehension and have argued that a feature-based theory is consistent with a view in which auditory speech recognition involves the interplay between auditory cortical areas and posterior cortical areas (retrieve the item that connects auditory form and meaning – i.e., lexical access). We now turn to production. In that domain, the central role of features has been known for a long time. Indeed, the concept of distinctive feature has an articulatory origin and interpretation, as discussed above. When a word is selected for pronunciation, its featural composition must be known in order to provide the correct commands to the articulators. The intuition is illustrated in Figure 6.4, which summarizes the last few steps in the production process, phonological encoding and syllabification, phonetic encoding – a feature-based encoding – and articulation. For a detailed analysis of the steps in the production process, see Levelt (1989) and Indefrey and Levelt (2004). The cortical areas assumed to be involved in these final steps of production are, primarily, Broca's area (for syllabification) and motor cortical areas and other areas known for motor planning (e.g., SMA, cerebellum).

The basic model one might derive is that production is largely a frontal process and perception a purely posterior process. Some recent evidence has complicated this idea. The importance of left inferior frontal cortex in perceptual tasks has been documented in several neuropsychological and imaging studies. For example, Broca's area is reliably activated when subjects are asked to perform sub-lexical tasks involving auditorily presented speech. Recent work has suggested that this anterior activation is driven primarily by processes involved in segmentation (Burton *et al.*, 2000; Zatorre *et al.*, 1992, 1996).

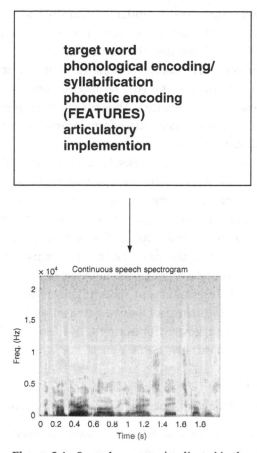

Figure 6.4   Several processes implicated in the planning of speaking a word.

6.3.4   *The coordinate frame problem: how to go from acoustic to articulatory space*

We have satisfactory evidence that frontal areas mediate production (and maybe also aspects of perception) and that temporal areas mediate perception. What, however, about the connection? The challenge is intuitively straightforward: acoustic information is specified in time-frequency coordinates (as shown in the spectrograms in Figures 6.3 and 6.4), but articulatory commands must be specified in motor coordinates, or joint space. It is with respect to this issue that the distinctive feature concept is particularly useful. Because distinctive features have an acoustic and an articulatory interpretation, they may be the currency that can be traded in "brain space" to allow for coordinate transformations. To illustrate why coordinate transformations may be necessary independent operations, consider the task of repeating nonwords. An experimenter provides the auditory stimulus "blicket" or "Krk" and you are asked to repeat it. To execute this trivial task, you cannot turn to lexical information (because there is no lexical entry; in fact, one can repeat items for which there are no similar items at all). Therefore, to execute the task, you must analyze the signal and turn it into units that can provide instructions for pronunciation. Because the input is in time–frequency coordinates and the output in time–articulator coordinates, there must be a representation that allows you to connect the two representational variants. Features appear to have the right kind of properties. They may be the representational substrate that allows the speaker/listener to transform information in ways to execute both perceptual and motor tasks.

Recent brain imaging data support this hypothesis. Specifically, the role of a temporal/parietal area has been studied. The data show that at least one critical region is deep within the posterior aspect of the Sylvian fissure at the boundary between the parietal and temporal lobes, a region referred to as "area Spt" (Sylvian–parietal–temporal) (Buchsbaum *et al.*, 2001; Hickok & Poeppel, 2004). Area Spt appears to be a crucial part of the network that performs a type of coordinate transformation suggested above, mapping between auditory representations of speech and motor representations of speech. This network could provide a mechanism for the maintenance of parity between auditory and motor representations of speech, as suggested, for example, by the motor theory of speech perception (Liberman & Mattingly, 1985).

6.3.5   *The functional anatomy of the speech processing system*

The functional-anatomic model that emerges has the following properties:

(1) The primary cortical substrate in which sound-based representations of speech are constructed is the bilateral superior temporal cortex (Binder *et al.*, 2000; Hickok & Poeppel, 2000, 2004; Norris & Wise, 2000).

(2) These areas must be organized such that the differentiation between different levels of representation (specifically acoustics, phonetics, and phonology) is maintained (Phillips, 2001; Poeppel, 2001).

(3) Sound-based representations interface (in task-dependent ways) with other systems. An acoustic-phonetic-articulatory "coordinate transformation" occurs in a temporal–parietal–frontal pathway (Buchsbaum *et al.*, 2001; Hickok & Poeppel, 2004) that links auditory representations to motor representations in superior temporal/parietal areas. A second, superior temporal to inferior temporal pathway interfaces speech-derived representations with lexical semantic representations.

(4) Anterior cortical regions play a role in specific perceptual speech segmentation tasks (Burton, 2001). This functional neuroanatomic model is shown in Figure 6.5 and accounts well for activation data as well as the clinical profiles from fluent aphasics (for detailed discussion, see Hickok & Poeppel, 2004).

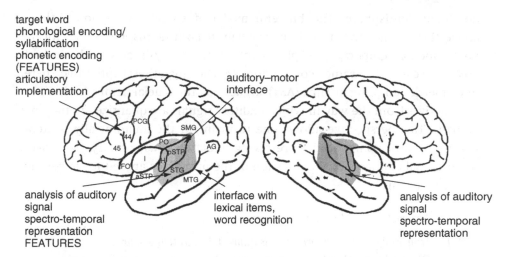

target word
phonological encoding/
syllabification
phonetic encoding
(FEATURES)
articulatory
implementation

auditory–motor
interface

analysis of auditory
signal
spectro-temporal
representation
FEATURES

interface with
lexical items,
word recognition

analysis of auditory
signal
spectro-temporal
representation

Figure 6.5   The functional anatomy of speech sound processing. The left and right hemispheres are "unfolded" at the Sylvian Fissure to permit visualization of auditory areas. Areas 44/45 are typically taken to be Broca's area. PCG – pre-central gyrus; SMG – supramarginal gyrus; AG – angular gyrus; MTG – middle temporal gyrus; STG – superior temporal gyrus; H – Heschl's gyrus; STP – superior temporal plane; PO – parietal operculum; FO – frontal operculum; I – insula.

6.3.6   Maintaining functional asymmetry in the auditory areas: the AST model

Whereas the majority of processes associated with speech and language processing are lateralized, there is an undeniable component to the process that is bilateral. We now turn to the question of what the two hemispheres are doing concurrently in the speech perception process. A growing body of evidence suggests that the right temporal lobe (superior temporal gyrus and superior temporal sulcus, in addition to primary auditory projection areas) plays a role in the analysis of the speech signal (Belin *et al.*, 2000; Binder *et al.*, 2000; Buchman *et al.*, 1986; Burton *et al.*, 2000; Hickok & Poeppel, 2000; Scott *et al.*, 2000) and it is now uncontroversial that an integrated model of the anatomy and physiology of speech perception needs to account for the contribution of both temporal cortices.

It is important to remember, in this context, that the lateralization characteristic of language processing is also well established. The data are consistent with the position that language processing *beyond* the analysis of the input signal is lateralized (Poeppel *et al.*, 2004). The computations that constitute the speech interface are mediated bilaterally, but the "central" computational system (generative engine) that we associate with phonological, morphological, syntactic, and semantic computation is (for the most part) lateralized to the dominant hemisphere. The bilateral model of speech perception outlined above then brings up an obvious problem: if both hemispheres, specifically both superior temporal gyri, play a role in the analysis of speech, do both areas execute the same computations? The hypothesis proposed here, Asymmetric Sampling in Time (AST), argues that the crucial hemispheric difference derives from the way in which auditory signals are quantized in the time domain. This perspective allows one to maintain the anatomically bilateral nature of processing while preserving functional asymmetry. Moreover, the proposal connects to the question of the primitives argued for in psycholinguistic research.

6.3.7   Asymmetric sampling in time: the premises

6.3.7.1   Temporally evolving information is chunked: integration windows

We typically think of the passage of time as an arrow, a continuous variable. The central nervous system, on the other hand, takes ongoing events and chunks them in time. Indeed, both psychophysical and electrophysiological data show that perceptual information is analyzed in temporally delimited windows (Näätänen, 1992; Theunissen & Miller, 1995). The importance of the concept of a temporal integration window is that it highlights the discontinuous processing of information in the time domain. The CNS, on this view, treats time not as a continuous variable but as a series of temporal windows, and extracts data from a given window. Recent perspectives on the concept of temporal windows, temporal processing, and temporal integration are provided by Hirsh and Watson (1996), Pöppel (1997), Viemeister and Plack (1993), and Warren (1999).

The link between "temporal integration window" and physiological mechanisms are hypothesized to be oscillatory neuronal activity: the period of an oscillation is assumed to be the duration of the temporal window. Gamma band activity ($\sim$40 Hz) is, thus, associated with temporal windows on the order of $\sim$25 ms, theta activity with $\sim$200 ms windows. Neurophysiological data support the idea of "temporal windows" or "sampling". Theunissen and Miller (1995) outline temporal coding in nervous systems and provide physiological definitions of integration windows. Several windows receive support from a neurophysiological perspective, a window associated with a short sampling period (25 ms or 40 Hz) and a window associated with a longer sampling period (200 ms or $\sim$5 Hz); but there are also other integration constants ($\sim$2–3 ms and 1000+ ms) that will not be discussed here. Moreover, many electrophysiological recordings in animal preparations have documented sampling at these rates in the form of stimulus-induced or stimulus-related rhythmic brain activity (oscillations) and other physiologic indicators. The short integration window concept is supported by the data on 40 Hz oscillations in perception. Llinas and colleagues (Joliot *et al.*, 1994) and Singer and colleagues (Singer, 1993) have made arguments for 40 Hz oscillations and synchronization, respectively, as time-based mechanisms to coordinate information. Moreover, high frequency (e.g., gamma) activity has been documented noninvasively in the auditory and visual systems.

Supporting evidence for longer windows comes, for example, from EEG and MEG studies. In particular, Näätänen and colleagues (Näätänen, 1992; Yabe *et al.*, 1997) have argued for long (200 ms/5 Hz) temporal integration windows in auditory cognition. Overall, the notion of temporal integration is motivated by a range of auditory research, both psychophysical and neurophysiological, and very short duration (<5 ms), short-duration (~25 ms), and long-duration (~200 ms) windows have received empirical and theoretical support. Recent psychophysical evidence that shows the relevance of a ~150–300 ms window comes from studies of audiovisual speech desynchronization; it is observed that AV speech tolerates asynchronies within these ranges without serious percep-tual degradation (Grant *et al.*, 2004).

One important qualification is that the AST model assumes that there is ongoing gamma band activity, which reflects the cortical "sampling rate." The larger gamma bursts, in this model, occur when the ongoing sampling activity is enhanced during the processing of some stimulus; from the AST perspective, these two aspects of gamma band activity are related but independent.

6.3.7.2   *Sensitivity to time structure*

Numerous hypotheses have been proposed to account for the demon-strable lateralization of function seen across many experimental tasks. For lower-level perceptual processes, there has been some convergence: auditory and visual psychophysical tasks that require fine-grained temporal information for their execution typically implicate the left hemisphere. For example, experiments probing the detection or discrimination of temporal order, temporal sequencing, gap detection, and masking have, on balance, implicated the left hemisphere (for review, see Nicholls, 1996). Recent brain imaging evidence supports the basic notion that there is a leftward bias for the analysis of rapid spectral changes (Zatorre & Belin, 2001; Zatorre *et al.*, 2002).

A frequently articulated view of speech perception argues that the neural mechanisms for speech are lateralized to the left hemisphere. Specifically, it is argued that (1) since the left hemisphere appears to be suited for processing rapid changes and (2) since the speech stream contains many rapid temporal changes there is a natural connection between rapid temporal information and the left hemisphere (e.g., Tallal *et al.*, 1993). If this hypothesis is on the right track, it is necessary to account for a variety of facts that are problematic on this view; for example: why does the imaging literature on speech perception consistently implicate both hemispheres? Why do neuropsychological data, for example data from pure word deafness, implicate both hemispheres? How are slow spectral changes and small frequency changes analyzed? The model outlined here attempts to capture some of these observations in a unified manner. The model suggests that there may be a bias in left-hemisphere mechanisms for rapidly changing spectral information but (1) there is a stronger bilateral contribution to speech perception than previously assumed and (2) there is a slight bias for spectrally fine-grained and slowly varying information in right-hemisphere mechanisms.

6.3.7.3   *Time scales in speech*

The critical information contained in speech occurs on multiple time scales. At an intuitive level one can appreciate the temporal (duration) difference between formant transitions, a syllable ("bar"), a multi-syllabic word ("barkeeper"), and a phrase or sentence ("barkeepers listen to drunks"). Rosen (1992) provides a summary of the acoustic and linguistic aspects of the temporal information in speech signals. He shows how the temporal envelope, periodicity, and spectral fine structure are differentially weighted in the encoding of segmental and supra-segmental linguistic contrasts.

Two time scales are relevant to develop the AST hypothesis: the short-duration time constant relevant for encoding formant transitions in stop consonants, approximately 20–40 ms; and the medium-duration time constant relevant for encoding syllables, approximately 150–300 ms. The role of the rapid formant transitions in the encoding of place-of-articulation differences has been appreciated for a long time (Liberman *et al.*, 1967). More recent work has emphasized the importance of syllables. For example, Greenberg has recently argued for the critical importance of syllables in speech recognition (e.g., Greenberg, 1998), and Mehler and colleagues (e.g., Mehler, 1981) have argued for a long time for the primacy of syllables in speech acquisition.

One contrast that is often cited as illustrating time-scale differences is the contrast between consonants (especially stop consonants) and vowels. There exist demonstrable distinctions between vowel and consonant processing. Pisoni (1973), for instance, has shown that short-term memory for vowels is different than short-term memory for consonants in a way that leads to appreciable processing differences. The model we are outlining here is not based on that distinction but on a purely timing-based distinction. The reason the vowel–consonant distinction is not sufficient to capture the relevant differences is that there is considerable overlap in time/duration between these classes. For example, many consonants can be long (consider /s/ /f/ /sh/ /m/) in the context of short vowels.

6.3.8   *The AST hypothesis and its characteristics*

The AST hypothesis posits that left (nonprimary) auditory areas, perhaps in the superior temporal gyrus, preferentially extract information from short (20–50 ms) temporal integration windows. The right-hemisphere homologues extract information from long (150–250 ms) integration windows. Why these windows? On the one hand, human listeners can resolve the rapid frequency changes typical of formant-transitions. Moreover, listeners have no problem distinguishing temporal order in words (say, e.g., pets vs. pest). This requires a high temporal resolution, at least on the order of 20–50 ms. On the other hand, listeners are able to distinguish among very small frequency changes (say on the order of 5 Hz), for example in the context of prosodic information and music perception. This requires high-frequency resolution. If we assume a frequency resolving power of about 5 Hz, a 200 ms window of analysis is required. By contrast, an analysis window of 25 ms allows a resolution of at best 40 Hz. If we attribute to normal listeners a frequency resolving power of 5 Hz and a temporal resolving power of 25 ms (order threshold), the multiple integration window proposal provides a way to maintain both types of information.

We assume that the initial representation of spectro-temporal receptive fields in primary (core) auditory cortex is bilaterally symmetric. The input signal (heavily preprocessed in the ascending auditory pathway) is analyzed – maybe a multiscale cortical decomposition is performed (Shamma, 2001) – but no strong lateral asymmetry is introduced in core auditory cortex. Subsequently, a "temporally asymmetric" elaboration of the cortical representation occurs in nonprimary areas. The hypothesized mechanism for this is that the proportion of neuronal ensembles with a temporal integration constant of ~25 ms is somewhat larger in left nonprimary areas; in contrast, the proportion of neuronal ensembles with a temporal integration constant of ~200 ms is somewhat larger in the right. As schematized in Figure 6.6, left and right cortical fields contain ensembles with multiple associated scale, but the slight asymmetry in proportion or preference leads to compelling functional asymmetry. Recent work by Zatorre and colleagues (Zatorre & Belin, 2001; Zatorre *et al.*, 2002) as well as by Ivry and colleagues (Ivry & Lebby, 1998; Ivry & Robertson, 1998) addresses similar problems, attempting to account for the lateralization of perceptual phenomena in speech and vision.

The figure also illustrates how to conceptualize the different information types related to the different integration windows. The same input signal will be

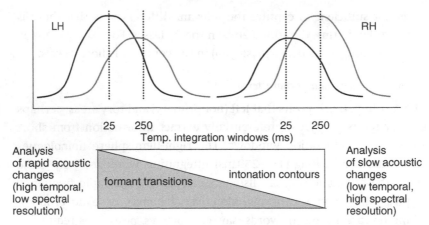

Figure 6.6 Elements of the asymmetric sampling in time (AST) model. The distributions illustrated in the black and gray curves represent the proportion of neuronal circuits with a preferred integration time. The black distributions of neuronal ensembles have a modal integration constant of ~20–50 ms, the gray ensembles a constant of ~150–300ms. Both populations of cells are represented bilaterally in the superior auditory cortex, but by hypothesis, their distribution is asymmetric; the right hemisphere predominately integrates over long-time constants, and the left hemisphere over short-time constants. This asymmetry in temporal integration windows leads to functional asymmetries, as indicated in the bottom panel of the figure.

subjected to two types of analysis that yield complementary information types. If rapidly changing information is relevant, left cortical regions provide the more appropriate neuronal substrate; more gradually changing information or information that requires fine-grained spectral distinctions will be predominantly analyzed by the right auditory cortex. An alternative way to think about this is that there is a "global," lower time–resolution analysis at the syllabic scale and a "local," high temporal resolution analysis at the sub-syllabic scale.

A physiologically motivated way to characterize the AST model is to view it as a sampling issue: the sampling rate of nonprimary auditory areas differs. Left-hemisphere areas sample the spectro-temporal cortical representations built in core auditory cortex at higher frequencies (~40 Hz; gamma band) and right-hemisphere areas at lower frequencies (4–10 Hz; theta and alpha bands).

6.3.9   Empirical support and challenges

The model makes a variety of predictions, some of which are unambiguously supported, others of which are problematic. For example, (1) linguistic and affective prosody (at the level of intonation contour) should be associated with right-hemisphere mechanisms. Neuropsychological data investigating the comprehension of affective prosody support this prediction (Ross *et al.*, 1997). However, experiments on linguistic prosody are problematic. Gandour *et al.* (2000) have shown that at least some aspects of prosody are clearly driven by left-anterior areas. (2) Phonetic phenomena occurring at the level of syllables should be more driven by right-hemisphere mechanisms. This prediction is difficult to examine because syllables by definition contain their phonemic constituents, and the experiments require selective processing of syllables vs. their constituent phonemes. However, there does exist support for the prediction: a recent dichotic listening study. Meinschaefer *et al.* (1999) showed that there was a rightward lateralization when the task demanded a focus on syllabicity rather than the phonemic structure of a given syllable. (3) Music perception should lateralize to the right for most musical attributes (including pitch). Work by Zatorre and colleagues supports this proposal (e.g., Zatorre *et al.*, 1994).

One very specific prediction, the connection between temporal integration windows and oscillatory activity, has been tested. If temporal integration is physiologically reflected as oscillatory activity, shorter time windows associated with the left hemisphere should yield oscillations in the gamma band that have more power in the left. Using whole-head MEG we tested this hypothesis using presentation of auditory stimuli of varying spectral complexity, ripples (dynamic broadband stimuli). High-frequency responses were robustly different for left and right regions, with gamma activity (25–60 Hz) being more pronounced in left temporal cortex (Poeppel *et al.*, 2000). This observation is consistent with the prediction that sensory input is analyzed on different timescales in the left and right.

Zatorre and colleagues have presented some very persuasive work on functional segregation and lateralization in auditory cognition. For example, in the seminal PET study by Zatorre *et al.* (1992) the same consonant–vowel–consonant stimulus set was associated with a strong leftward (frontal) lateralization when subjects made judgments requiring place-of-articulation analysis and a rightward lateralization when subjects judged pitch differences among the stimuli. In work on music perception, Zatorre has shown an association between melodic analysis and rightward lateralization, both using imaging and neuropsychological techniques (Zatorre, 1997; Zatorre *et al.*, 1994). Zatorre discusses the hemispheric differences observed from a perspective that is very comparable to ours: he argues that left-temporal cortex is specialized for temporal analysis and right-auditory cortex for spectral analysis. What we offer in addition is a proposed mechanisms that builds on the time constants of neuronal ensembles. Importantly, recent fMRI evidence supports various aspects of the model. Boemio *et al.* (2005), using nonspeech signals inspired by certain auditory properties of speech, tested the AST hypothesis rather directly and report a timing-induced asymmetry. An anatomic model is offered to account for the activations and their distributional differences as a function of stimulus timing. Hesling *et al.* (2005) use a speech-derived stimulus and also support the hypothesized generalizations.

6.4   Conclusions

Speech perception is the process of extracting information from an acoustic signal and constructing the appropriate representation that can interface with the stored items in your mental lexicon and the linguistic computational system (Blumstein, 1995; Chomsky, 1995). In the first part of the article we showed why speech perception is hard – for example, because there is no one-to-one mapping from stretches of sound to phonemes and because there are no (obvious) invariant properties in the signal. That these difficulties are not trivial is attested by the fact that automatic speech recognition technology is not particularly far along. Nevertheless, the human brain deals with the problems effectively. We suggest that the efficacy of the system derives from at least three properties of the speech processor. First, a speaker's *knowledge* of phonology significantly helps the process. Second, the problem is broken down in *space*: multiple areas contribute to different aspects of the problem (much like in vision). Third, the problem is broken down in *time* by analyzing signals on different time scales.

A prerequisite for the development of a model of the cognitive neuroscience of speech is theoretical agreement on what the appropriate linguistic units of study are. Here, we built on the assumption that the basic unit of speech that makes sense of neuronal data is the distinctive feature. It is the concept that best connects linguistic theory to biological data.

Notes

1. The predictability claim has to be qualified somewhat. There are cases of larger expressions whose particular form – meaning combination is not (entirely) predictable from their components. Well-known examples are idiomatic expressions like *kick the bucket*, whose meaning [die] is not predictable from the meaning of the components and their combination. Unpredictability is often taken to be a defining property of items that are stored in the lexicon.

2. Of course this is not always true. Morphological derivatives of words such as compounds or inflectional derivatives are typically not signaled by blank spaces. On the other hand, phrasal idioms like the ones mentioned in the previous footnote are often treated as basic lexical units. Nevertheless, the orthographic rules demand the use of blank spaces inside those idioms.

3. A plausibility argument can be given as follows:

imagine that there was no internal structure to speech sounds or to the phonology of a word. Each word in a language would therefore have a unique acoustic exponent. These acoustic signals would be simply listed without any inherent organization expressible for instance through a similarity matrix. Such a system would show an effect of the lexicon size on the efficacy of speech perception. For example, we estimate the average lexicon size of an English speaker at 10 000 to 20 000 words, while speakers of some Southeast Asian languages are estimated to have a vocabulary size of over 100 000 words. Given this difference, it should be much harder for speakers of one of these Southeast Asian languages to identify any word in the signal, no matter what its phonological form or acoustic exponent is simply because the search space is an order of magnitude larger. However, while it is well-known that the size of the lexicon matters locally, that is, if there are many similar sounding words it takes longer to identify one specific word within this set, it has never been reported that the lexicon size has a global effect.

4. Writing systems such as the one used to transcribe English represent relatively closely the intuitions of speakers that words are made of segments.

5. The space is determined by the phoneme inventory and prosodic constraints on words.

6. Feet and higher prosodic units like phonological word and phrase are the relevant unit for assignment of stress and intonation patterns.

7. The term "allophone" describes a particular realization of a phoneme. Since languages have different phoneme inventories, what is an allophone in one language can be a phoneme in another.

8. The term "coronal" appeals to the corona (tip and blade) of the tongue. Distinctive features are typically but not always assumed to be equipollent, that is specified for ±.

References

Belin, P., Zatorre, R. J., Lafaille, P., Ahad, P., and Pike, B. (2000). Voice-selective areas in human auditory cortex. *Nature*, **403**(6767), 309–12.

Binder, J. R., Frost, J. A., Hammeke, T. A., *et al.* (2000). Human temporal lobe activation by speech and nonspeech sounds. *Cerebral Cortex*, **10**, 512–28.

Binder, J. R., Frost, J. A., Hammeke, T. A., Rao, S. M., and Cox, R. W. (1996). Function of the left planum temporale in auditory and linguistic processing. *Brain*, **119**, 1239–47.

Blumstein, S. (1995). The neurobiology of the sound structure of language. In M. Gazzaniga, ed., *The Cognitive Neurosciences*. Cambridge, MA: MIT Press.

Boatman, D., Hart, J., Lesser, R. P. *et al.* (1998). Right hemisphere speech perception revealed by amobarbital injection and electrical interference. *Neurology*, **51**(2), 458–64.

Boemio, A., Fromm, S., Braun, A., and Poeppel, D. (2005). Hierarchical and asymmetric temporal sensitivity in human auditory cortices. *Nature Neuroscience*, **8**, 389–95.

Buchman, A., Garron, D., Trost-Cardamone, J. E., Wichter, M. D., and Schwartz, M. (1986). Word deafness: one hundred years later. *Journal of Neurol Neurosurgery Psychiatry*, **49**(5), 489–99.

Buchsbaum, B. R., Hickok, G., and Humphries, C. (2001). Role of left posterior superior temporal gyrus in phonological processing for speech perception and production. *Cognitive Science*, **25**, 663–78.

Burton, M. W. (2001). The role of inferior frontal cortex in phonological processing. *Cognitive Science*, **25**, 695–709.

Burton, M. W., Small, S. L., and Blumstein, S. E. (2000). The role of segmentation in phonological processing: an fMRI investigation. *Journal of Cognitive Neuroscience*, **12**, 679–90.

Chomsky, N. (1995). *The Minimalist Program*. Cambridge, MA: MIT Press.

Damasio, A. R. (1992). Aphasia. *The New England Journal of Medicine*, **326**(8), 531–9.

Dehaene-Lambertz, G., Dupoux, E., and Gout, A. (2000). Electrophysiological correlates of phonological processing: a cross-linguistic study. *Journal of Cognitive Neuroscience*, **12**, 635–47.

Dupoux, E., Kakehi, K., Hirose, Y., Pallier, C., and Mehler, J. (1999). Epenthetic vowels in Japanese: a perceptual illusion? *Journal of Experimental Psychology: Human Perception and Performance*, **25**, 1568 –78.

Gandour, J., Wong, D., Hsieh, L., *et al.* (2000). A crosslinguistic PET study of tone perception. *Journal of Cognitive Neuroscience*, **12**(1), 207–22.

Grant, K. W., van Wassenhove, V., and Poeppel, D. (2004). Detection of auditory (cross-spectral) and auditory-visual (cross-modal) synchrony. *Speech Communication*, **44**, 43–53.

Greenberg, S. (1998). A syllable-centric framework for the evolution of spoken language. *Brain and Behavioral Sciences*, **21**(4), 518.

Griffiths, T. D., Rees, A., and Green, G. G. R. (1999). Disorders of human complex sound processing. *Neurocase*, **5**, 365–78.

Halle, M. (1990). Phonology. In D. Osherson and H. Lasnik, eds., *Language. An Invitation to Cognitive Science*. Cambridge, MA: MIT Press.

Helenius, P., Salmelin, R., Service, E., and Connolly, J. E. (1998). Distinct time courses of word and context comprehension in the left temporal cortex. *Brain*, **121**, 1133–42.

Hesling, I., Dilharreguy, B., Clement, S., Bordessoules, M., and Allard, M. (2005). Cerebral mechanisms of prosodic sensory integration using low-frequency bands of connected speech. *Human Brain Mapping* **26**(3), 157–69.

Hickok, G. and Poeppel, D. (2000). Towards a functional neuroanatomy of speech perception. *Trends Cognitive Sciences*, **4**, 131–8.

Hickok, G. and Poeppel, D. (2004). Dorsal and ventral streams: a framework for understanding aspects of the functional anatomy of language. *Cognition*, **92**, 67–99.

Hirsh, I. and Watson, C. S. (1996). Auditory psychophysics and perception. *Annual Review of Psychology*, **47**, 461–84.

Indefrey, P. and Levelt, W. J. M. (2004). The spatial and temporal signatures of word production components. *Cognition*, **92**, 101–44.

Ivry, R. and Lebby, P. (1998). The neurology of consonant perception: specialized module or distributed processors? In M. Beeman and C. Chiarello, eds., *Right Hemisphere Language Comprehension: Perspectives from Cognitive Neuroscience*. Mahwah, NJ: Erlbaum, pp. 3–25.

Ivry, R. B. and Robertson, L. C. (1998). *The Two Sides of Perception*. Cambridge, MA: MIT Press.

Joliot, M., Ribary, U., and Llinas, R. (1994). Human oscillatory brain activity near 40 Hz coexists with cognitive temporal binding. *Proceedings of the National Academy of Sciences USA*, **91**(24), 11748–51.

Kaye, J. (1989). *Phonology: A Cognitive View*. Hillsdale, NJ: Lawrence Erlbaum Associates.

Kenstowicz, M. (1994). *Phonology in Generative Grammar*. Cambridge, MA: Blackwell.

Levelt, W. J. M. (1989). *Speaking*. Cambridge, MA: MIT Press.

Liberman, A. M., Cooper, F. S., Shankweiler, D. P., and Studdert Kennedy, M. (1967). Perception of the speech code. *Psychological Review*, **74**, 431–61.

Liberman, A. M. and Mattingly, I. G. (1985). The motor theory of speech perception revised. *Cognition*, **21**, 1–36.

Mazoyer, B. M., Dehaene, S., Tzourio, N., *et al.* (1993). The cortical representation of speech. *Journal of Cognitive Neuroscience*, **5**(4), 467–79.

Mehler, J. (1981). The role of syllables in speech processing – infant and adult data. *Philosophical Transactions of the Royal Society B* **295**, 333–52.

Meinschaefer, J., Hausmann, M., and Güntürkün, O. (1999). Laterality effects in the processing of syllable structure. *Brain and Language*, **70**, 287–93.

Näätänen, R. (1992). *Attention and Brain function*. Hillsdale, NJ: Lawrence Erlbaum Associates, Publishers.

Nicholls, M. E. (1996). Temporal processing asymmetries between the cerebral hemispheres: evidence and implications. *Laterality*, **1** (2), 97–137.

Norris, D. and Wise, R. (2000). The study of prelexical and lexical processes in comprehension: psycholinguistics and functional neuroimaging. *The New Cognitive Neurosciences*. G. M. Cambridge: MIT Press.

Phillips, C. (2001). Levels of representation in the electrophysiology of speech perception. *Cognitive Science*, **25**, 711–31.

Phillips, C., Pellathy, T., Marantz, A., *et al.* (2000). Auditory cortex accesses phonological categories: an MEG mismatch study. *Journal of Cognitive Neuroscience*, **12**, 1038–55.

Pisoni, D. (1973). Auditory and phonetic memory codes in the discrimination of consonants and vowels. *Perception and Psychophysics*, **13**, 253–60.

Poeppel, D. (2001). Pure word deafness and the bilateral processing of the speech code. *Cognitive Science*, **25**, 679–93.

Poeppel, D., Boemio, A., Simon, J., *et al.* (2000). *High-frequency Response Asymmetry to Auditory Stimuli of Varying Spectral Complexity*. New Orleans: Society for Neuroscience.

Poeppel, D., Wharton, C., Fritz, J., *et al.* (2004). FM sweeps, syllables, and word stimuli differentially modulate left and right non-primary auditory areas. *Neuropsychologia*, **42**, 183–200.

Poeppel, D., Yellin, E., Phillips, E., *et al.* (1996). Task-induced asymmetry of the auditory evoked M100 neuromagnetic field elicited by speech sounds. *Cognitive Brain Research*, **4**, 231–42.

Pöppel, E. (1997). A hierarchical model of temporal perception. *Trends Cognitive Sciences*, **1**(2), 56–61.

Price, C. (2000). The anatomy of language: contributions from functional neuroimaging. *Journal of Anatomy*, **197**, 335–59.

Pylkkanen, L., Stringfellow, A., and Marantz, A. (2002). Neuromagnetic evidence for the timing of lexical activation: an MEG component sensitive to phonotactic probability but not to neighborhood density. *Brain and Language*, **81**, 666–78.

Rosen, S. (1992). Temporal information is speech: acoustic, auditory, and linguistic aspects. *Philosophical Transactions of the Royal Society London B*, **336**, 367–73.

Ross, E. D., Thompson, R. D., and Yenkosky, J. (1997). Lateralization of affective prosody in brain and the callosal integration of hemispheric language functions. *Brain and Language*, **56**(1), 27–54.

Scott, S. K., Blank, C. C., Rosen, S., and Wise, R. J. (2000). Identification of a pathway for intelligible speech in the left temporal lobe. *Brain*, **123**, 2400–6.

Shamma, S. (2001). On the role of space and time in auditory processing. *Trends Cognitive Sciences*, **5**, 340–8.

Singer, W. (1993). Synchronization of cortical activity and its putative role in information processing and learning. *Annual Review Physiology*, **55**, 349–74.

Tallal, P., Miller, S., and Fitch, R. (1993). Neurobiological basis of speech: a case for the preeminence of temporal processing. *Annals New York Academy of Science*, **682**, 27–47.

Theunissen, F. and Miller, J. P. (1995). Temporal encoding in nervous systems: a rigorous definition. *Journal of Computational Neuroscience*, **2**, 149–62.

van Wassenhove, V., Grant, K., and Poeppel, D. (2005). Visual speech speeds up the neural processing of auditory speech. *Proceedings of the National Academy of Sciences USA*, **102**, 1181–6.

Viemeister, N. F. and Plack, C. J. (1993). Time analysis. In W. A. Yost, A. N. Popper, and R. R. Fay, eds., *Human Psychophysics*. New York: Springer.

Warren, R. M. (1999). *Auditory Perception*. Cambridge, UK: Cambridge University Press.

Yabe, H., Tervaniemi, M., Reinikainen, K., and Näätänen, R. (1997). Temporal window of integration revealed by MMN to sound omission. *Neuroreport*, **8**, 1971–4.

Zatorre, R. J. (1997). Cerebral correlates of human auditory processing: perception of speech and musical sounds. In J. Syka, ed., *Acoustical Signal Processing in the Central Auditory System*. New York: Plenum Press, pp. 453–468.

Zatorre, R. and Belin, P. (2001). Spectral and temporal processing in human auditory cortex. *Cerebral Cortex*, **11**, 946–53.

Zatorre, R., Belin, P., and Penhune, V. B. (2002). Structure and function of auditory cortex: music and speech. *Trends in Cognitive Sciences*, **6**(1), 37–46.

Zatorre, R. J., Evans, A. C., and Meyer, E. (1994). Neural mechanisms underlying melodic perception and memory for pitch. *Journal of Neuroscience*, **14**, 1908–19.

Zatorre, R. J., Evans, A. C., Meyer, E., and Gjedde, A. (1992). Lateralization of phonetic and pitch discrimination in speech processing. *Science*, **256**, 846–9.

Zatorre, R. J., Meyer, E., Gjedde, A., and Evans, A. C. (1996). PET studies of phonetic processing of speech: review, replication, and reanalysis. *Cerebral Cortex*, **6**(1), 21–30.

7

Varieties of silence: the impact of neuro-degenerative diseases on language systems in the brain

KARALYN PATTERSON, NAIDA L. GRAHAM, MATTHEW A. LAMBON
RALPH, AND JOHN R. HODGES

7.1   Introduction

The human faculty of language is a breathtaking skill. It allows us to communicate observations, thoughts, wishes, intentions, emotions, etc., to another person in the same room (by speaking), to a person in the next room (by shouting), to someone thousands of kilometers away (by speaking on the telephone or sending a fax), and even to future generations (by writing stories, poems, books, or scientific articles). Language is characterized by almost infinite variation and creativity. Every person alive today (with the exception of pre-verbal infants and people with severely impaired language skills) probably utters a number of sentences every day that he or she has never produced before. What other form of behavior could compete with this for degree of novelty and originality?

Language is typically considered to involve a set of interacting, but somewhat separate, domains of ability or knowledge. These include the sound structure of the language (*phonology*); word meanings (*semantics*); the ways in which individual morphemes combine to create complex words (*morphology*); the ways in which morphologically simple or complex words combine to create phrases and sentences (*syntax*); and finally, at least in the relatively brief time since a substantial proportion of the world's population has become literate, knowledge of how words are written in the speaker's language (*orthography*).

How and where does the brain represent and process this complex set of abilities? Because language is unique to humans, we can only learn about this topic by studying humans. As is clear from chapters in other parts of this book, substantial information about the brain structures involved in other forms of cognitive ability (such as vision, hearing, spatial skills, motor control, attention,

Topics in Integrative Neuroscience: From Cells to Cognition, ed. James R. Pomerantz. Published by Cambridge University Press. © Cambridge University Press 2008.

memory, etc.) has been acquired through research with nonhuman animals; but there are no animal models of language. And because our societies do not condone brain-invasive experimentation on humans, most of what we have learned in the past about the neural basis of language derives from nature's accidental and unfortunate experiments: damage or disease to the human brain resulting in language deficits.

Sources of information on this topic are no longer quite so restricted. We now have relatively noninvasive techniques of functional brain imaging that can be applied to normal speakers: Positron Emission Tomography (PET) and functional Magnetic Resonance Imaging (fMRI); both the techniques themselves and the design of experiments utilizing these techniques are rapidly becoming more sensitive and sophisticated. Nevertheless, our knowledge about the neural basis of language comes mainly from research on its impairments. Furthermore, even in the current climate of excitement about functional imaging, many researchers believe that aphasia – language disorders from brain injury or disease – will continue to provide one of the vital sources of evidence in this area. This is because functional imaging studies of language in normal individuals typically produce activation in multiple brain regions, some of which might reflect incidental aspects of the paradigm rather than the component of language under investigation (Price, 1998). Lesions to well-specified brain regions that are consistently correlated with specific language deficits seem more likely to reflect essential parts of the language system, although of course this form of evidence is not free from problems of interpretation either.

Modern history of the study of brain and language begins with two European neurologists: Paul Broca (1824–1880) in France and Carl Wernicke (1848–1905) in Germany. These two pioneers made careful observations of the language deficits in individual aphasic patients who had suffered a cerebrovascular accident (stroke). Broca and Wernicke then managed to perform post-mortem dissections on the brains of these patients after their deaths, and identified the regions that had been damaged by the stroke. Broca's research focused on a patient with a severe disorder of expressive language; combining the behavioral observations with his subsequent neuroanatomical discoveries, Broca concluded that the ability to produce speech relied on a specific area in the posterior, inferior frontal lobe of the left hemisphere (Broca, 1861). This is approximately the region labeled 44/45 in Figure 7.1. Wernicke's key research concerned a patient with severely impaired speech comprehension; the post-mortem examination revealed focal damage to the posterior part of the superior temporal lobe in the left hemisphere (area 22 in Figure 7.1). He equated this region with a centre for the "sound images" of words or, as we might now say, spoken word recognition (Wernicke, 1874).

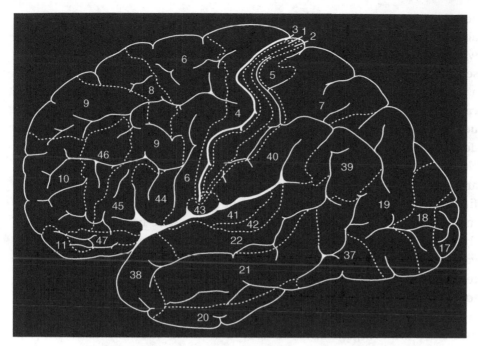

Figure 7.1   The lateral surface of the left hemisphere (based on a figure from Pulvermüller & Preissl, 1991), numbered with cortical areas defined by Brodmann (1909).

The 100+ years since these studies have been accompanied by great advances in techniques for lesion localization: there are not only more sophisticated post mortem analyses than those available to Broca and Wernicke, but we have structural and functional imaging techniques applicable to the living brain. We also have more systematic procedures for assessing and describing language deficits. On the basis of these developments, present-day brain and language stories are more complicated than the ones told by Broca and Wernicke; nevertheless, our current understanding of the neural basis of language is an expansion of theirs rather than a whole new story. Furthermore, even if not all of the details were correct, the basic associations between language function and brain location identified by Broca and Wernicke are compatible with other aspects of brain function (Blumstein, 1994). For example, it is well established from studies of humans and other animals that auditory perception, a critical component of speech recognition, relies on regions of the temporal lobe near Wernicke's area. Likewise, it is known that motor function, a critical component of speech production, relies on brain structures in the frontal lobe near Broca's area.

The conclusions about brain and language drawn by Broca and Wernicke were based on patients who had suffered cerebrovascular incidents. Vascular aetiology as a cause of aphasia continued to be the primary source of evidence about language organization in the brain for most of the twentieth century, with neurodegenerative diseases being largely neglected. The reasons for this selective focus are not entirely obvious, but one major factor seems to have been a belief that vascular lesions are focal and circumscribed while the damage caused by degenerative conditions is widespread and patchy. This view continued to dominate despite reports early in the twentieth century (Pick, 1904) that degenerative disease could yield strikingly specific cognitive impairments. Now, early in the twenty-first century, views are at long last changing; in fact, at least some current researchers would argue that while the earlier belief may fit the physical characteristics of lesions, the impact on functional brain systems may be more circumscribed in the case of progressive brain disease. Lesions from cerebrovascular accidents – which are determined by the geography of the vascular system – are quite likely to cut across functionally organized subsystems in the brain. Pathological processes, on the other hand, may be more likely to follow lines of functional neural connectivity.

The last decade has seen a particular surge of interest in the cognitive deficits associated with degenerative diseases that cause relatively focal atrophy (shrinkage due to loss of neural tissue) of the frontal and/or temporal lobes of the brain. Snowden *et al.* (1996) distinguished three major syndromes in this sphere. One of these, called "frontotemporal dementia" (or often just "frontal dementia") will not be considered further here, as it does not appear to have any specifically linguistic consequences but rather disrupts aspects of behavior such as problem-solving, judgement, decision-making, emotional and social appropriateness, etc. The remaining two syndromes are the focus of this chapter: progressive fluent and progressive nonfluent aphasia.

7.2   Progressive fluent aphasia, aka semantic dementia

Seen from the perspective of language ability, and specifically speech production, "progressive fluent aphasia" is a good label for this syndrome: the patients are aphasic, and increasingly so with time, but their spontaneous speech remains relatively fluent. It is now more standard, however, to refer to the syndrome as "semantic dementia," a label created by Snowden *et al.* (1989). The appropriateness of this name is due to the fact that, at least by hypothesis and yet to be disproven, the language deficits and all other impairments documented in this condition are attributable to a progressive deterioration of semantic memory (Hodges *et al.*, 1992; Patterson, Lambon Ralph *et al.*, 2006; Rogers *et al.*, 2004; Schwartz *et al.*, 1979; Warrington, 1975). Semantic memory is the component of human memory that encompasses not only knowledge of the meanings of words, but also knowledge about (nonlinguistic) concepts, objects, and people.

The most prominent language deficit in semantic dementia is a progressive loss of expressive and receptive content–word vocabulary. This is hardly surprising: of the various components of language processing, the ability to produce and to comprehend content words relies most obviously on activation of semantic representations. Before we consider the ways in which the vocabulary impairment is manifested, it is useful to have a brief summary of the aspects of language processing that function reasonably well in semantic dementia: phonology and syntax.

7.2.1   Phonology

Virtually all aphasic patients with vascular aetiology, whatever their classification in the terminology of aphasic syndromes, make errors in both spontaneous speech and in object naming that are phonological approximations to the correct word/name (Blumstein, 1994; Martin & Saffran, 1997). As discussed towards the end of this chapter, the same is true of patients with nonfluent progressive aphasia (Croot et al., 1998, 1999; Nestor et al., 2003). In contrast, it is rare to encounter phonological errors in the spontaneous speech of patients with semantic dementia and progressive fluent aphasia. In fact, although this has not yet been quantified, it is possible that errors of this sort do not occur significantly more often in the speech of these patients than in normal individuals' speech. Furthermore, in object-naming tasks, where (unlike spontaneous speech) the experimenter knows what the intended target word should be, these patients' failures to produce the correct target name take the form of single-word semantic errors (prototypical category coordinates or superordinate labels), circumlocutions (often with very impoverished content), and omissions ("I don't know"), but almost never phonological errors (Hodges & Patterson, 1996). The speech-production deficit in semantic dementia is therefore probably the result of the patient having insufficient semantic information to activate the correct, or often any, phonological representation, rather than a disruption of the phonological system itself. Similarly, assessments of receptive phonological processing such as minimal pair judgements (i.e., judging that two spoken tokens of the same word are the same, but that two spoken words differing by only a single phonetic feature – e.g., "blank/plank" – are different) yield reasonably normal levels of performance in patients with semantic dementia (Knott et al., 1997), suggesting that problems in comprehending speech arise centrally.

The skills of reading aloud and writing to dictation in semantic dementia are well preserved for stimuli consisting of high-frequency words and/or words with

typical correspondences between spelling and pronunciation. The great majority of patients, however, show a striking pattern of surface dyslexia and surface
dysgraphia, making "regularization" errors to lower-frequency words with an
unpredictable relationship between spelling and sound (e.g., reading aloud the
word *blood* as "blude" and spelling the word *cough* as COFF). According to one
theoretical interpretation, these "surface" patterns of reading and spelling disorder are attributable to a reduction in the normal semantic constraints on
deriving the correct pronunciation or spelling of words, combined with relatively preserved phonological processing (Graham *et al.*, 2000; Plaut *et al.*, 1996).
Acquired surface dyslexia in semantically impaired patients has been frequently
reported not only in English-speaking cases (McCarthy & Warrington, 1986;
Parkin, 1993; Patterson & Hodges, 1992), but also in patients speaking other
languages, characterized by widely varying degrees of consistency in spelling–
sound correspondences (see Chiacchio *et al.*, 1993 for Italian; Fushimi *et al.*, 2003
and Patterson *et al.*, 1995 for Japanese kanji). One of the intriguing features of
cross-language research on such a phenomenon is that it manifests itself in
different ways in various languages, which can be predicted once one knows
which aspects of the correspondence between spelling and sound are unpredictable in each language. Thus, regularization errors in English occur for words
with segmental atypicalities in the spelling–sound relationship; in Italian, by
contrast, where segmental correspondences between orthography and phonology are completely predictable, the reading errors occur in response to supra-
segmental atypicality (stress pattern). In Japanese, patients with semantic
dementia are very error-prone when reading words written in Kanji, the
Japanese writing system based on Chinese characters, in which the relationship
between character and pronunciation is highly context/word-specific. Reading
aloud in Kana, where each character is associated with a consistent spoken
syllable or mora of the language, is typically flawless.

7.2.2   Syntax

Receptive processing of the syntactic aspects of language is largely
intact, at least until late in the course of semantic dementia. For example, on a
test of sentence–picture matching designed to assess processing of various
syntactic structures (the Test for the Reception of Grammar: Bishop, 1989),
patients typically score within the normal range; where the number of errors
exceeds normal limits, the errors are usually lexical rather than syntactic in
nature (Hodges *et al.*, 1992). There have even been some striking empirical
demonstrations that patients with semantic dementia use syntactic structure
to disambiguate reference to lexical terms which they no longer understand
(Breedin & Saffran, 1999). Also, patients with semantic dementia have been

assessed in tasks where the subject is asked to listen to spoken speech and to monitor for a specific target word, under three stimulus conditions: (1) normal utterances (both syntactically and semantically acceptable); (2) syntactically well-formed but meaningless utterances; and (3) scrambled word order. The patients' response times in this monitoring task reveal the facilitation characteristic of normal listeners for condition (2) relative to (3), even though they fail to benefit further (as normal listeners do) from the semantic appropriateness of condition (1) (Hodges *et al.*, 1994).

On the expressive side, there has as yet been little formal attempt to assess the syntactic quality of speech output in semantic dementia; but on the basis of both other researchers' reports and our own experience of listening to dozens of patients with this disorder, it seems clear that the striking abnormality of speech is always word-finding difficulty and almost never any major syntactic anomaly. On the other hand, given the interactive nature of lexical/semantic with syntactic processes, the patients' profound disorder of the former can have consequences for the latter (Patterson & MacDonald, 2006). For example, one of the patients with semantic dementia in our clinic recently replied to a query with "I want to *say* you right now that . . .". We interpret this as an utterance that began with the intention to retrieve the word *tell*; when he reached that point in the sentence, *tell* was unavailable, and so he replaced it with *say*, which is an appropriate substitute except that it requires a different syntactic structure ("I want to say *to* you right now . . .") but he failed to adjust his output accordingly.

7.2.3   The nature of the vocabulary loss in speech production

Patients with semantic dementia are significantly (and, with progression, profoundly) impaired in any task that requires the production of content words in "self-generated" speech. As indicated above, they have no significant phonological or articulatory deficits, so that if the word-form is provided for them, they can reproduce it easily. Thus, they perform normally in tasks of word repetition or reading aloud (with the already-noted proviso that if the word has an unpredictable spelling–sound relationship, the patients are at risk of producing it with a regularized pronunciation). By contrast, in all language tasks where the speaker must generate the word form on the basis of some conceptual specification, patients with semantic dementia are seriously impaired. Category fluency is one task typically used in neuropsychological testing. The subject is given the name of a common conceptual category (e.g., *animals* or *birds* or *vehicles*) and asked to generate as many exemplars of this category as possible in one minute. Normal speakers can generate dozens of exemplars in 60 seconds for categories of this sort. But these patients manage only a few (Hodges *et al.*, 1992) and, with disease progression, often reach a stage where their response to a prompt like *birds* is "well, there are big ones and little ones," or even "I can't remember what a bird is."

In spontaneous speech, the profound anomia of these patients may not be so apparent to the casual observer, because the patients sometimes succeed in steering around unavailable content words. Nevertheless, and again especially with disease progression, spontaneous speech is revealingly "empty," and also demonstrates the patients' impaired comprehension of content words. Below is an example from patient IF, in conversation with Professor John Hodges. Note IF's perfect repetition of words that he fails to understand (like *hobbies* and *comprehension*). Also, harking back to the previous section, note the fact that his syntactic constructions are mostly adequate but sometimes rather odd (as in his sad response to the question about his main difficulties), which probably results from his inability to find the substantive words needed to express himself.

JH: What kind of job did you do after you left school?

IF: I like to do it, 10 times 20 times 50 ... [*Note: he was an accountant*]

JH: Do you have any hobbies?

IF: Hobbies, what are they?

JH: Things you like to do.

IF: Oh, I like to play golf.

JH: What are your main difficulties?

IF: Difficulties ... well, some of my friends have given myself away from them, because I can't speak to them.

JH: How long have you been having trouble finding words?

IF: In 1989, there was one word I couldn't think about, and then later there were three words I couldn't think about ...

JH: How's your comprehension?

IF: What's comprehension?

Probably the most frequently used task to assess content–word vocabulary in aphasic patients is object naming, usually conducted with pictures of common objects (e.g., from the Snodgrass & Vanderwart, 1980, corpus of 260 pictures, for which normal speakers essentially always produce the same conventionally correct label). Our research group has reported extensive data on object naming in semantic dementia, including a longitudinal study of the dramatic decline in this ability (Hodges *et al.*, 1995). Table 7.1 presents a subset of previously unpublished naming results from case DG.

There are many interesting observations to be made from this data set, including the following five. First is the sheer level of deficit: DG succeeded in naming fewer than 10% of pictures for which normal speakers score essentially

Table 7.1. *Patient DG's naming responses to a subset of the pictures in the Snodgrass and Vanderwart corpus. On the entire test, she scored 24/260, correctly naming:* dog, cow, chicken; tree, flower; arm, foot, hand; car, aeroplane, lorry, motorcycle, bicycle; house, bed, box, cup, fork, scissors, clock, glasses; hat, coat, shoe

DG's Response	Mammals: Stimulus pictures yielding response
correct	dog, cow
"dog"	cat, horse, pig, squirrel, sheep, deer, goat, fox, leopard, tiger, giraffe, camel, skunk, raccoon
"big dog"	rhinoceros, bear, gorilla, elephant
"little dog"	mouse, rabbit, monkey
"nice dog"	kangaroo
"horse"	lion, zebra
"little horse"	donkey

DG's Response	Birds: Stimulus pictures yielding response
correct	chicken
"bird"	eagle, penguin
"chicken"	(generic) bird
"dog"	swan
"little dog"	duck, rooster
"little thing"	owl
"don't know"	peacock

DG's Response	Insects: Stimulus pictures yielding response
"dog"	beetle
"little dog"	bee, spider
"bird"	ant
"long thing"	caterpillar
"don't know"	fly, butterfly

DG's Response	Other animals: Stimulus pictures yielding response
"dog"	turtle, seal
"little dog"	alligator
"cat"	snail
"long thing"	snake
"little thing"	seahorse
"big thing"	lobster
"don't know"	fish, frog

DG's Response	Manmade things: Stimulus pictures yielding response
"box"	bread, door, watering can, suitcase, kettle, spinning wheel, top, bowl, pot, fridge, stove, toaster, ashtray, envelope, thimble
"little box"	accordion, frying pan, vase, nut, record player, salt shaker, whistle, basket
"big box"	garbage can, desk, barn, window, barrel, television, dresser
"round thing"	button, football, helmet, ring, ball, ear
"long thing"	guitar, nail, paintbrush, ladder, sled, broom, plug, chain, ruler, flute, tie, key, pipe

100%. Second is the strong modulation of success by frequency or familiarity of the concept and name: her only correct responses were to very common, every-day objects. Third is the severe restriction on the variety of names/labels available to DG. We know from other semantic tasks involving no speech production that the naming deficit is not *just* a name-finding problem; that is, this profound anomia is the result of degraded conceptual knowledge about objects – knowledge of the kind that enables normal individuals to distinguish between different but somewhat similar objects such as a *rhinoceros* and an *elephant*, or a *beetle* and a *spider*. It is also clear, however, that one of the consequences of this semantic deterioration is a gradual loss of vocabulary, such that only high-frequency terms remain available. Thus the patient, no longer knowing the defining features of a *rhinoceros*, does not call it "elephant" either, but instead can only fall back on the higher-frequency term "horse" that corresponds to a much more prototypical animal. Fourth is the vitally important fact that the "loss" of conceptual knowledge in semantic dementia is not all or none but partial. The fact that DG's knowledge was degraded rather than totally lost is illustrated, for example, by the fact that she still had some approximate knowledge about the size of some animals (all of these things are roughly the same size as depicted in the Snodgrass and Vanderwart line drawings). Thus she used "big dog" for large animals like *elephant* and *rhinoceros*, but "small dog" for exemplars like *mouse* and *rabbit*. Fifth, and of considerable theoretical significance, there is a prototypicality effect: DG assigned an animal name like "dog" or "horse" to most of the rather standard animals; she only used nonanimal labels like "little thing" or "long thing" for the rather nontypical-looking animals like *seahorse* and *caterpillar*.

Although the majority of experiments on vocabulary deficits in aphasia have employed picture-naming tasks, we have also assessed content–word voca-bulary in connected speech by patients with semantic dementia (Bird *et al.*, 2000; Patterson & MacDonald, 2006), using a picture-description task (the "Cookie Theft" picture from Goodglass & Kaplan, 1983). Relative to the narra-tives generated by age-matched normal speakers, the patients' descriptions, as expected, reveal a striking reduction in production of specific content words that grows worse with increasing disease severity. For example, in the picture, a boy is standing on a stool that is obviously just about to tip over. Virtually every control subject uses the word "stool" in describing this aspect of the picture; but in the Patterson and MacDonald study, none of the 21 patients with semantic dementia produced the word "stool." They either called it by the higher-frequency term "chair" or by the even more general and higher-frequency word "thing"; some of the most severe patients did not refer to the stool at all. Likewise, almost every normal participant uses the word "overflowing" to comment on the water pouring over the edge of the kitchen sink at which a woman is standing. Only 2/21 patients produced the word "overflowing." Others used more common words/phrases (such as "come down") or again, in severe cases, used no verb at all to comment on the water overflowing, which is highly abnormal language behavior. Bird *et al.* (2000) noted that although specific nouns and verbs were both vulnerable to progression of semantic dementia, the simple quantity of verbs remained within, or near to, normal limits for longer than the nouns. This might be the predicted pattern on the basis of what is known or hypothesized about neuroanatomical correlates of noun and verb processing, which is an association of noun deficits with left inferior temporal lesions and of verb deficits with damage to frontal regions (Bak *et al.*, 2001; Gainotti *et al.*, 1995; Pulvermüller *et al.*, 2001). Perhaps the most important outcome of the Bird *et al.* study, however, was the demonstration that the slight preponderance of verbs over nouns in the speech of patients with semantic dementia is likely to find an adequate explanation in frequency differences between these two word classes. Since the verbs used by normal speakers to describe the Cookie Theft scene are of significantly higher frequency than the nouns occurring in these descriptions, and since the patients' speech is increasingly restricted to higher-frequency words, it is unsurprising that verbs are slightly more resilient.

7.3   The neuroanatomy of semantic representations

Impairment to a specific cognitive function A combined with a clearly identified neuroanatomical locus of lesion X in a sufficiently large number of patients has traditionally been accepted as evidence that function A "resides" in region X. On this logic, which is certainly an oversimplification, the residence of amodal semantic memory (i.e., not just the semantic aspect of language) is the anterior region of the inferior/middle temporal lobe (areas 38, 21 and 20 in Figure 7.1), because this is consistently the location of the earliest and most severe atrophy in patients with semantic dementia (Levy *et al.*, 2004; Mummery *et al.*, 2000; Seeley *et al.*, 2005). Initially, this atrophy is often quite asymmetrical, but with disease progression there is always bilateral temporal atrophy. This anterior portion of the temporal lobe is a plausible neuroanatomical location from which to predict a cross-modality semantic memory deficit, because neurophysiological studies of nonhuman primates (Gloor, 1997) suggest that this region has white matter connections from higher-order cortex associated with every sensory modality (vision, audition, touch, and olfaction).

It is also vital to note that brain regions which do not exhibit significant abnormalities under standard structural brain-imaging techniques may do so

Table 7.2. *Patient PP: absolute values for regional oxygen consumption (ml/100 ml/min) and as a percentage of the mean for six age-matched controls, for areas of the left temporal lobe (area numbers correspond to those in Figure 7.1). From Patterson et al. (1994)*

	Absolute	%
Inferior Temp. [area 20]	1.67	56[***]
Middle Temp. [area 21]	1.85	57[***]
Superior Temp. [area 22]	2.39	74
Posterior Temp. [area 37]	1.89	56[***]

[***] = 3 s.d. below control mean.

either (i) with measures of brain metabolism, (ii) in functional imaging studies that measure activity in selective brain regions in response to a cognitive task, or indeed (iii) when more sensitive, sophisticated structural techniques are employed. All three of these techniques have suggested that in addition to the highly prominent atrophy in the anterior, inferior temporal lobe, there may be additional though less striking abnormalities in more posterior (still inferior) regions of the temporal lobe. Examples of this finding from the three different techniques just described are as follows.

Table 7.2 shows PET measurements of regional oxygen consumption during a resting state in a patient with semantic dementia; this technique gives a general indication of the brain regions that are functioning normally/abnormally. As expected, there was substantial and statistically significant hypometabolism in the inferior and middle temporal regions where the patient had very obvious atrophy on MRI structural scanning; and slightly but insignificantly reduced metabolism in the superior temporal area where there was no serious structural damage. The important thing to note is the very significantly reduced metabolism in the posterior temporal region where there was also no major atrophy. This is what is meant by a "functional" lesion, that is an undamaged region that fails to function adequately, presumably because of reduced neural input from the damaged areas to which it is normally connected.

Secondly, in the first PET activation study of semantic dementia (Mummery *et al.*, 1999), four patients and six age-matched normal control subjects performed a semantic judgement task based on the Pyramids and PalmTrees test (Howard & Patterson, 1992), in which the subject looks at a target item (a concrete noun presented as either a picture or a word) and chooses one of two response items (also concrete concepts represented as either words or pictures) that is semantically related to the target. There is no perceptual similarity between the target and the correct response and the two response choices belong to the same semantic category so that there is also no category clue to the correct choice. An example is the target *tree* (in the picture, just a generic deciduous tree with leaves) paired with the response choices *onion* and *apple*. There is no physical resemblance between a tree and an apple; and both apples and onions are round-ish shaped growing things that people eat. One simply has to know that apples grow on trees but onions do not. The network of regions for which the normal controls showed significantly increased activation in the semantic task relative to a control condition followed the usual pattern for this sort of contrast, including temporal, temporo-parietal, and frontal areas in the left hemisphere. The patients with semantic dementia showed at least some semantic activation in many of the same regions as the controls, with the striking exception of area 37 (Figure 7.1) on the left: striking because, once again, none of the four cases revealed any significant structural abnormality here. The consistently documented structural atrophy more anteriorly in the temporal lobe is therefore only evidence that this region is one essential component of the brain's network for semantic memory.

Finally, Studholme *et al.* (2004) performed structural MRI scans on 20 patients with semantic dementia and then applied the recently developed technique of deformation tensor morphometry, which measures focal tissue contraction in brain atrophy. Once again, although by far the most dramatic abnormalities were at the very front of the temporal lobe, the posterior left temporal regions did exhibit significant contraction.

Do the areas of significant structural and functional lesion in these patients, who have a profound deficit in producing content–word vocabulary (and in conceptual knowledge more generally), correspond to the cortical areas activated in other functional imaging experiments when normal speakers are asked to generate content–word vocabulary or perform other semantic tasks? With careful selection from the functional imaging literature, one can probably find results that either match or conflict with almost any function–location pairing identified by lesion data. Despite that rather pessimistic caveat, the answer to the question posed in the first sentence of this paragraph is fairly positive. For example, in a PET study concerned not with language processes per se but with a contrast between general semantic memory (e.g., facts about dogs) and the subject's own autobiographical memory (a specific episode involving a dog), activation in area 21 of the left temporal lobe (see Figure 7.1) was associated with the retrieval of nonperceptual semantic knowledge (Lee *et al.*, 2002).

Focusing more specifically on language, Warburton *et al.* (1996) measured regional blood flow with PET while normal adults retrieved either nouns or verbs. In the noun task, the cue was a superordinate category label (e.g., "furniture") and the subject was to generate as many exemplars as possible from this category (e.g., *table, chair, cabinet, bed*, etc.) in a 15-second period before the next category label was presented. Note that although the period is shorter than that typically used in the standard category fluency task administered to patients (60 seconds), these two tasks are otherwise highly parallel. In the PET verb retrieval task used by Warburton and many other researchers (e.g., Tatsumi *et al.*, 1999), the cue was a common concrete noun (e.g., "apple") and the subject was to generate verbs or actions appropriate to this word (e.g., *eat, pick, slice, peel*, etc.). Each of these two central activation tasks was contrasted, in the standard PET subtraction analysis, with various other conditions, including rest, listening to spoken words, and the other part-of-speech condition (e.g., nouns minus verbs). This design results in a very rich data set which cannot be presented in full here. The result to be highlighted is that, in most of the contrasts of interest, content–word retrieval yielded peak activation in regions of the inferior-to-middle left temporal lobe (e.g., again, area 21 in Figure 7.1). This outcome is of interest (i) because it corresponds to a region of consistent atrophy in patients with semantic dementia, and (ii) because – with minor variations – the PET regional activation was the same for nouns and verbs. Of course this does not mean that there are no differences in the neural representations of these two major parts of speech; but patients with semantic dementia are significantly impaired in their ability to produce both, and it is therefore noteworthy that there is a brain region activated in common when normal speakers produce either nouns or verbs.

One puzzle is that functional imaging studies of semantic memory in normal individuals, even studies employing no explicit verbal task (e.g., semantic judgements on pictures of objects: Mummery *et al.*, 1999), often produce a significant increase in activation for semantic relative to control tasks only in left hemisphere regions. This is puzzling because the results from semantic dementia are most compatible with the hypothesis that conceptual knowledge is represented across left *and* right temporal lobes. There are not yet enough cases in the literature with the combination of neuropsychological and neuroradiological data necessary to illuminate the roles of the two hemispheres in semantic memory. The fact that there are to date more reported cases with predominantly left- than right-temporal atrophy also limits any current clear perspective on this question. Furthermore, we do not even know yet how to interpret this asymmetry in presentation of the disease. Does it represent a genuine differential vulnerability of the two sides of the brain, or are left temporal structures more crucial to semantic representations? Another factor may be that the greater anomia that typically accompanies major left-sided damage (discussed further below) simply makes the cognitive deficit more apparent.

Our hypothesis of bilateral representation for general conceptual knowledge is based on the observation that deficits on semantic tests (such as object naming, word–picture matching, sorting of pictures or words into semantic categories, associative semantic judgements, etc.) are seen not only in patients with predominantly left temporal atrophy but also in those with mainly right-sided damage. It seems, on the face of it, implausible that there would be substantial duplication across left and right temporal lobes in their "responsibility" for knowledge of the same concepts or features; and sources of evidence other than semantic dementia (e.g., patients with vascular lesions: Tranel et al., 1997) suggest at least a degree of specialization between the conceptual systems in the two hemispheres. Some kind or extent of dual representation is not, however, an idea that can be ruled out; and it is compatible with the observation that serious degradation of general conceptual knowledge seems not to occur without at least a degree of bilateral atrophy. For example, a number of patients have now been reported (Graham et al., 1995, 1999; Papagno & Capitani, 2001) whose semantic dementia began with a phase of unilateral left anterior temporal changes, accompanied cognitively by increasing anomia but by performance on semantic tests that was just within or only minimally outside normal limits. Longitudinal assessments revealed that subsequently, in parallel with the appearance of additional structural abnormalities in anterior right temporal regions, semantic memory declined sharply in these cases.

The most dramatic difference in language performance that has emerged from our analyses of patients with greater left than right atrophy (referred to here as L > R) in contrast to those with greater abnormality on the right (R > L) is in the impact of semantic degradation on expressive vocabulary, as measured by picture naming. We assessed this relationship in a combined cross-sectional and longitudinal analysis in which we plotted each patient's naming score for pictures of 48 concrete concepts as a function of the corresponding level of semantic deficit – defined for this purpose as the patient's score on a word-to-picture matching test for the same 48 items (Lambon Ralph et al., 2001). This analysis reveals that, for a given level of semantic impairment (except near ceiling or floor), the L > R patients are significantly more anomic on average than the R > L cases (see Figure 7.2). The nature of the naming errors is also rather different across the two sub-groups: although all patients make some of each of the three main naming-error types seen in semantic dementia (which, as noted earlier, are

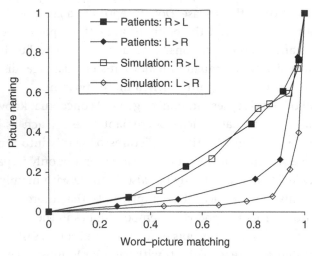

Figure 7.2   Performance of patients with varying degrees of severity of semantic dementia, and of a connectionist network with varying degrees of damage to its semantic system, for picture naming (*Y* axis) and word-to-picture matching (*X* axis) for the same set of 48 items. From Lambon Ralph *et al.* (2001).

(1) semantic errors [category superordinates and coordinates], (2) circumlocutions, and (3) omissions), there are relatively more semantic errors in the R > L patients and relatively more failures to respond at all in the L > R group.

Our account of this pattern is that semantic representations of concrete concepts are distributed across left- and right-temporal regions, but that – because speech production is so strongly lateralized to the left hemisphere – the semantic elements on the left side are much more strongly connected to the phonological representations required to name the concepts. This explains how a patient in the early stages of semantic dementia with atrophy exclusively on the left side can be significantly anomic with only minor deficits on semantic tasks that do not require naming (e.g., Graham *et al.*, 1995; Papagno & Capitani, 2001). We have developed a connectionist network based on this proposal, in which (1) the elements of semantic representations are spread equally across simulated left- and right-hemisphere components, (2) items from the same semantic category share a significant proportion of their semantic elements, and (3) the connection weights between semantic and phonological representations are much stronger for left-sided semantic elements due to a higher learning rate imposed on those connections during training. After training, the network settles on the correct semantic and phonological patterns for all items in the training set. With subsequent partial "lesions" to the semantic layer, a given degree of damage on the left yields both poorer naming accuracy (see Figure 7.2) and fewer semantic naming errors than the same degree of lesion to the right side.

7.4   Progressive nonfluent aphasia

Despite the fact that the nonfluent form of progressive aphasia was the first to be described under the label of progressive aphasia (Mesulam, 1982), cases of this type have received substantially less empirical and theoretical attention than the fluent, semantically impaired patients. This might relate to the fact that the phonological and syntactic disorders associated with the non-fluent variant have (in some form or another) been the focus of a substantial literature on aphasia due to cerebrovascular accident. The profound semantic disorder observed in fluent progressive aphasia, by contrast, is of a form and a severity that does not occur in cases of stroke, and is therefore more novel. There has consequently been considerable theoretical excitement about seman-tic dementia, while research on nonfluent progressive aphasia has languished somewhat. Because our research group, too, has largely concentrated on the fluent variant, and also due to limited space, this section will be short; but the language phenomena in nonfluent progressive aphasia are just as fascinating and deserving of attention.

Patients of both varieties often complain that they cannot talk (recall IF's comment, when being interviewed by Professor Hodges, that he cannot speak to his friends). At an impressionistic level, one might say that the fluent patients can speak perfectly well except that they have no conceptual vocabulary to talk with, but that the nonfluent patients – despite having a fairly good vocabulary – genuinely do lose the ability to speak. With disease progression, connected speech with any semblance of normal grammatical structure becomes utterly beyond their capabilities. And even before that, phonological distortions on the speech produced become prominent.

Below is an example from an interview by Professor John Hodges with patient WK, who at this point was in the rather early stages of nonfluent progressive aphasia, with speech that, although slow and effortful, had reasonable syntactic structure. What is so striking about this speech sample is (1) its fairly sophisti-cated content–word vocabulary, including words like *spoonerism* (the term coined to describe the speech errors associated with Dr. Spooner, the famous English scholar who apparently made many amusing transposition errors such as "You hissed my mystery lecture" instead of "You missed my history lecture"), combined with (2) the phonologically distorted form in which these content words tended to emerge in WK's speech. It seems particularly ironic that WK produced a phonological speech error (though not a spoonerism) on the word *spoonerism* which refers to a type of phonological speech error! The mispronounced words are in bold type with the inferred intended target in parentheses following the error.

JH: What's troubling you about your speech?
WH: Getting twisted, you know, **spoozerizm** (spoonerism).
JH: What about talking with other people?
WK: If other people are talking, they go quickly, and I can't get **behond** (behind) them, I mean I can't get in front of them, I can't get my **wads** (words). It's very **deficult** (difficult).
JH: So, when you want to speak, what happens exactly?
WK: I can't get started. When I've **constracted** (constructed) it . . .

These phonological errors, although easy enough to spot in spontaneous speech, are even more plentiful when the patients attempt production of experimenter-selected target words in the task of picture naming. Below are six examples of classical phonological errors from WK's picture naming, followed by two even more extraordinary naming errors that represent phonological errors superimposed on other response/error types.

trumpet→   **trambet**
cucumber→   **kewfedent**
volcano →   **volkako**
skeleton →   **skelekon**
pagoda →   **pagolo**
sextent →   **santinet**
indian →   **emiko** (intended target must have been "eskimo")
snail →   **eskarto** (intended target must have been "escargot," the French word for snail!)

It is important to remember that these are responses not in a task of word reading or repetition but of picture naming. Since a picture of an object offers only semantic information and no clues to the phonology of its name, these responses indicate that – in stark contrast to what we observe in (and infer from) picture naming performance in semantic dementia – WK's language system is successfully retrieving enough semantic information to activate low-frequency phonological representations. The degradation occurs further along in the process, in the phonological representations themselves or in the process whereby these get translated into articulation. There are, to date, relatively few studies where patients with this language disorder have also been assessed on demanding receptive phonological tasks, such as judging whether a spoken word presented by the experimenter is the precisely correct name for a simultaneously presented picture (example = a picture of a coherent assemblage of bones, accompanied on a "correct" trial by the spoken word "skeleton"; but on an "incorrect" trial by "skelekon," which differs from the correct name by only one distinctive phonetic feature, place of articulation). Where such probing receptive tasks have been given (e.g., Croot *et al.*, 1999), nonfluent progressive aphasic patients have typically been impaired, suggesting a central phonological deficit and not just one of translating phonological representations into speech; but it is possible that both of these aspects of language are affected.

One year after the sample of WK's conversation reproduced above, his speech had deteriorated significantly in terms of syntactic structure. For example, in describing the Cookie Theft picture mentioned earlier (in the section on vocabulary loss in semantic dementia), WK said:

> "The sink is next to the lady, and she does do stop the ... letting the **wotting** (wetting?) the floor ...
> Stay ... the water, got to find to on the floor.
> Boy's on a **spool** (stool) to get jar cookie"

And another nonfluent progressive patient HK, at a more advanced stage than WK's, described the Cookie Theft thus:

> "Plates"
> "Washing it and drying up"
> "Coming out" (pointing to the water). "Little boy ... and ..."

This is a total of 11 words, produced over a period of about 5 minutes!

Like cases with semantic dementia, nonfluent progressive aphasic patients have a higher success rate for word production in tasks of repetition and reading aloud, where they are provided with a spoken or written version of the target, than in naming or fluency tests or any form of self-generated production (Croot *et al.*, 1998). This task differential in terms of completely accurate production of individual words is not, however, as great for the nonfluent cases, since in repetition and reading they are still at risk of phonological errors, especially on longer words. Furthermore, they are rarely as severely anomic as the semantically impaired patients. In some of the more impaired nonfluent cases, while the advantage for reading and repetition over self-generated speech is observable with single-word stimuli, it all but disappears once whole sentences are required; that is, relatively severe nonfluent patients not only fail to produce whole sentences in conversation or picture description, but also cannot repeat or read these materials either. They paraphrase and indeed miss out words or whole chunks of the sentence, including both content and function words that they would easily produce in single-word repetition or reading (Graham *et al.*,

2004; Patterson, Graham *et al.*, 2006). We have been very struck by some of these patients' performance on a small task designed to answer the following question. Suppose that English words with an irregular spelling-to-sound correspondence (like *pint* or *blood* or *gauge*), which tend to yield regularization errors in single-word reading by surface dyslexic patients, are embedded in text: does the availability of a syntactic and semantic context reduce the rate of regularizations? We have administered this test to patients with nonfluent progressive aphasia. To our surprise, the result for a few cases has been neither of the two alternative outcomes that one might expect (either equal performance on the set of irregular words in isolation and in context, or better performance in context); but instead significantly worse performance on these words in text. This is not because the patients necessarily make errors of commission when reading meaningful sentences: they just leave many words out altogether. The demands of producing connected speech under any conditions seem to be too great.

We have explored some of the challenging theoretical issues surrounding this language deficit with regard to single content–word production in a study of two brothers with nonfluent progressive aphasia (Croot *et al.*, 1999). Apart from the probable genetic link in these two cases, which is always of interest to medical science, the linguistic issues addressed in these experiments included the relationship between performance on expressive and receptive word tasks (as mentioned above), and the relationship of impaired speech production to the working memory deficit that is prominent in all of these patients. Virtually no research has yet been addressed to the severe inability of these patients to produce connected speech, and this is one focus of our current research in Cambridge. The patients are certainly impaired in syntactic tasks, both expressive and receptive (e.g., they perform poorly on the Test for the Reception of Grammar on which fluent progressive aphasics do well). At least at an impressionistic level, however, it seems unlikely that the devastation of connected speech will find a satisfactory answer in these syntactic problems as it is usually thought to do in Broca's aphasia following stroke. For example, the grammatical elements of speech (such as function words and inflections in English) tend to be conspicuously lacking in the speech of Broca's aphasics, and indeed such patients have significant difficulty producing small grammatical words even in single-word reading tasks. In a dramatic characterization of this phenomenon, Gardner and Zurif (1975) described how such patients may successfully read aloud the content words *bee* and *inn* but fail to read their exact phonological equivalents in function word vocabulary, *be* and *in*. This pattern does not hold for nonfluent progressive patients, at least not the ones in our series, all of whom score just as highly in reading function words as content words (Patterson, Graham *et al.*, 2006).

The neuroanatomy of nonfluent progressive aphasia is also less well understood than that of semantic dementia, partly because the atrophy tends to be more diffuse and less focal than the atrophy centred on the anterior temporal lobe in the fluent patients. Functional imaging in some cases (the resting metabolic scans mentioned above, in Table 7.2) has revealed considerable hypometabolism in the anterior insula of the frontal lobe, around Brodmann areas 44/45 in Figure 7.1 (Nestor *et al.*, 2003). It may therefore turn out to be relevant that although the patients' neuropsychological deficits are certainly most prominent in the language domain, most of these cases are also impaired on tests of planning and flexibility that are considered to be functions of the frontal lobe. It is.possible that even beyond the known association with syntactic processing, frontal structures play an essential role in managing connected speech.

7.5   Concluding remarks

This chapter has reviewed a number of the salient features that characterize the two major forms of acquired language disorder (aphasia) that occur in neurodegenerative disease: fluent and nonfluent progressive aphasia. Because both types of patients eventually lose almost all ability to communicate by speaking, we have described these two conditions as resulting in two different "varieties of silence" (a phrase borrowed from an old radio skit by the British comedy team of the *Goons*: in this skit, they are evaluating different varieties or qualities of silence; when they open one "box of silence" from which a loud roar emerges, one Goon observes to another that this is the variety of silence that one can get free on the National Health Service!). Although we are a long way from a satisfactory understanding of either condition, our interim and simplified conclusions are as follows. The features of fluent progressive aphasia seem to be entirely explicable in terms of progressive degradation of the semantic or conceptual component of the language system, resulting in profound deterioration of both expressive and receptive content–word vocabulary. Structural and functional brain imaging of patients with this condition suggest that, within a widespread cortical network representing conceptual knowledge, one critical area comprises bilateral, but perhaps especially left, anterior and inferior temporal lobes. The features of nonfluent progressive aphasia seem to be partially explicable in terms of progressive degradation of the phonological and syntactic components of the language system, but we suspect that an additional underlying deficit will be necessary to account for the profound deterioration in producing connected speech. Neuroanatomically speaking, this additional deficit seems likely to depend on frontal-lobe structures which may or may not be language specific.

The research fields of neuropsychology and neurolinguistics have barely begun to tap the rich vein of data that can be obtained from studies of progressive aphasia. One aspect that has not been emphasized here is that the progression itself can be extremely informative, both about the purely linguistic features (e.g., which symptoms emerge first?) and in the quest for an understanding of the neural basis of language (how does the linguistic progression map onto the spread of the disease process?). It is sometimes a rather heart-breaking enterprise to study these cases and to measure the inexorable decline of their communicative abilities. Whether one studies language acquisition, skilled language function, or language deficits, however, it is also a privilege to have the opportunity to learn about this most fascinating and complex of human abilities.

References

Bak, T. H., O'Donovan, D. G., Xuereb, J. H., Boniface, S., and Hodges, J. R. (2001). Selective impairment of verb processing associated with pathological changes in Brodmann areas 44 and 45 in the motor neurone disease/dementia/aphasia syndrome. *Brain*, **124**, 102–24.

Bird, H., Lambon Ralph, M. A., Patterson, K., and Hodges, J. R. (2000). The rise and fall of frequency and imageability: noun and verb production in semantic dementia. *Brain and Language*, **73**, 17–49.

Bishop, D. (1989). *Test for the Reception of Grammar*. London: Medical Research Council.

Blumstein, S. E. (1994). Impairments of speech production and speech perception in aphasia. *Philosophical Transactions of the Royal Society of London* B, **346**, 29–36.

Breedin, S. and Saffran, E. M. (1999). Sentence processing in the face of semantic loss: a case study. *Journal of Experimental Psychology: General*, **128**, 547–62.

Broca, P. (1861). Remarques sur la siege de la faculté du langage articule, suivies d'une observation d'aphemie (perte de la parole). *Bulletin de la Societé d'Anatomie (Paris)*, **36**, 330–57.

Brodmann, K. (1909). *Vergleichende Lokalisations lehre der Grosshirnrinde in ihren Prinzipien dargestellt auf Grund des Zellenbaues*. Leipzig: Barth. English version: *Localisation in the Cerebral Cortex*. London: Smith-Gordon, 1994.

Chiacchio, L., Grossi, D., Stanzione, M., and Trojano, L. (1993). Slowly progressive aphasia associated with surface dyslexia. *Cortex*, **29**, 145–52.

Croot, K., Patterson, K., and Hodges, J. R. (1998). Single word production in nonfluent progressive aphasia. *Brain and Language*, **61**, 226–73.

Croot, K., Patterson, K., and Hodges, J. R. (1999). Familial progressive aphasia: insights into the nature and deterioration of single word processing. *Cognitive Neuropsychology*, **16**, 705–47.

Fushimi, T., Komori, K., Ikeda, M., *et al.* (2003). Surface dyslexia in a Japanese patient with semantic dementia: evidence for similarity-based orthography-to-phonology translation. *Neuropsychologia*, **41**, 1644–58.

Gainotti, G., Silveri, M. C., Daniele, A., and Giustolisi, L. (1995). Neuroanatomical correlates of category specific semantic disorders: a critical survey. *Memory*, **3**, 247–64.

Gardner, H. and Zurif, E. (1975). BEE but not BE: oral reading of single words in aphasia and alexia. *Neuropsychologia*, **13**, 181–90.

Gloor, P. (1997). *The Temporal Lobe and Limbic System*. New York/Oxford: Oxford University Press.

Goodglass, H. and Kaplan, E. (1983). *The Assessment of Aphasia and Related Disorders*. Philadelphia: Lea and Febiger.

Graham, K. S., Patterson, K., and Hodges, J. R. (1995). Progressive pure anomia: insufficient activation of phonology by meaning. *Neurocase*, **1**, 25–39.

Graham, K. S., Patterson, K., Pratt, K., and Hodges, J. R. (1999). Relearning and subsequent forgetting of semantic category exemplars in a case of semantic dementia. *Neuropsychology*, **13**, 359–80.

Graham, N. L., Patterson, K., and Hodges, J. R. (2000). The impact of semantic memory impairment on spelling: evidence from semantic dementia. *Neuropsychologia*, **38**, 143–63.

Graham, N. L., Patterson, K., and Hodges, J. R. (2004). When more yields less: speaking and writing in nonfluent progressive aphasia. *Neurocase*, **10**, 141–55.

Hodges, J. L., Graham, N., and Patterson, K. (1995). Charting the progression in semantic dementia: implications for the organisation of semantic memory. *Memory*, **3**, 463–95.

Hodges, J. R. and Patterson, K. (1996). Nonfluent progressive aphasia and dementia: a comparative neuropsychological study. *Journal of the International Neuropsychological Society*, **2**, 511–24.

Hodges, J. R., Patterson, K., Oxbury, S., and Funnell, E. (1992). Semantic dementia: progressive fluent aphasia with temporal lobe atrophy. *Brain*, **115**, 1783–806.

Hodges, J. R., Patterson, K., and Tyler, L. K. (1994). Loss of semantic memory: implications for the modularity of mind. *Cognitive Neuropsychology*, **11**, 505–42.

Howard, D. and Patterson, K. (1992). *Pyramids and Palm Trees: A Test of Semantic Access from Pictures and Words*. Bury St Edmunds, UK: Thames Valley Test Company.

Knott, R., Patterson, K., and Hodges, J. R. (1997). Lexical and semantic binding effects in short-term memory: evidence from semantic dementia. *Cognitive Neuropsychology*, **14**, 1165–216.

Lambon Ralph, M. A., McClelland, J. L., Patterson, K., Galton, C. J., and Hodges, J. R. (2001). No right to speak? The relationship between object naming and semantic impairment. *Journal of Cognitive Neuroscience*, **13**, 341–56.

Lee, A. C. H., Graham, K. S., Simons, J. S., *et al.* (2002). Regional brain activations differ for semantic features but not categories. *NeuroReport*, **13**, 1497–501.

Levy, D. A., Bayley, P. J., and Squire, L. R. (2004). The anatomy of semantic knowledge: medial vs. lateral temporal lobe. *Proceedings of the National Academy of Sciences*, **101**, 6710–15.

Martin, N. and Saffran, E. M. (1997). Language and auditory verbal short-term memory impairment: evidence for common underlying processes. *Cognitive Neuropsychology*, **14**, 641–82.

McCarthy, R. and Warrington, E. K. (1986). Phonological reading: phenomena and paradoxes. *Cortex*, **22**, 359–80.

Mesulam, M. M. (1982). Slowly progressive aphasia without generalized dementia. *Annals of Neurology*, **11**, 592–8.

Mummery, C. J., Patterson, K., Price, C. J., *et al.* (2000). A voxel-based morphometry study of semantic dementia: relationship between temporal lobe atrophy and semantic memory. *Annals of Neurology*, **47**, 36–45.

Mummery, C. J., Patterson, K., Wise, R. J. S., *et al.* (1999). Disrupted temporal lobe connections in semantic dementia. *Brain*, **122**, 61–73.

Nestor, P. J., Graham, N. L., Fryer, T. D., *et al.* (2003). Progressive non-fluent aphasia is associated with hypometabolism centred on the left anterior insula. *Brain*, **126**, 2406–18.

Papagno, C. and Capitani, E. (2001). Slowly progressive aphasia: a four-year follow-up study. *Neuropsychologia*, **39**, 678–86.

Parkin, A. (1993). Progressive aphasia without dementia: a clinical and cognitive neuropsychological analysis. *Brain and Language*, **44**, 201–20.

Patterson, K., Graham, N., and Hodges, J. R. (1994). The impact of semantic memory loss on phonological representations. *Journal of Cognitive Neuroscience*, **6**, 57–69.

Patterson, K., Graham, N. L., Hodges, J. R., and Lambon Ralph, M. A. (2006). Progressive non-fluent aphasia is not a progressive version of non-fluent (post-stroke) aphasia. *Aphasiology*, **20**, 1018–34.

Patterson, K. and Hodges, J. R. (1992). Deterioration of word meaning: implications for reading. *Neuropsychologia*, **30**, 1025–40.

Patterson, K., Lambon Ralph, M. A., Jefferies, E., *et al.* (2006). "Pre-semantic" cognition in semantic dementia: six deficits in search of an explanation. *Journal of Cognitive Neuroscience*, **18**, 169–83.

Patterson, K. and MacDonald, M. C. (2006). Sweet nothings: narrative speech in semantic dementia. In S. Andrews, ed., *From Inkmarks to Ideas: Current Issues in Lexical Processing*. Hove: Psychology Press, pp. 299–317.

Patterson, K., Suzuki, T., Wydell, T., and Sasanuma, S. (1995). Progressive aphasia and surface alexia in Japanese. *Neurocase*, **1**, 155–65.

Pick, A. (1904). Zur Symptomatologie der linksseitigen Schläfenlappenatrophie. *Monatschrift für Psychiatrie und Neurologie*, **16**, 378–88. English translation: Girling, D. M. and Berrios, G. E. [1997]. On the symptomatology of left-sided temporal lobe atrophy. *History of Psychiatry*, 8, 149–59.

Plaut, D. C., McClelland, J. L., Seidenberg, M. S., and Patterson, K. (1996). Understanding normal and impaired word reading: computational principles in quasi-regular domains. *Psychological Review*, **103**, 56–115.

Price, C. J. (1998). The functional anatomy of word comprehension. *Trends in Cognitive Sciences*, **2**, 281–8.

Pulvermüller, F., Haerle, M., and Hummel, F. (2001). Walking or talking? Behavioural and electrophysiological correlates of action verb processing. *Brain and Language*, **78**, 143–68.

Pulvermüller, F. and Preissl, H. (1991). A cell assembly model of language. *Network: Computation in Neural Systems*, **2**, 455–68.

Rogers, T. T., Lambon Ralph, M. A., Garrard, P., *et al.* (2004). The structure and deterioration of semantic memory: a neuropsychological and computational investigation. *Psychological Review*, **111**, 205–35.

Schwartz, M. F., Marin, O. S. M., and Saffran, E. M. (1979). Dissociations of language function in dementia: a case study. *Brain and Language*, **7**, 277–306.

Seeley, W. W., Bauer, A. M., Miller, B. L., *et al.* (2005). The natural history of temporal variant frontotemporal dementia. *Neurology*, **64**, 1384–90.

Snodgrass, J. S. and Vanderwart, M. (1980). A standardized set of 260 pictures: norms for name agreement, image agreement, familiarity, and visual complexity. *Journal of Experimental Psychology: Human Learning and Memory*, **6**, 174–215.

Snowden, J. S., Goulding, P. J., and Neary, D. (1989). Semantic dementia: a form of circumscribed cerebral atrophy. *Behavioural Neurology*, **2**, 167–82.

Snowden, J. S., Neary, D., and Mann, D. M. A. (1996). *Frontotemporal Lobar Degeneration: Frontotemporal Dementia, Progressive Aphasia, Semantic Dementia*. New York: Churchill Livingstone.

Studholme, C., Cardenas, V., Blumenfeld, R., *et al.* (2004). Deformation tensor morphomotry of semantic dementia with quantitative validation. *NeuroImage*, **21**, 1387–98.

Tatsumi, I., Fushimi, T., Sadato, N., *et al.* (1999). Verb generation in Japanese – a multicenter PET activation study. *NeuroImage*, **9**, 154–64.

Tranel, D., Damasio, H., and Damasio, A. R. (1997). A neural basis for the retrieval of conceptual knowledge. *Neuropsychologia*, **35**, 1319–27.

Warburton, E., Wise, R. J. S., Price, C. J., *et al.* (1996). Noun and verb retrieval by normal subjects: studies with PET. *Brain*, **119**, 159–79.

Warrington, E. K. (1975). Selective impairment of semantic memory. *Quarterly Journal of Experimental Psychology*, **27**, 635–57.

Wernicke, C. (1874). *Der aphasische Symptomencomplex. Eine psychologische Studie auf anatomischer Basis*. English translation: Eggert, G. H. [1977]. *Wernicke's Works on Aphasia: A Sourcebook and Review*. New York: Mouton.

8

Why is language unique to humans?

JACQUES MEHLER, MARINA NESPOR, AND MARCELA PEÑA

8.1   Introduction

Linguists, psychologists, and neuroscientists have studied language acquisition with the tools and models available to their respective fields. Linguists elaborated some of the most sophisticated theories to account for how this unique human competence arises in the infants' brains. Chomsky (1980) formulated the parameter setting theory (hereafter, PS) to account for how infants, on the basis of partial and noisy language input, acquire grammar. PS assumes that infants are born with "knowledge" of Universal Grammar (UG). This includes both genetically determined universal principles and binary parameters. Universal principles describe the properties common to all natural languages. Binary parameters capture the grammatical properties on which natural languages differ from one another. The linguistic input determines the particular value of a parameter. PS postulates that exposure to the surrounding language determines how the parameters of UG are set.[1]

We acknowledge that PS has many virtues. It addresses the problem of language acquisition without making unjustified but common simplifications, for example, that imitation is the privileged mechanism responsible for the emergence of linguistic competence. The theory, furthermore, is quite appealing because it assumes, realistically, a biological perspective, namely, that the child is equipped with a species-specific mechanism to acquire natural language. Moreover, the PS theory has been formulated with sufficient detail and precision as to make it easy to falsify. In contrast, proposals that assume that language is acquired by means of a general learning device appear more difficult to support. Criticisms of proposals according to which general learning mechanisms are sufficient to explain language acquisition have been given by many

Topics in Integrative Neuroscience: From Cells to Cognition, ed. James R. Pomerantz. Published by Cambridge University Press. © Cambridge University Press 2008.

theoreticians (see Chomsky, 1959; Fodor, 1975; Lenneberg *et al.*, 1964; Pinker, 1984).

All theories agree that at least parts of grammar have to be learned. What distinguishes the different positions is the scope and nature of learning. How does the learning proceed? PS assumes an initial state characterized by knowledge specific to language. In contrast, theoreticians who favor a general learning mechanism, assume that the initial state is characterized by learning principles that apply to all areas in which the organism gains knowledge. PS has the advantage that it is rather easy to falsify. If syntax cannot be acquired given the normal input, then PS would have to be abandoned. Indeed, if PS turns out to be misguided, badly informed, or incorrect, another theory will have to be formulated and evaluated. This is far from being an exceptional situation. Rather, it is one that is obtained in all scientific domains. In contrast, recent generic learning accounts (see Plunkett, McClelland, and many others) have not yet been presented in sufficient detail to be falsifiable. In this chapter, we ignore the generic learning account and focus on some aspects of PS.

So far, we have highlighted the positive aspects of PS. However, a problem resides in the hidden assumptions that investigators have made when trying to explicate the learning of grammar. PS was formulated with syntax acquisition in mind and investigators generally assumed that infants have already gained, in one way or another, knowledge of the lexicon, including the phonological information it carries, before setting grammatical parameters. If this were the case, both the lexical and the phonological properties of the language could be learned without having to consider syntax. Only if one believes that infants store the sounds in the surrounds ignoring any additional information that they contain, could one understand why researchers interested in the acquisition of syntax have ignored the first year of life: during this period, babies would only memorize the sounds in their surrounds and acquire the first few words. If one makes such presuppositions, it seems also reasonable to assume that infants set grammatical parameters after acquiring a basic vocabulary. By and large, scholars working in the PS tradition have assumed that the first year of life can be neglected without missing essential aspects of the acquisition process. In fact, if syntax is the crux of language and there is nothing syntactic being learned during the first year of life, why should one study that period at all? The presupposition that acquisition starts with the first linguistic productions, roughly at 8 months of age or later, explains why PS investigators have exclusively reported data on language production.

Supporting the PS position may have been justified by data on animal behavior. Indeed, animals with auditory systems similar to our own tend to respond to speech patterns much like infants younger than 8 months (see Kuhl, 1987;

Ramus *et al.*, 2000 among many others). Apes, but also dogs, have "lexicons" that can attain a few dozen words (see Premack, 1971, 1986). Tamarins, chinchillas, and several other animals treat and respond to sounds much like humans (see Doupe, this book). However, their perceptual and mnemonic abilities are not sufficient to enable them to construct a grammar comparable to that of human languages. In contrast to the assumption that the first years of life is irrelevant to the acquisition of syntax, we show below that language acquisition begins with the onset of life. Indeed, recent data supports the view that the sound pattern of language plays an important role in the learning of syntax.

Psychologists have explored general learning accounts of knowledge acquisition, including language. Most of those studies have tried to understand how productive a model of language acquisition entirely based on associations can be. Within this stream of research, the brain is regarded as a huge network that works in a Hebbian fashion.[2] This explains why many psychologists, as well as many neuroscientists, though by no means all, have adopted a contrasting viewpoint from that of linguists. Their tendency has been to neglect syntax and assume that by focusing exclusively on speech perception and production, a functional theory of language will ensue. Undeniably, behavioral scientists have achieved great success studying perception and production. Some of them believe that it is sufficient to study how language production and perception unfold during development to understand how syntax (or semantics) is computed by the mind. This stance was strengthened because, while it is easy to study how babies or animals perceive speech sounds, it is very hard to study the acquisition of syntax in the laboratory. Psychologists who work assuming a generic learning mechanism behave as if the mystery of syntax acquisition will disappear by observing how infants learn to conform to the structure of language (see Seidenberg & MacDonald, 1999; Tomasello, 2000, among many others).

We believe that true progress will be accomplished once the above divide of research strategies is overcome. Losing sight of the uniqueness of syntax is dangerous and so is neglecting how signals are processed and represented by the very young infant. Indeed, the linguistic input can be viewed as speech signal (or hand gestures for the deaf) that contains information about different aspects of grammar, syntax included; that is, the triggers of different parameters may be present in some shallow acoustic form in the input the child receives. However, unlike many reflexes that are triggered by a sensorial stimulus even the first time the organism encounters it, it seems highly probable that speech signals do not trigger the setting of a syntactic parameter the first time the infant listens to a sentence. Rather, it seems more likely that the child would gather enough information to draw a conclusion about the appropriate value of a parameter. In fact, many infants (maybe even a majority) are exposed to two languages from birth onwards. The two languages might require that a single parameter be set in two different ways. Will the information that is necessary to fix a parameter in one language of exposure be masked by noise from the other language? Will there be two files, one for each of the two languages? Or rather will there be a single noisy file that will result in utter confusion to the child? These are some of the issues that are essential for linguists and cognitive neuroscientists to confront together to bring their theoretical stances in closer harmony with one another and with the facts.

Fortunately, the polarity we described above is already diminishing. The interaction between the fields began to increase when scholars began to realize that grammar acquisition, even in a tradition like the one defined by PS, remains rather vague. Indeed, even though linguists studied the influence of syntax on the phonological shape of speech (see Nespor & Vogel, 1986; Selkirk, 1984, among others), they have not explored how speech signals trigger the fixation of parameters in infants. As will be argued below, we believe that the time is ripe to explore how humans sample information from the surrounds to discover the abstract properties of language. Only then will we be able to understand what the essential difference is between the human and the evolved ape's brain. That will be the time when a new impulse will be given to the study of the biological foundations of language.

Studies by Chomsky (1980, 1986), Wexler and Culicover (1980), Pinker (1984), and others have lucidly argued for a PS conception of language acquisition. However, the PS formulation may have been seriously under-specified making it hard to judge its adequacy. In fact, Mazuka (1996) has argued that, in its usual formulation, PS contains a fatal paradox. Of course, solutions to most of these problems might turn up in the years to come. Morgan *et al.* (1987), Cutler (1994), and Nespor *et al.* (1996), among others, have proposed some putative solutions. However, few proposals have explored how the infant evaluates and computes the triggering signals. Some recent results suggest that nearly 2-month-olds are sensitive to the prosodic correlates of the different values of the head-complement parameter (Christophe *et al.*, 1997; Christophe *et al.*, 2003).

In the early 1980s, some psychologists and some linguists like Wanner and Gleitman (1982) already foresaw some of the difficulties in existing theories of grammar acquisition and proposed that phonological bootstrapping may help the infant out of its quandary. Wanner and Gleitman (1982) held that some properties of the phonological system that the child is learning may help uncover lexical and syntactic properties. Some years later, Morgan and Demuth (1996) added that specifically prosody might contain signals that can act as triggers helping the child to learn syntax. Indeed, these authors conclude, as we do above, that the study of the speech signals that can act as triggers is essential to understand the first steps into language. A better understanding of the speech signal might also uncover whether PS is a solution to the problem highlighted by learnability theorists: the poverty of the stimulus (see Wexler & Culicover, 1980; and many others). The postulation of innate structure was the way chosen to overcome the poverty of the stimulus problem. Today, we see that this proposal is not sufficiently specific. Indeed, if an important part of the endowment comes as binary parameters, we still need to understand how these are set to the values adequate for the surrounding language. The general assumption was that by understanding a few words, simple sentences like *drink the juice*, *eat the soup*, will allow the child to generalize the fact that, in his/her language, objects follow verbs. As Mazuka (1996) pointed out, this assumption is unwarranted. Indeed, how does the child know that soup means *soup* (Noun) rather than *eat* (Verb)? Even if Mom always says *eat* in front of diverse foods, the child could understand that what she means is *food*! If the signals were to inform the child about word order, one could find a way out of this paradox. Before we know if this is a true solution, we need to ask whether such signals exist and if they do, whether the infant can process them.

The prosodic bootstrapping hypothesis arose from linguistic research that focused on the prosodic properties that are systematically associated with specific syntactic properties (see Nespor & Vogel, 1986; Selkirk, 1984, among many others). These authors found interesting associations between these two grammatical levels, making plausible the notion that signals might cue the learner to postulate syntactic properties in an automatic, encapsulated fashion.

Let us assume that babies are born with Universal Grammar. It still is essential to understand how they learn their maternal language. We know that the properties of the speech signals are processed very precociously; and if one believes, as we do, that speech signals contain the information that is necessary to set the main parameters, we still have to explain what happens during the first 18 months of life. What is the baby doing that takes it so long to get going? What is the infant learning throughout this period? Since infants perceive the cues that can set triggers and since these are supposed to function in an automatic and encapsulated way, we are committed to the view that infants have "learned" many aspects of the language before they begin to produce speech. We have the responsibility, however, to give an account of the specific processes that happen during the first months of life. As we argued above (p. 4), a parameter will not be set after listening to a single utterance. Rather, properties of utterances are stored and only when the information becomes "reliable" will it be used to set a parameter. Since some parameters can only be set after other grammatical properties have already been acquired (and each of them requiring considerable information storage), we might understand the "slow" pace of learning. Learning the outstanding properties of grammar is just one aspect of language acquisition. In addition, the child has to learn a great deal of arbitrary linguistic properties. The sound of words is arbitrary. One should also not forget that most words are heard in connected speech. Thus, we must investigate how the infant parses the input to identify words. A proposal made by Saffran *et al.* (1996) is that this requires the inspection of the statistical properties of the incoming speech signals.

Let us now spell out the purpose of the present chapter. While we assume that UG is part of the infant's endowment and that it guides language acquisition, we also acknowledge that statistical properties of the language spoken in the surrounds inform and guide learning. This is in contrast to the position of some theorists as MacWhinney (1987) and Seidenberg and MacDonald (1999) who argue that it is unnecessary to pay attention to grammar learning, since all that is required is to explain how the child learns to comprehend and produce language. The authors, and many others, believe that it is possible to explain linguistic performance exclusively on the basis of the infant's sensitivity to the statistical properties of signals. Generally, this position is defended on the basis of rather simplified scenarios in which each solution is proposed for the acquisition of just one aspect of grammar. How would their model stand up in the real setting in which infants learn language, not to mention bilingual settings, or the creolization of pidgin languages.

The above presentation makes it clear that more data and research are needed to understand how the biological human endowment interacts with the learning abilities during the first months of life. We are in a rather good position, because during the last few years, new and fascinating results have been secured allowing us to start having a coherent picture of language acquisition.

8.2   Innate dispositions for language?

Before and after birth, infants experience speech in noisy environments. A conjecture that is often made by pediatricians and naïve observers is that this cacophony that infants experience is not a problem because they had learned to attend to speech during gestation. The womb, however, is not such a quiet place. Indeed, experiments carried out with pregnant quadrupeds and also on volunteer pregnant women reveal that intra-uterine noise tends to be even more important than the noise that the infant encounters after birth. The bowels, blood circulation, other body movements, to mention a few sources, generate noise with considerable energy (Querleu *et al.*, 1988). Thus, acoustic stimulation in the womb will not explain how infants segregate speech from background noise. How does the infant identify the signals that carry linguistic information? Why are music, telephone rings, animal sounds, etc. segregated during language acquisition?

Psycholinguists have explored experimentally this difficult question. Colombo and Bundy (1983) have reported that infants respond preferentially to speech streams as compared to other noises. This result, however, is difficult to evaluate, since it is always conceivable that infants would prefer a nonspeech stimulus different from the one used by Colombo and Bundy (1983). Maybe, a melody might be found that is equally attractive as the speech stream. Few experimenters have explored this question in a more convincing way. Mehler *et al.*, 1988 found that neonates behave differently when they are exposed to normal utterances as compared to the same utterances played backward. These authors interpret their finding as showing that infants attend to speech rather than to other stimuli even when they are matched for pitch, intensity, and duration.

More evidence is needed to be convinced that the neonate's brain responds specifically to speech sounds rather than to the human voice (regardless of whether it is producing speech or coughs, cries, sneezes, etc.). Humans are incapable to produce backward speech. The impossibility of the vocal tract to produce backward speech might be an alternative explanation of Mehler *et al.*'s results mentioned above. The contrast between a natural utterance (producible by the human vocal tract) and a machine-made rearrangement of the same utterance (that no human vocal tract could produce) may be the relevant factor, rather than the contrast between speech and nonspeech that the authors invoke. Belin *et al.* (2000) have recently claimed that there is a brain area that is devoted to processing conspecific vocal productions. He examined adult subjects in an fMRI imaging experiment while they were listening to various speech and nonspeech sounds all made by the human vocal tract (i.e., speech but also laughs, sighs, and various onomatopoeia). In response to all these stimuli, he found bilateral activation along the upper banks of the STS (Superior Temporal Sulcus). However, vocal sounds elicit greater activation than nonvocal sounds bilaterally in nonprimary auditory cortex. If Belin *et al.*'s results are corroborated, one might explain the speech vs. backward speech results mentioned above because only speech can be produced by the human vocal tract.

Belin and his colleagues have argued that the brain is organized to process human voices much like other parts of the brain are organized to process human faces. Indeed, Kanwisher *et al.* (1997) have proposed that faces are processed in a specific area, the FFA (fusiform face area). According to Belin *et al.*, human voice is processed in the STS. This conclusion may be premature since we do not yet know the set of stimuli that activate the voice recognition area.[3]

Our own outlook is that it is essential to study the specificity of cortical areas devoted to process different information types, before any prior learning has occurred. Establishing whether certain areas of the brain are organized in specific ways is essential for the study of infancy and also for the construction of theories of development. Thus, in contrast to the above-described investigations our research focuses mainly on the initial state of the cognitive system. Adults may have already learned how to process and encode faces or human vocal tract production, and as a result have taken possession of cortical tissue for this purpose. Therefore, to distinguish what is due to our endowment and what arises as a consequence of learning, it is necessary to investigate very young infants and whenever possibly neonates since in the first months many acquisitions have already been documented (for some investigations that bear mostly on language, see Jusczyk, 1997; Kuhl et al., 1992; Mehler & Dupoux, 1994; Werker & Tees, 1984).

Standard neurological science has gathered evidence that the left hemisphere (LH) is more involved with language representation and processing than the right hemisphere (RH). Are infants born with specific LH areas devoted to speech processing or is the LH specialization the sole result of experience? The response to this question is still tentative. Numerous investigations have reported that infants are born with speech processing abilities similar to those displayed by experienced adults. For instance, infants discriminate all the phonetic contrasts that arise in natural languages, (see Jusczyk, 1997, Mehler & Dupoux, 1994). At first, this finding was construed as showing that humans are born with specific neural machinery devoted to speech. Subsequent investigations, however, demonstrated that basic acoustic processes are sufficient to explain these early abilities that humans share with other organisms (see Jusczyk, 1997; Jusczyk et al., 1977; Kuhl & Miller, 1975). Thus, it is reasonable to postulate a species-specific disposition to acquire natural language, but we still lack data to ground the view that we are born with cortical structures specifically dedicated to the processing of speech.

As we mentioned above, functional asymmetries, in particular a superiority of the LH, seem to be related to speech processing. A great deal of neuropsychological evidence points in that direction (see Bryden & Allard, 1981; Dronkers, 1996; Geschwind, 1970). Likewise, experimental studies carried out on normal adult volunteers suggest that LH dominance characterizes speech processing (see Bertelson, 1982 among many others). We still ignore whether such LH superiority is the consequence of language acquisition or whether language is mastered because of this tissue specialization. Developmental psychologists investigated this issue in some detail. Most behavioral studies found an asymmetry in very young humans (see Bertoncini *et al.*, 1989; Best *et al.*, 1982; Segalowitz & Chapman, 1980). A few ERP studies have also found trends for LH superiority in young infants (see Dehaene-Lambertz & Dehaene, 1994; Molfese & Molfese, 1979). Both the behavioral and the ERP data suggest that LH superiority exists in the infant's brain but more evidence is desirable to strengthen and to further understand the cortical organization of the immature brain. Fortunately, we are entering a new era and it is becoming possible to use more advanced imaging methods to study the functional brain organization in newborn infants. A number of methods are being pursued in parallel. Numerous groups have begun to study healthy infants using fMRI (G. Dehaene-Lambertz, personal communication). In the following section, we focus on recent results we obtained with Optical Topography (OT).

8.3   Brain specialization in newborns: evidence from OT

Optical Topography is a method derived from Near Infrared technology developed in the early 1950s (see Villringer & Chance, 1997 for an excellent review of the field). This technology allows us to estimate the vascular response of the brain following stimulation.[4] In particular, it allows to estimate the concentration of oxyhemoglobin (oxyHb) and deoxyhemoglobin (deoxyHB) over a given area of the brain.

We used a prototype device produced by Hitachi and modified by us. This device allowed us to place two sets of optic fibers on each side of the infant's head. We first studied the simultaneous activation of two areas of the brain. These areas were located to be, as nearly as possible, homologous to each other on the LH and the RH. We assume that we have placed the probes so as to measure activity over the RH and the LH temporal and parietal areas. Each infant was tested with three kinds of blocks of stimuli. In one condition (Forward Speech, FW), infants hear sequences of 15 seconds of connected French utterances separated from one another by periods of silence of variable duration (from 25 to 35 seconds). In another condition (Backward Speech, BW), infants are tested like in the FW condition but with the speech sequences played backward (the signal was converted from FW to BW using a speech editor). Ten such blocks are presented in the FW and in the BW conditions for each infant. Finally, in another condition, infants are exposed to silence for a duration comparable to the average duration of the above conditions. The latter is a comparison measure for the other two conditions.

Not all infants completed the ten blocks in each condition. In order for an infant to be kept in the final data analysis, the subject had to complete at least

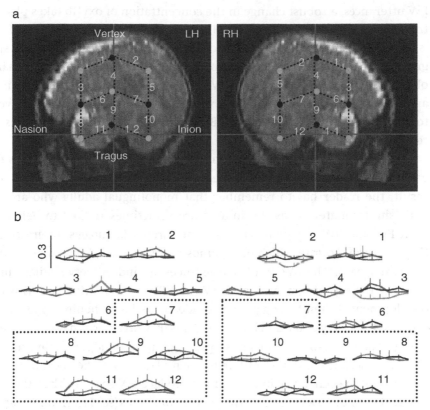

Figure 8.1 Positioning of the OT probes and observed results. (a) OT channels projected on an MR image of a 2-month-old infant. Red dots correspond to emitter and blue dots to detector optical fibers. The numbers on the black dotted lines, between adjacent emitter–detector pairs of fibers, correspond to the channels from which changes in Hb concentration were estimated. Indicated skull landmarks (inion, nasion, tragus, and vertex) were used to place the probes. (b) The numbers above the plots correspond to channel numbers in a. The plots show the grand average of the mean of total Hb (mmol.mm) for successive 5-s windows. The first window begins 5 s before the onset of a block. The vertical black line in channel 1 of the LH indicates the range of total Hb concentration in mmol.mm valid for all of the channels. Total Hb is plotted in red for FW, in light green for BW, and in blue for SIL. Ascending bars indicate SDs. The six channels enclosed within dotted lines (7–12) cover the temporal regions below the Sylvian fissure (lower channels). Channels 1–6 were placed over the frontoparietal regions above the Sylvian fissure (upper channels); (with permission from PNAS) (for color image please see www.cambridge.org/9780521143400).

three blocks in each one of the three conditions – FW, BW, and Silence. The preliminary results suggest that like in adults, the hemodynamic response begins 4 to 5 seconds after the infant receives the auditory stimulation. This time-locked response appears more clearly for the oxyHB than for the deoxyHB. The pattern of results shows that roughly 5 seconds after the presentation of the

FW utterances, a robust change in the concentration of oxyHb takes place over the temporo-parietal region of the LH. Interestingly, the concentration of oxyHB is relatively stable both in the BW and in the Silence conditions. Forward speech gives rise to a significant increase in oxyHb over the LH. No significant change is observed when BW speech is used. While the energy is identical in FW and BW, and their spectral properties are mirror images of each other, only FW gives rise to a significant increase of deoxyHB over the LH. Figure 8.1 illustrates these results.

These results suggest that the brain of the newborn infant responds differently to natural and backward speech. To understand the singularity of this result, the reader has to remember that monolingual adults who are tested with similar materials as the infants are sometimes tricked to believe that both FW and BW are sentences in some foreign languages. Interestingly, if they are asked to rate which one sounds more "natural," they tend to choose forward speech. The BW and FW utterances are indeed very similar but they differ at the suprasegmental level. FW and BW speech differ in terms of the development of their timing patterns. Indeed, final lengthening appears to be a universal property of natural language. Thus, BW utterances have initial lengthening. In addition, some segments (stops i.e., [p], [t], [k], [b], [d], and [g] and affricates, like [ts] or [dz]) become very different when played BW. The vocal tract cannot produce BW speech. Since infants cannot produce FW speech either, they might ignore the contrast between the BW and FW conditions (see Liberman & Mattingly, 1985). Since the neonate's brain responds in a different way to FW and BW utterances, we suggest that babies, in some sense of "know," know the difference between utterances that can and cannot be articulated by humans. We might tentatively attribute this result to the specialization of certain cortical areas of the neonate's brain for speech. Humans might have, like many other vertebrates, specialized effectors and receptors for a species-specific vocalization, which in our case is speech. This possibility needs to be studied in greater detail.

The above results have to be evaluated with care. Results from the work we have carried out with nonhuman organisms show that they display a behavior similar to that of infants, when confronted with FW and BW speech. In a series of studies comparing the newborn infant and the tamarin monkey behavioral responses, Ramus *et al.* (2000) showed that like infants, tamarins discriminate two languages when the utterances are played forward but fail to do so when the utterances are played backward. Tamarins will never develop speech, yet they notice the change from FW to BW speech. This ought to temper any desire to conclude that the above results are based on a species-specific system to process natural speech. They may also suggest that the specialization may be more basic, that is, not for speech as such but for sounds produced by vocal tracts that emit air through a narrow passage. Higher vertebrates produce sounds in this way.

In an attempt to replicate and expand the above experiment, a new device was used to measure simultaneously activation over 12 positions on the RH and 12 on the LH (see Peña, Maki, Dehaene-Lambertz, Bouquet, Koizumi & Mehler, 2003). The design of the experiment was otherwise identical to the one described above. The outcome shows that the overall pattern of activation mimics that already observed with the more primitive device. Indeed, we found that the infant's brain is activated by acoustic stimuli, regardless of whether these are FW or BW speech as compared to no stimulation. However, we also found that the total HB response to FW is larger on the LH than on similar areas of the RH. This is not the case for BW. Indeed, for BW speech, the total HB response is comparable on the RH and the LH. These results suggest that normal speech is differently processed to a very well-matched control, namely BW speech.

Obviously, the advent of imaging studies with neonates will permit new and more precise investigations to establish whether the specialization for speech is really present at birth or whether there is activation for streams of sounds that can be produced by a vertebrate's vocal tract. We believe that these kinds of study will set in motion new investigations that will clarify the validity of many of our current views. In the meantime, these studies have shed some light into complex issues that were hard to study with more traditional behavioral methods.

8.4   Neonates use rhythm to tune into language

Rhythm is a percept that relates to the relative duration of constituents in a sequence. What are the elements responsible for rhythm in language? Three constituents have been proposed to be roughly isochronous in different languages, thus giving rise to rhythm: syllables, feet, and morae (see Abercrombie, 1967; Ladefoged, 1975; Pike, 1945). Syllables have independently been construed as a basic constituent or atom in speech production and comprehension (see Cutler *et al.*, 1983; Levelt, 1989; Mehler, 1981). Infants begin to produce syllables several months after birth, with the onset of babbling. However, the infant may process syllables before he/she produces them. If so, we ought to find precursors illustrating that neonates process syllables in linguistic-like ways.[5] Bertoncini (1981) explored this issue using the nonnutritive sucking technique showing that very young infants distinguish a pair of syllables that differ only in the serial order of their constituents segments, for example, *PAT* and *TAP*. The infants, however, fail to distinguish a pair of items derived from the previous ones by replacing the vowel [a] by the consonant [s]. This renders the items *TSP* and *PST*, impossible syllables. To understand the infant's failure to distinguish this pair, in a control experiment, infants were presented with the same items but surrounded by a vocalic context. When the same sequences are presented in a syllabic context, as when they are surrounded by a vowel (as in *UPSTU* and *UTSPU*), the infant's discrimination ability is restored. This experiment suggests that the infant makes distinctions in linguistic-like contexts that are neglected in other acoustic contexts.

As we mentioned in Note 6, some languages (e.g., Croatian, some varieties of Berber, etc.) allow specific consonants to occupy the syllabic nuclear position. For instance, in Croatian, *Trieste*, the Italian city, is named *Trst* where [r] is the nucleus. This is not an exceptional case in the language. Indeed, the word for "finger" is *prst* and the word for "pitcher" is *vrč*. Why then were the results reported in the previous experiment obtained? Why did the infants neglect to treat *PST* and *TSP* as syllables? Maybe we tested infants who were already rather old, i.e., 2 months, and thus had already considerable exposure to the surrounding language. Since they are all raised in a French environment, it is possible that the stimuli were already considered extraneous to their language and thus their differences neglected. Alternatively, PST and TSP are impossible syllables in any language. To the best of our knowledge, in fact, there is no language that allows [s] as a syllabic nucleus. We are currently exploring means to choose between these two alternative explanations. We predict that infants have no difficulties in distinguishing pairs in which [r] or [l] figure as nuclei (e.g. [prt] vs. [trp] or [plt] vs. [tlp]) since such syllables occur in a few languages but that they will have difficulty distinguishing sequences in which the nuclear position is occupied by [s] or [f] (e.g. [pst] vs. [tsp] or [pft] vs. [tfp]). To insure that the infant has not become familiar with the syllable repertoire in the surrounding language, we are testing neonates in their first week of life.

That infants are attending to speech using syllabic units has also been claimed by Bijeljac-Babic *et al.* (1993). These authors showed that infants distinguish lists of bi-syllabic items from a list of tri-syllabic ones. They used CVCV items (e.g., *maki, nepo, suta, jaco*) and CVCVCV items (e.g., *makine, posuta, jacoli*). This result is observed regardless of whether the items differ or are matched for duration. Indeed, some of the original items were compressed and others expanded to match the mean durations of the two lists. Infants discriminated the lists equally well, suggesting that it is the number of syllables or just the number of vowels in the items that counts for their representation. We have had to focus on syllables rather than feet or morae because few studies have explored whether neonates represent these units. Below we are going to explain why we believe that syllables, or possibly vowels, play such an important role during the early steps of language acquisition.

The results described above fit well together with recent evidence showing that neonates are born with remarkable abilities to learn language. For instance, in the last decade numerous studies have uncovered the exceptional abilities of babies to process the prosodic features of utterances (see Mehler *et al.*, 1988; Moon *et al.*, 1993). Indeed, for many pairs of languages, infants tend to notice when a speaker switches from one language to another. What is the actual cue that allows infants to detect this switch? The essential property appears to be linguistic rhythm, defined as the proportion that vowels occupy in the utterances of a language (see Ramus *et al.*, 1999). If two languages have different rhythms (an important change in %V), the baby will detect a switch from one language to the other. If languages have similar rhythms, as for instance, English and Dutch or Spanish and Italian, very young infants will fail to react to a switch (see Nazzi *et al.*, 1998).

The variability of the inter-vocalic interval (i.e., ΔC, the standard deviation of the intervocalic intervals) also plays an important role in explaining the infants' behavior. In fact, ΔC in conjunction with %V provides an excellent measure of language rhythm that fits well with the intuitive classification of languages that phonologists have provided. Indeed, their claim is that there are basically three kinds of rhythm depending on which of three possible units maintains isochrony in the speech stream: stress-timed rhythm, syllable-timed rhythm and mora-timed rhythm (see Abercrombie, 1967; Ladefoged, 1975; Pike, 1945). However, once exact measures were carried out, contrary to many an expectation, isochronous units were not found (see Dauer, 1983; Manrique & Signorini, 1983; but see Port *et al.*, 1987). This does not mean, as one might have argued, that the classification linguists proposed on the basis of their intuitions has to be dismissed. Rather, Ramus *et al.*'s definition of rhythm on the basis of ΔC and %V divides languages exactly into those three intuitive classes, as shown in Figure 8.2.

A language with a high %V and a small ΔC (like Japanese or Hawaiian) is likely to have a small syllabic repertoire. Mostly, such languages allow only CVs, and Vs giving rise to the typical rhythm of the mora-class. Moreover, intervocalic intervals cannot be very variable since consonant clusters are avoided and codas are in general disallowed. In Japanese, for instance, codas generally contain /n/ (as in the word *Honda*).[6] Romance languages, as depicted in Figure 8.2, have a smaller value of %V because their syllabic repertoires are larger. Indeed, these languages allow both onsets and codas. Moreover, onsets may contain consonant clusters and occasionally also codas contain more than one consonant (e.g., *prêt*, *sparo*, *tact*, *parc*, etc.). However, fewer syllable types are allowed in Romance languages than in stress-timed languages as Dutch and English. Indeed, while in

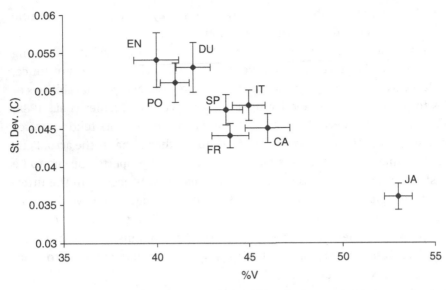

Figure 8.2 %V is the mean proportion of the utterances in a language that is occupied by vowels and ΔC or St. Dev. (C) is the standard deviation of the consonantal intervals. The plot incorporates eight languages spoken by four female speakers. Each speaker utters 20 sentences (each language is represented by 80 utterances). The distribution of the languages is compatible with the notion that they can be grouped into three classes as predicted by phonological intuitions (from Ramus *et al.*, 1999).

Romance languages the typical syllabic repertoire ranges from 6 to 8 syllables, Germanic languages have over 16 syllable types. This conception of rhythm relates to Dauer (1983) and also Nespor (1990) who claim that linguistic rhythm is a side effect of the syllabic repertoire that languages instantiate. Languages such as Japanese have a very restricted syllable repertoire, and thus a relatively high proportion of utterances is taken up by vowels. In contrast, languages with a large number of syllable types, thus many consonant clusters, tend to have a smaller proportion of utterances taken up by vowels. Interestingly, one could conclude that after a larger number of languages is included in Figure 8.2, it might turn out that some more classes or even a continuum is obtained rather than the clustering of languages into the few classes that we now observe. However, if the notion of rhythm is really related to the claim according to which the number of syllable types is what gives rise to the intuitive notion of linguistic rhythm, things will go in favor of a clustering. Indeed, the syllable repertoires come in groups. Up until now, we have languages that have 2 or 3 syllable types (Hawaiian, Japanese, etc.), 6 to 10 syllable types (Spanish, Greek, Italian, etc.) and languages that have 16 or more (English, Dutch, etc.) (see Nespor, 1990). Future scrutiny with a larger set of languages will determine whether the notion that languages fall into a restricted number of classes is born out or not; and if so, how many classes there are.

We are willing to defend the conjecture that languages cluster into a few classes, because rhythm, as defined by Ramus *et al.* (1999), is sufficient to explain the available behavioral results. Indeed, Ramus *et al.* (1999) simulated the ability to discriminate switches from one language to another in infants and adults. He showed that %V is sufficient to account for all the empirical findings involving neonates. This outcome sustains our resolve to pursue this line of investigation. Indeed, it is unlikely that linguistic rhythm would play such an important role in determining the neonate's behavior without having any further influence on how language is learned.

The first adjustment the neonate makes to the surrounding language concerns rhythm. The processing of linguistic rhythm appears to change over the first 2 months of life. Mehler *et al.* (1988) remarked that while American 2-month-olds fail to discriminate Russian from French, 1-week-old French infants successfully discriminate not only Russian from French but also English from Italian. The authors argued that by 2 months of age infants have encoded some properties of their native language and stop discriminating between two unfamiliar rhythms. Such a bias may explain the observed failure to discriminate a switch between two "unknown" languages. Christophe and Morton (1998) further investigated this same issue testing 2-month-old British infants. They found that the infants were able to discriminate a switch between English and Japanese but not a switch between French and Japanese. Presumably, the former pair of languages is discriminated because it entails one familiar and one novel rhythm. The second switch yields no response because neither language has a familiar rhythm. To buttress their interpretation, Christophe and Morton (1998) also tested the behavior of these same British infants with Dutch. First, they corroborated their prediction that these infants would fail to discriminate Dutch from English, because the two languages have a similar rhythm. Next, they showed that the infants discriminate Dutch from Japanese, two foreign languages for these infants. In fact, while Dutch differs from English, their rhythm is similar, and thus, although Dutch is not their native language it still catches the infants' attention.

Pure behavioral research may be insufficient to ground the above explanations. We hope, however, that adequate brain-imaging methods, used as indicators of processing, could provide more information to decide whether learning and development of language requires a passage through an attention-drawing device based on rhythm.

Why are infants interested in rhythm even before the segments of the utterances capture their curiosity?[7] What information does linguistic rhythm provide to render it so relevant for language acquisition? We have followed two procedures to answer these questions. First, we have tried to gather data using optical topography (see above pp. 214–217), to pursue the exploration of language processing in the neonate, as described above. Second, we have explored the potential role of rhythm in other areas of language acquisition. Specifically, we asked whether rhythm may play a role in the setting of syntactic parameters, and also whether it might be exploited in segmentation, as described in the following sections.

8.5   Segmenting the speech stream

Ramus *et al.* (1999) (see Section 3.4) conjectured that language rhythm provides the infant information about the richness of the syllabic repertoire of the language (cf. Dauer, 1983; Nespor, 1990).

For the sake of the argument, we assume that the infant gains this type of information from the rhythmic properties in the signal. What would then be the use of such information for the language-learning infant? What profit does the baby draw by knowing that the number of syllable types is 4, 6, or 16? Will such information facilitate perception of speech? Or will such information be essential to master the production routines or elementary speech acts? We cannot answer these questions in detail. However, there is yet no reason to believe that knowing the size of the syllabic repertoire facilitates perception of speech. Is there evidence that a learner performs better when he/she has prior knowledge of the number of types or items in the set to be learned? We can give an indirect answer by looking at lexical acquisition. Surely, infants learn the lexicon without ever knowing or caring whether they have to master 4000 or 40 000 words. Why would knowledge of the number of syllable types be useful compared to learning the syllables in the language much as one learns words? There is no ready answer to this question, which does not mean that in the future an answer will not be forthcoming. However, there is an explanation for the infant's precocious interest in rhythm. Rhythmic information may constrain lexical acquisition. Indeed, the size of the syllabic repertoire is inversely correlated with the mean length of words. Hence, gaining information about rhythm may provide through an indirect route a bias as to the average size of the lexical items in the language of exposure (Mehler & Nespor, 2004).

When listening to connected speech, the baby has to break up the input into constituent-like words. However, it is well known that speech signals do not afford reliable acoustic cues about the beginning and the end of words. The most naïve psycholinguistic explanation of parsing is to postulate that there are gaps between words but in fact there are none. Prosodic cues may signal the end of a word that is found at the right edge of larger constituents, such as phonological phrases or intonational phrases, but not every word of the speech stream. In fact, even when gaps are found, they are as likely to fall within words as between words, for example because the release of a voiceless stop is preceded by a constriction that very much looks like a pause.

How can rhythm help segmenting the continuous speech stream? Mehler and Nespor (2004) have proposed that infants who listen to a language with a %V that is higher than 50%, like in "mora-timed" languages, will tend to parse signals looking for long constituents while infants who listen to a language whose %V is below 40% will tend to search for far shorter units (see p. 00 for details). This follows from the fact that the syllabic repertoire in, for example, Japanese is very limited,[8] which entails that monosyllables will be rare and long words will be very frequent, unless speakers are willing to put up with polysemy to such an extent as to threaten communication. However, languages are designed to favor rather than to hinder communication. Hence, words turn out to be long in Japanese as well as in any other language with a restricted syllabic repertoire. In contrast, languages such as Dutch or English, which have a very rich syllabic repertoire (%V close to 45%), allow for a large number of different syllables; hence, without increasing ambiguity one can imagine that among the first 1000 words in the language many will be monosyllables (nearly 600 out of 1000). Languages like Italian, Spanish, or Catalan, whose %V lies between that of Japanese and that of English, also have an intermediate number of syllable types. As expected, the length of the most common words falls between two and three syllables.

Assuming that rhythmic properties are important during language acquisition and, furthermore, that very young infants extract the characteristic rhythm of the language of exposure, it would be nice to know the computational processes that allow such an extraction to take place. Unfortunately, at this time, we have no concrete results that would allow us to explain how these computations are performed. Hopefully, future studies will clarify whether the auditory system is organized to extract rapidly and efficiently the rhythmic properties of stream of speech, and/or whether we are born to be powerful statistical machines so that small differences in rhythm between classes of languages can be ascertained. Independent of how the properties that characterize the rhythmic classes are identified, our conjecture is that the trigger that biases the infant to expect words of a certain length is determined by rhythm. Once rhythm has set or fixed this bias, one may find that infants segment speech, relying on other mechanisms. For example, the statistical computations that Saffran and her colleagues have invoked (see below) may be an excellent tool to segment streams of speech into constituents. However, it is possible that the rhythm in the stream will bias the learner to go for longer or shorter items depending on the language they are learning.

Saffran *et al.* (1996) and Morgan and Saffran (1995) have revived the view that statistical information plays a central role in language acquisition. Indeed, information theorists (Miller, 1951) had already postulated that the statistical properties of language could help process signals and acquire parts of language. Connectionism has also highlighted the importance of statistics for language learning. They have even gone as far as viewing the language learner as a powerful statistic machine. Without going as far as those investigators have gone, we recognize that the advantage of statistics is that it can be universally applied to unknown languages, and thus pre-linguistic infants may also exploit it.

Saffran *et al.* (1996) have shown that adults and 9-month-old infants confronted with unfamiliar monotonous artificial speech streams tend to infer word boundaries through the statistical regularities in the signal. A word boundary is postulated in positions where the transitional probability (hereafter TP) drops between one syllable and the next.[9] Participants familiarized with a monotonic stream of artificial speech recognize tri-syllabic items delimited by dips in TP. As an example, imagine that *puliko* and *meluti* are items with high TPs between the constituent syllables. If Ss are asked which of *puliko* or *likome* (where *liko* are the last two syllables of the first word and *me* the first syllable of the second word) is more familiar, they tend to select the first well above chance. Among a large number of investigations that have validated Saffran *et al.*'s findings, we have found that, by and large, French and Italian adult speakers perform as the English speakers of the original experiment.[10]

Let us summarize what we have tried to suggest this far. We have noticed that linguistic rhythm can be captured as suggested by Ramus *et al.* (1999) by measuring the amount of time/utterance occupied by vowels and by the variability of the intervocalic intervals. This proposal presupposes that our processing system makes a categorical distinction between consonants and vowels. In the following section, we expand on the notion that there is a basic categorical distinction between Vs and Cs, and we go on to propose a view of language acquisition based on the consequences of this divide.

8.6   Rhythm, signals, and triggers

Developmental psycholinguists and students of adult language perception and production considered the possibility that different phonological units are highlighted depending on the rhythmic class to which a language belongs, as described above. More recently, linguists and psycholinguists started exploring whether the different phrasal phonological properties related to syntax can guide the infant in the setting of parameters that are essential to acquire language. We are presently exploring to what extent linguistic rhythm can help the learner discover some of the nonuniversal properties of syntax. It is in this research area that the investigation of the syntax–prosody interaction might offer a link between an exclusively syntactic approach to PS and the cognitive neuroscience approach, which concentrates on the perception and production of speech.

The acquisition of some aspects of language is facilitated by the statistical properties encoded in the speech signal (see p. 224). For most classical association accounts of acquisition, the more a property is transparently encoded in the signal, the easier it will be to learn, regardless of the domain - including language. Such theories assume that the signals are rich enough to inscribe structure in the head of the learner. No innate knowledge is postulated over and beyond the ability to associate signals. In contrast to classical learning, linguists have argued that in order to learn to speak a language one must learn grammar. For this to happen, they argue, innate knowledge has to be postulated because general learning mechanisms are not sufficient to allow the infant to acquire grammar directly from the signal. The nature of this knowledge is roughly spelled out in the PS theory. We believe that this is the richest account of language acquisition we are aware of because it relates universal principles to aspects of grammar that are language specific. As we stated before, this theory might be correct or not. However, it is the only theory that can be explored in sufficient detail as to allow its dismissal if it does not mesh well with observation.

Our proposal is to integrate PS with a general theory of learning. While it is commonly taken for granted that general learning mechanisms play a role in the acquisition of the lexicon (Bloom, 2000), their role in the actual setting of the parameters has not been sufficiently explored. In fact, while signals might give a cue to the value of a certain parameter, general learning mechanisms might play a role in establishing the validity of such a cue for the language of exposure. For instance, in order to decide whether in a language complements precede or follow their head, it is necessary to establish whether the main prominence of its phonological phrases is rightmost or leftmost, as we will see below. Within a language, syntactic phrases, by and large, are of one type or another: that is they are either Head–Complement (HC) or Complement–Head (CH). There are languages, however, in which a specific phrase might have a word order different from the standard word order of the language. Since the pre-lexical infant ignores whether this exception weakens the relation of prominence with the underlying parameter, it needs a mechanism to cope with the presence of this confusing information. In all likelihood, statistical computations allow the infant to discover and validate the most frequent phonological pattern that can then be used as a cue to the underlying syntax (see Nespor *et al.*, 1996). Even if such exceptional patterns did not exist in a language, the need for statistics remains plausible. Indeed, even an infant that is exposed to a regular language (as to the HC order) might occasionally hear irregular patterns, for example foreign locutions or speech errors. In this case, the frequency distribution difference between the occasional and the habitual patterns will allow the infant to converge to the adequate setting.

Let us focus in more detail on the case of the HC parameter. This is a central parameter for learning the syntax of one's language. Indeed, in the great majority of languages, the setting of this parameter simultaneously specifies the relative order of heads and complements and of main clauses with respect to subordinate clauses. That children start the two-word stage without making mistakes in the word order suggests that this parameter is set precociously (see Bloom, 1970; and also Meisel, 1992). In addition, before that, they react differently to the appropriate, as compared to the wrong, word order (Hirsh-Pasek & Golinkoff, 1996). These facts suggest that children must set this parameter quite early in life.

Given our viewpoint, it would be quite desirable to imagine a scenario in which the infant finds ways and means to set basic parameters prior or at least independently of the segmentation of the speech stream into words. If the child sets parameters before learning the meaning of words, prosodic bootstrapping would become immune to the paradox pointed out by Mazuka (1996). She observes that to understand the word order of, say, heads and complements in the language of exposure, an infant must first recognize which is the head and which is the complement. But once the infant has learned to recognize in a pair of words which one functions as head and which as complement, it already knows how they are ordered. If you know how they are ordered, the parameter becomes pointless. Without syntactic knowledge, word meaning cannot be learned and without meaning, syntax cannot be acquired either.

How can a child overcome this quandary and get information about word order just by listening to the signal? What is there in the speech stream that might give a cue to the value of this parameter? Rhythm, in language as in music, is hierarchical in nature (see Liberman & Prince, 1977; Selkirk, 1984). We have seen above that at the basic level, rhythm can be defined on the basis of %V and ΔC. At higher levels, the relative prominence of certain syllables (or the vowels that form their nucleus) with respect to other syllables reflects some aspects of syntax. In particular, in the phonological phrase,[11] rightmost main prominence is characteristic of head–complement languages, like English, Italian, or Croatian while leftmost main prominence characterizes complement–head languages, like Turkish, Japanese, or Basque (Nespor & Vogel, 1986). A speech stream is thus an alternation of words in either weak–strong or strong-weak chunks. Suppose that this correlation between the location of main prominence within phonological phrases and the value of the HC parameter is indeed universal. Then we can assume that by hearing either a weak–strong or a strong–weak pattern, an infant becomes biased to set the parameter to the correct value for the language of exposure. The advantage of such a direct connection between signal and syntax (see Morgan & Demuth, 1996) is that the only prerequisite is that infants hear the relevant alternation. To see whether this is the case, Christophe *et al.* (1997) and Christophe *et al.* (2003) carried out a discrimination task using resynthetized utterances drawn from French and Turkish sentences. These languages have similar syllabic structures and word final stress but they differ in the locus of the main prominence in the phonological phrase, an aspect that is crucial for us.[12] The experiment used delexicalized sentences pronounced by the same voice.[13] Infants 6- to 12-weeks-old discriminate French from Turkish. It is concluded that infants discriminate the two languages only on the basis of the different location of the main prominence. Knowing that infants discriminate these two types of rhythmic patterns opens a new direction of research to assess whether infants actually use this information to set the relevant syntactic parameter.

8.7 The C/V distinction and language acquisition

Why does language need to have both vowels and consonants? According to Plato, rhythm is "order in movement." But why, at one level of the rhythmic architecture, is the order established by the alternation of vowels and consonants? Why do all languages have both Cs and Vs? Possibly, as phoneticians and acousticians argue (see Stevens, 2000), this design structure has functional properties that are essential for communication. Indeed, vowels have considerable energy, allowing them to carry the signal, while consonants are modulations that allow increasing the number of messages with different meaning that can be transmitted. Even if one believes that this explanation is correct, it may not be the only one of the reasons why languages necessarily include both vowels and consonants.

Nespor *et al.* (2003) has proposed that vowels and consonants, because of their different phonetic and phonological properties, play a different functional role in language acquisition and language perception. The main role of consonants is to be intimately involved with lexical structure, while that of vowels is to be linked to grammatical structures.

The lexicon allows the identification of thousands of lemmas, while grammar organizes the lexical items in a regular system. There is abundant evidence that consonants are more distinctive than vowels. For instance, cross-linguistically there is a clear tendency for Cs to outnumber Vs: the segmental system most frequent in the languages of the world has 5 vowels and around 20 consonants. But languages with just 3 vowels are also attested and historical linguists working on common ancestors of different languages have posited two or even one vowel for proto-Indo-European.

A widespread phenomenon in the languages of the world is to reduce vowels in unstressed positions. Languages like English, in which unstressed vowels are centralized to schwa, thereby losing their distinctive power, represent an extreme case. No comparable phenomenon affects consonants. The pronunciation of Cs is also less variable (thus more distinctive) than that of Vs. Prosody is responsible for the variability of vowels within a system: both rhythmic and intonational information (be it grammatical or emotional) is by and large carried by vowels. Acoustic-phonetic studies have documented that while the production of vowels is rather variable, consonants are more stable. Moreover, experimental studies have shown that while consonants are perceived categorically, vowels are not (Kuhl *et al.*, 1992; Werker *et al.*, 1984). These different reasons for the variability of vowels, of course, make them less distinctive. Evidence for the distinctive role of consonants is also attested by the existence of languages (e.g., Semitic languages) in which lexical roots are composed uniquely by consonants. To the best of our knowledge, there is no language in which lexical roots are composed just of vowels.

The above noted asymmetry between Vs and Cs in linguistic systems is reflected in language acquisition. The first adjustments infants make to the maternal language are related to vowels rather than to consonants. Indeed, several pieces of evidence can be advanced to buttress this assertion. In a study, Bertoncini *et al.* (1988) showed that very young infants presented with four syllables in random order during familiarization react when a new syllable is introduced, provided that it differs from the others by at least its vowel. If the new syllable differs from the other syllables only by the consonant, its addition will be neglected.[14] However, 2-month-olds show a response to both, that is whether one adds a syllable that differs from a member of the habituation set by its vowel or by its consonant. We must remember, however, that the above results are not due to limitations in discrimination ability but rather to the way in which the stimuli are represented.[15] We can conclude that the first representation privileges vowels but that by 2 months of age vowels and consonants are sufficiently well encoded as to yield a similar phonological representation. In fact, by 6 months of age infants respond preferentially to the vowels of their native language.[17] In contrast, Werker and her colleagues have shown that consonant contrasts that are discriminated before 8 months are neglected a few months later if they are not used in the maternal language (Werker & Tees, 1984); that is, when the infant goes from phonetic to phonological representations, vowels seem to be adjusted to the native values before consonants. This observation is yet another indication that vowels and consonants are categorically distinct from the onset of language acquisition. Our suggestion is that these two categories have a different function in language and in its acquisition.

As we mentioned above (see p. 227), vowels and consonants, even when they are equally informative from a statistical point of view, are not exploited in similar ways. Newport & Aslin (2004) used a stream of synthetic speech consisting of CV syllables of equal pitch and duration in which the vowels change constantly and "words" are characterized only by high TPs between the consonants. Participants successfully segment such a stream.[18] We replicated this robust finding with Italian and French-speaking subjects (Bonatti et al., 2005). In a similar experiment in which the statistical dependences were carried by vowels while the intervening consonants vary, the participant in our experiment failed to segment the stream into constituent "words." Thus, a pre-lexical infant (or an adult listening to an unknown language) identifies word candidates on the basis of TP dips between either syllables or consonants, but not between vowels. However, see FN ... Why should this be so? As pointed out above, consonants change little when the word is pronounced in different emotional or emphatic contexts while vowels change a lot. Moreover, a great number of languages introduce changes in the vowels that compose a group of morphologically related words, that is *foot–feet* in English, and more conspicuously, in Arabic: *kitab* "book," *kutub* "books," *akteb* "to write." In brief, consonants rather than vowels are mainly geared to insure lexical functions. Vowels, however, have an important role when one attempts to establish grammatical properties. We argued above that the rhythmic class of the first language of exposure is identified on the basis of the proportion of time taken up by vowels. Identifying the rhythm, we argued, provides information about the syllable repertoires, that is a part of the phonology. Moreover, it gives information about the mean length of words in the language. Also, a piece of information carried by vowels relates to the location of the main prominence within the phonological phrase. As was argued above, prominence is related to a basic syntactic parameter.

8.8   Conclusion

In this chapter, we have argued that both innate linguistic structure and general learning mechanisms are essential to our understanding of the acquisition of natural language. Linguists have paid a lot of attention to universal principles or constraints that delimit the nature of our endowment for language. Psychologists, in contrast, have focused on how the child acquires the language of exposure, without being concerned with the biological underpinnings of this achievement. After scrutinizing the limitations of both positions, we have pleaded for an integration of the two approaches to the study of language acquisition. Currently, there is a growing consensus that biologically realistic models have to be elaborated in order to begin understanding the uniqueness of the human mind and in particular of language.

In our research, we have highlighted the importance of exploring how signals relate to the fixation of parameters. We have tried to demonstrate that signals often contain information that is related to unsuspected properties of the computational system. We laid out a proposal of how rhythm can guide the learner toward the basic properties of the language's phonology and syntax. We have also argued that basic phonological categories, namely vowels and consonants, play different computational roles during language acquisition. These categories play distinctive roles across languages and appear to be sufficiently general for us to conjecture that they are a part of the species' endowment.

Another aspect that we highlighted concerns the attested acoustic capacity of vertebrates to discriminate and learn phonetic distinctions (see Kluender *et al.* 1998; Ramus *et al.*, 2000, etc.). They also have the ability to extract and use the statistical properties of the stimulating sequences in order to analyze and parse them into constituents (M. Hauser, personal communication). These results suggest that humans and other higher vertebrates can process signals much in the same way. However, the fact remains that only humans, and no other animals, acquire the language spoken in the surrounds. Moreover, simple exposure is all that is needed for the learning process to be activated. Thus, we must search for the prerequisites of language acquisition in the knowledge inscribed in our endowment.

The fact that cues contained in the speech stream directly signal nonuniversal syntactic properties of language makes it clear that to understand how the infant attains knowledge of syntax precociously and in an effortless fashion, attention must be paid to the very cues that the signals provide. How can this argument be sustained when we have just acknowledged that human and nonhuman vertebrates process acoustic signals in a similar fashion? Because, a theory of language acquisition requires not only an understanding of signal processing abilities but also of how these cues affect the innate linguistic endowment. The nature of the language endowment, once precisely established, will guide us toward an understanding of the biological foundation of language, and thus will clarify why we diverge so significantly from other primates. This in turn will hopefully lead us to formulate a testable hypothesis about the origin and evolution of natural language.

Notes

1. To illustrate this, consider a child who hears mostly sentences with a Verb–Object order. The child, putatively, obtains automatically information from the linguistic input to set the relevant word-order parameter. If this were so, it would constitute a great asset, since fixing the word-order parameter may greatly facilitate the acquisition of grammar and also the acquisition of the lexicon. Likewise, the child exposed to a language that can have sentences without an overt subject, for example Italian ("piove," "mangiano arance," etc.), or to a language whose sentences require overt mention of subjects, for example English ("it rains," "they eat oranges"), supposedly gets information from the linguistic input to set the relevant parameter.

2. See Hebb, D. O. (1949). *Organization of Behavior*. New York: Wiley.

3. To establish that the FFA is an area that is specifically triggered by faces, Kanwisher and also others had to test many other stimuli and conditions. Even so, Gauthier and her collaborators have challenged the existence of the FFA showing that this area is also activated by other sets whose members belong to a categorized ensemble even though they are not faces. Moreover, Gauthier and her colleagues showed that when Ss learn a new set before the experiments, its members then activate the FFA activation. Gauthier argued that her studies show that the FFA is not uniquely a structure devoted to face processing. Without denying the validity of Gauthier's results, Kanwisher still thinks that the FFA is a *bona fide* face area. We think that although we understand much better the FFA than the Belin's voice, we still have to be very careful before we accept the proposed locus as a voice-specific area. A fortiori we need equal parsimony before we admit that we do have a specific voice-processing area. Future research will clarify this issue.

4. This device uses near-infrared light to evaluate how many photons are absorbed in a part of the brain following stimulation. The device is light and non-invasive. In this sense, it is comparable to most Evoked Response Potential devices currently in use. The difference is that like fMRI it estimates the vascular response in a given area of the cortex. Another difference is that like fMRI its time resolution is poorer than that of ERP. Our device uses bundles of fiber optics that are applied to the infants' head. These light bundles contain a fiber that delivers near-infrared light of two wavelengths. The other fiber, which is placed 3 cm away from the irradiating one, is a light-collector fiber. One of the wavelengths is absorbed by oxyHb while the other is absorbed by deoxyHb. When one measures the changes in emerging light for each wavelength, it is possible to estimate precisely the functional organization of the underlying cortical areas.

5. A universal property of syllables is that they have an obligatory *nucleus* optionally preceded by an *onset* and followed by a *coda*. While onset and coda are occupied by consonants (C), the nucleus is generally occupied by a vowel (V). In some languages, the nucleus can be occupied by a sonorant consonant (as [m], [n],

[l], and [r], in particular [r]). Thus, a syllable may not contain more than one vowel. CV is the optimal syllable, that is the onset tends to be present and the coda absent. All natural languages have CV syllables. There is a hierarchy of increasing complexity in the inclusion of syllable types in a given language. Thus, a language that has V will also have CV, but not vice versa. A language that has V, instead, does not necessarily have VC. That is, in some languages all syllables end in a vowel. Similarly, a language that has CVC will also have a CV in its repertoire. A language that includes a CCV in its repertoire will have CV and a language that includes CVCC also has CVC. The prediction then is that while CVC is a well-formed potential syllable in many languages, CCC is not, in particular if none of the consonants is sonorant.

6. Or geminates as in the word *Sapporo*.

7. Werker and Tees (1983) were the first to point out that the first adjustment to the segmental repertoire of the language of exposure becomes apparent at the end of the first year of life.

8. Syllable types in Japanese are CV and V. Coda consonants are limited to be either an [N] or a geminate consonant shared with the following syllable.

9. Saffran, *et al.* use streams that consist of artificial CV syllables that are assembled without leaving a pause between one another. All syllables have the same duration, loudness, and pitch. TPs between adjacent syllables (in any trisyllable) range from 0.25 to 1.00. The last syllable of an item and the first syllable of the next one have TPs ranging from 0.05 to 0.60.

10. One divergence between the results reported by the Rochester group and our own concerns the computation of TPs on the consonantal and vocalic tiers. Apparently, native English speakers can use both tiers to calculate TPs (see Section 8.7). Our own Ss, regardless of whether they are native French or native Italian speakers, can only use the consonantal tier, see p. 27 for more details.

11. The phonological phrase is a constituent of the phonological hierarchy that includes the head of a phrase and all its function words. It also includes some complements and modifiers under specific syntactic conditions as well as conditions concerned with weight (Nespor & Vogel, 1986).

12. The effect of the resynthesis is that all segmental differences are eliminated.

13. Sentences were synthetized using Dutch diphones with the same voice.

14. Two kinds of habituation were used, [bi], [si], [li], and [mi] or [bo], [bae], [ba], and [bo]. The introduction of [bu] causes the neonate to react to the modification regardless of the habituation. The introduction of [di] after the neonate is habituated with the first set of syllables neglected and so is the introduction of [da] after habituation with the second set.

15. In discrimination experiments, one evaluates whether infants react when a repeated syllable suddenly changes. In the present study, one evaluates whether the infant reacts when a set of four repeated syllables suddenly includes a novel syllable. In this case, one tests the details with which the initial set of syllables was represented

rather than a simple discrimination.

16. American infants respond preferentially to American vowels as compared to Swedish vowels while Swedish infants respond preferentially to Swedish vowels compared with English ones (see Kuhl, P. K., Williams, K. A., et al., 1992. Linguistic experience alters phonetic perception in infants by 6 months of age. *Science*, **255**, 606–8).

17. Thus, if a word has the syllables C-, and C'-, C'' with the consonants that predict the next one exactly, regardless of the vowels that appear between them, it will be preferred to a part word like C''-, C*-, and C**, where the stars illustrate that the two last syllables come from another "word." Of course, words have no probability dip between the consonants but part words enclose a TP dip between C'' and C*.

References

Abercrombie, D. (1967). *Elements of General Phonetics*. Chicago: Aldine.

Belin, P., Zatorre, R. J., Lafaille, P., Ahad, P., Pike, B. (2000). Voice-selective areas in human auditory cortex. *Nature*, **403**(20 January), 309–12.

Bertelson, P. (1982). Lateral differences in normal man and lateralization of brain function. *International Journal of Psychology*, **17**, 173–210.

Bertoncini, J. (1981). Syllables as units in infant speech perception. *Mehler, Journal of Infant Behavior and Development*, **4**, 247–60.

Bertoncini, J., Bijeljac-Babic, R., Jusczyk, P. W., Kennedy, L. J. and Mehler, J. (1988). An investigation of young infants' perceptual representations of speech sounds. *Journal of Experimental Psychology: General*, **117**, 21–33.

Bertoncini, J., Morais, J., Bijeljac-Babic, R., McAdams, S., Peretz, I. and Mehler, J. (1989). Dichotic perception and laterality in neonates. *Brain and Cognition*, **37**, 591–605.

Best, C. T., Hoffman, H. and Glanville, B. B. (1982). Development of infant ear asymmetries for speech and music. *Perception and Psychophysics*, **31**, 75–85.

Bijeljac-Babic, R., Bertoncini, J. and Mehler, J. (1993). How do four-day-old infants categorize multisyllabic utterances? *Developmental Psychology*, **29**, 711–21.

Bloom, L. (1970). *Language Development: Form and Function in Emerging Grammars*. Cambridge, MA: MIT Press.

Bloom, P. (2000). *How Children Learn the Meanings of Words*. Cambridge, MA: MIT Press.

Bonatti, L. L., Peña, M., Nespor, M. and Mehler, J. (2005). Linguistic constraints on statistical computations: the role of consonants and vowels in continuous speech processing. *Psychological Science*, **16**, 451–9.

Bryden, M. P. and Allard, F. A. (1981). Do auditory perceptual asymmetries develop? *Cortex*, **17**, 313–18.

Chomsky, N. (1959). A review of B. F. Skinner's Verbal Behavior. *Language*, **35**, 26–58.

Chomsky, N. (1980). *Rules and Representations*. New York: Columbia University Press.

Chomsky, N. (1986). *Knowledge of Language*. New York: Praeger.

Christophe, A., Guasti, M. T., Nespor, M., Dupoux, E. and van Ooyen, B. (1997). Reflections on prosodic boot strapping: its role for lexical and syntactic acquisition. *Language and Cognitive Processes*, **12**, 585–612.

Christophe, A. and Morton, J. (1998). Is Dutch native English? Linguistic analysis by 2-month-olds. *Developmental Science*, **1**(2), 215–19.

Christophe, A., Guasti, M. T., Nespor, M. and van Ooyen, B. (2003). Prosodic structure and syntactic acquisition: the case of the head-complement parameter. *Developmental Science*, **6**, 213–22.

Colombo, J. and Bundy, R. S. (1983). Infant response to auditory familiarity and novelty. *Infant Behavior and Development*, **6**, 305–11.

Cutler, A. (1994). Segmentation problems, rhythmic solutions. *Lingua*, **92**, 81–104.

Cutler, A., Mehler, J., Norris, D. and Segui, J. (1983). A language specific comprehension strategy. *Nature*, **304**, 159–60.

Dauer, R. M. (1983). Stress-timing and syllable-timing reanalyzed. *Journal of Phonetics*, **11**, 51–62. Le coup de grâce porté à la théorie de l'isochronie des intervalles inter-stress, et la mise en évidence d'une base phonétique et phonologique pour la sensation de rythme syllabique ou à stress.

Dehaene-Lambertz, G. and Dehaene, S. (1994). Speed and cerebral correlates of syllable discrimination in infants. *Nature*, **370**, 292–5.

Dronkers, N. F. (1996). A new brain region for coordinating speech articulation. *Nature*, **384**(14 November), 159–61.

Fodor, J. (1975). *The Modularity of Mind*. Cambridge, MA: MIT Press.

Geschwind, N. (1970). The organization of language and the brain. *Science*, **170**, 940–4.

Hebb, D. O. (1949). *Organization of Behavior*. New York: Wiley.

Hirsh-Pasek, K. and Golinkoff, R. M. (1996). *The Origins of Grammar: Evidence From Early Language Comprehension*. Cambridge, MA: MIT Press.

Jusczyk, P. W. (1997). *The Discovery of Spoken Language Recognition*. Cambridge, MA: MIT Press.

Jusczyk, P. W., Rosner, B. S., Cutting, J. E., Foard, F. and Smith, L. B. (1977). Categorical perception of non-speech sounds by two-month old infants. *Perception and Psychophysics*, **21**, 50–4.

Kanwisher, N., McDermott, J. and Chun, M. M. (1997). The fusiform face area: a module in human extrastriate cortex specialized for face perception. *Journal of Neuroscience*, **17**(11), 4302–11.

Kluender, K. L., Lotto, A. J., Holt, L. L. and Bloedel, S. L. (1998). Role of experience for language-specific functional mapping of vowel sounds. *The Journal of the Acoustical Society of America*, **104**(6), 3568–82.

Kuhl, P. (1987). The special-mechanisms debate in speech research: categorization tests on animal and infants. In S. Harnad, ed., *Categorical Perception: The Groundwork of Cognition*. Cambridge: Cambridge University Press, 355–86.

Kuhl, P. K. and Miller, J. D. (1975). Speech perception by the chinchilla: voiced-voiceless distinction in alveolar plosive consonants. *Science*, **190**, 69–72.

Kuhl, P. K., Williams, K. A., Lacerda, F., Stevens, K. N. and Lindblom, B. (1992). Linguistic experience alters phonetic perception in infants by 6 months of age. *Science*, **255**, 606–8.

Ladefoged, P. (1975). *A Course in Phonetics*. New York: Harcourt Brace Jovanovich.

Lenneberg, E. (1967). *Biological Foundation of Language*. New York, NY: Wiley.

Levelt, W. J. M. (1989). *Speaking: From Intention to Articulation*. Cambridge, MA: MIT Press.

Liberman, A. M. and Mattingly, I. G. (1985). The motor theory of speech revised. *Cognition*, **21**, 1–36.

Liberman, M. and Prince, A. (1977). On stress and linguistic rhythm. *Linguistic Inquiry*, **8**, 240–336.

MacWhinney, B. (1987). *Mechanisms of Language Acquisition*. Hillsdale, NJ: Erlbaum.

Manrique, A. M. B. D. and Signorini, A. (1983). Segmental durations and rhythm in Spanish. *Journal of Phonetics*, **11**, 117–28.

Mazuka, R. (1996). How can a grammatical parameter be set before the first word? In J. L. Morgan and K. Demuth, eds., *Signal to Syntax: Bootstrapping from Speech to Grammar in Early Acquisition*. Mahwah, NJ: Lawrence Erlbaum Associates, pp. 313–30.

Mehler, J. (1981). The role of syllables in speech processing: infant & adult data. *Philosophical Transactions of the Royal Society*, **B295**, 333–52.

Mehler, J. and Dupoux, E. (1994). *What Infants Know*. Cambridge, MA: Blackwell.

Mehler, J. and Nespor, M. (2004). Linguistic rhythm and the development of language. In A. Belletti (ed.) *Structures and Beyond. The Carthography of Syntactic Structures*. Vol. 3. Oxford: Oxford University Press, pp. 213–22.

Mehler, J., Jusczyk, P., Lambertz, G., Halsted, N., Bertoncini, J. and Amiel-Tison, C. (1988). A precursor of language acquisition in young infants. *Cognition*, **29**, 143–78.

Meisel, J. M., (ed.) (1992). *The Acquisition of Verb Placement. Functional Categories and V2 Phenomena in Language Acquisition*. Dordrecht: Kluwer Academic Press.

Miller, G. A. (1951). *Language and Communication*. New York: McGraw-Hill Book Company Inc.

Molfese, D. L. and Molfese, V. J. (1979). Hemisphere and stimulus differences as reflected in the cortical response of newborn infants to speech stimuli. *Developmental Psychology*, **15**, 501–11.

Moon, C., Cooper, R. P. and Fifer, W. P. (1993). Two-day-olds prefer their native language. *Infant Behavior and Development*, **16**, 495–500.

Morgan, J. L. and Demuth, K. (1996a). Signal to Syntax: an overview. In J. L. Morgan and K. Demuth, eds., *Signal to Syntax: Bootstrapping from Speech to Grammar in Early Acquisition*. Mahwah, NJ: Lawrence Erlbaum Associates, pp. 1–22.

Morgan, J. L. and Demuth, K. (1996b). *Signal to Syntax: Bootstrapping from Speech to Grammar in Early Acquisition*. Mahwah, NJ: Lawrence Erlbaum Associates.

Morgan, J. L., Meier, R. P. and Newport, E. L. (1987). Structural packaging in the input to language learning: contributions of prosodic and morphological marking of phrases to the acquisition of language. *Cognitive Psychology*, **19**, 498–550.

Morgan, J. L. and Saffran, J. R. (1995). Emerging integration of sequential and suprasegmental information in preverbal speech segmentation. *Child Development*, **66**, 911–36.

Nazzi, T., Bertoncini, J. and Mehler, J. (1998). Language discrimination by newborns: towards an understanding of the role of rhythm. *Journal of Experimental Psychology: Human Perception and Performance*, **24**(3), 756–66.

Nespor, M. (1990). On the rhythm parameter in phonology. In I. M. Roca, ed., *Logical Issues in Language Acquisition*. Dordrecht: Foris, pp. 157–75.

Nespor, M., Guasti, M. T. and Christophe, A. (1996). Selecting word order: the Rhythmic Activation Principle. In U. Kleinhenz, ed., *Interfaces in Phonology*. Berlin: Akademie Verlag, pp. 1–26.

Nespor, M., Mehler, J., and Peña, M. (2003). On the different role of vowels and consonants in language processing and language acquisition. *Lingue e Linguaggio*, 221–47.

Nespor, M. and Vogel, I. (1986). *Prosodic Phonology*, Dordrecht: Foris.

Newport, E. L. and Aslin, R. N. (2004). Learning at a distance I. Statistical learning of non-adjacent dependencies. *Cognitive Psychology*, **48**, 127–62.

Peña, M., Maki, A., Kovacic, D., Dehaene-Lambertz, G., Koizumi, H., Bouquet, F. and Mehler, J. (2003). Sounds and silence: an optical topography study of language recognition at birth. *Proceedings of the National Academy of Sciences USA*, **10**, 11702–5.

Pike, K. L. (1945). *The Intonation of American English*. Ann Arbor, Michigan: University of Michigan Press.

Pinker, S. (1984). *Language Learnability and Language Development*. Cambridge, MA: Harvard University Press.

Port, R. F., Dalby, J. and O'Dell, M. (1987). Evidence for mora-timing in Japanese. *Journal of the Acoustical Society of America*, **81**(5), 1574–85.

Premack, D. (1971). Language in chimpanzee. *Science*, **172**, 808–22.

Premack, D. (1986). *Gavagai!* Cambridge, MA: MIT Press.

Querleu, D., Renard, X., Versyp, F., Paris-Delrue, L. and Creprin, G. (1988). Fetal hearing. *European Journal of Obstetrics and Gynecology and Reproductive Biology*, **29**, 191–212.

Ramus, F., Hauser, M. D., Miller, C., Morris, D. and Mehler, J. (2000). Language discrimination by human newborns and by cotton-top tamarin monkeys. *Science*, **288**, 349–51.

Ramus, F., Nespor, M. and Mehler, J. (1999). Correlates of the linguistic rhythm in the speech signal. *Cognition*, **73**(3), 265–92.

Saffran, J. R., Aslin, R. N. and Newport, E. L. (1996). Statistical learning by 8-month-old infants. *Science*, **274**, 1926–8.

Segalowitz, S. J. and Chapman, J. S. (1980). Cerebral asymmetry for speech in neonates: a behavioral measure. *Brain and Language*, **9**, 281–8.

Seidenberg, M. S. and MacDonald, M. C. (1999). A probabilistic constraint approach to language acquisition and processing. *Cognitive Science*, **23**(4), 569–88.

Selkirk, E. O. (1984). *Phonology and Syntax: The Relation Between Sound and Structure*. Cambridge, MA: MIT Press.

Stevens, K. (2000). *Acoustic Phonetics*. Cambridge, MA: MIT Press.

Tomasello, M. (2000). Do young children have adult syntactic competence? *Cognition*, **74**, 209–53.

Villringer, A. and Chance, B. (1997). Non-invasive optical spectroscopy and imaging of human brain function. *Trends in Neuroscience*, **20**(10), 435–42.

Wanner, E. and Gleitman, L. R. (1982). *Language Acquisition: The State of the Art*. Cambridge, UK: Cambridge University Press.

Werker, J. F. and Tees, R. C. (1983). Developmental changes across childwood in the perception of non-native speech sounds. *Canadian Journal of Psychology*, **37**, 278–86.

Werker, J. F. and Tees, R. C. (1984). Cross-language speech perception: evidence for perceptual reorganisation during the first year of life. *Infant Behavior and Development*, **7**, 49–63.

Wexler, K. and Culicover, P. (1980). *Formal Principles of Language Acquisition*. Cambridge, MA: MIT Press.

PART III   MEMORY SYSTEMS

Introduction to Memory Section

LARRY R. SQUIRE

Memory is a large topic, built on the fundamental idea that the experiences one has can change the nervous system, so that behavior and mental activity can later be different as a result of what came before. Yet, memory is more than a record of personal experience. Humans can learn and then teach what they have learned to others, thereby making it possible to transmit information from one generation to another.

In the twentieth century the study of memory became part of the domains of both biological and psychological science. Work has proceeded at several levels of analysis – from questions about the cellular and molecular events that underlie synaptic change to questions about complex behavior. Between these poles are other important questions, such as what brain systems are important for memory and how they operate to support memory. As we enter the new millennium, biology and psychology have converged on a number of fundamental questions about memory. Is memory one thing or many? If there are different kinds of memory, what are their operating characteristics? Where in the brain do the important events occur? Where is memory stored? What happens at the level of individual cells and synapses?

The modern era of memory research can be said to have begun in 1957 when the effects on memory of medial temporal lobe resection were described in a patient who became known as HM. HM exhibited profound forgetfulness against a background of largely intact intellectual and perceptual functions. This case showed that memory is to some extent a separable cognitive function and that the structures within the medial temporal lobe are important for memory. To identify which structures were important, an animal model of human memory impairment was needed to evaluate the effects on memory of selective damage to medial temporal lobe structures. An animal model of

Topics in Integrative Neuroscience: From Cells to Cognition, ed. James R. Pomerantz. Published by Cambridge University Press. © Cambridge University Press 2008.

human amnesia was first achieved in the monkey in the early 1980s, and systematic experiments with this model eventually identified the anatomical components of the medial temporal lobe memory system: the hippocampus and adjacent perirhinal, entorhinal, and parahippocampal cortices.

Three other important developments also occurred during this period. First, a number of new memory tasks were developed for the rat, and continuing study of memory with these tasks brought the work with rats into substantial agreement with the findings from humans and monkeys. Thus, by the early 1990s it developed that the three major species involved in research on memory systems and behavior appeared to be telling a rather consistent story about how the hippocampus and related structures contribute to memory functions.

A second important development was the emerging evidence for the idea that memory is not a single faculty of the mind but is composed of distinct systems. Although there had been a century of philosophical and psychological discourse about the classification of memory, it was now possible to reach a clearer, more concrete, and ultimately a more accurate account of memory by placing the work within a biological framework. The medial temporal lobe is involved in only declarative memory, which refers to the capacity for conscious recollections about facts and events. Declarative memory is the kind of memory referred to when the word "memory" is used in everyday language. Declarative memory can be contrasted with a collection of nondeclarative, nonconscious learning abilities where performance changes without requiring conscious memory content. Nondeclarative memory thus refers to several different systems important for memory formation and memory storage: classical conditioning of skeletal musculature (cerebellum), conditioning of emotional responses (amygdala), habit learning (neostriatum), and perceptual priming and perceptual learning (neocortex).

A third development was the increasing possibility of studying the cellular and molecular basis of synaptic plasticity and behavioral memory. Work on memory in the invertebrates *Aplysia* and *Drosophila* began in the 1960s and 1970s and has become a major resource. The sea hare *Aplysia* is advantageous because its central nervous system contains only about 20 000 cells. Many of the cells are distinctive and can be identified from animal to animal. The fruit fly Drosophila is advantageous because it has only four pairs of chromosomes. Mutations can be readily produced in single genes, and the animal can be reared by the thousands in the laboratory. The potential for cellular and molecular studies of memory improved dramatically in the early 1990s with the development of techniques for deleting or adding single genes and for studying the effects of these manipulations on behavioral learning and memory. Notably, it became possible to carry out such studies in the mouse using methods that restrict the expression of genes to specific brain regions and that allow gene expression to be turned on and off. These advances inaugurated the modern molecular study of memory in mammals.

Taken together, these three developments mean that it has become possible to approach the multiple memory systems of the mammalian brain as a coherent program of inquiry which bridges from molecules to behavior, from genes to cognition, in many cases similar aspects of memory can be studied in humans, monkeys, rodents, and other mammals. The four chapters in this part capture the promise and excitement of current work on the neuroscience of mammalian memory.

The first chapter ("Memory systems") considers the anatomy of declarative memory, animal models of declarative memory, and the structure and organization of nondeclarative memory. One important theme is that the structures in the medial temporal lobe have only a time-limited role in memory. Thus, the hippocampus and related medial temporal lobe structures are not the permanent repositories of either spatial or nonspatial memories. These conclusions draw on findings from both humans and experimental animals. A second theme is that an elemental form of declarative memory, recognition memory, depends on the integrity of the hippocampus in humans, monkeys, and rodents. The capacity for recognizing previously encountered material as familiar can be construed as depending on the same relational functions that many have proposed are at the heart of declarative memory and hippocampal function. Thus, successful recognition performance requires that a link be made at the time of learning between the to-be-remembered item and its context, or between the item and one's interaction with it.

The second chapter ("A brain system for declarative memory") begins with a historical treatment of how the medial temporal lobe memory system was identified. The chapter then summarizes progress in characterizing the operation of this system, drawing primarily from studies of the rat. Hippocampus-dependent memory is comprised of stored sequences of events and places, and the hippocampus has the capacity to link distinct episodes by their common features. Comparisons between the functions of the hippocampus and the adjacent parahippocampal region, based on neurophysiological data, suggest that the parahippocampal region has access to and maintains information about stimulus identity and that the hippocampus combines information across stimulus events and maintains information about conjunctions among events as well as more abstract information that is common to many events. These functions are contrasted with the function of neocortical association areas, where information is initially processed and ultimately stored.

The third chapter ("The role of the lateral nucleus of the amygdala in auditory fear conditioning") turns to the role of the amygdala in fear learning in the rat.

Fear conditioning is a form of nondeclarative memory, and in its simplest form is independent of hippocampal function. The lateral nucleus is critical for forming an association between the conditioned and unconditioned stimuli (CS and US; typically a tone and footshock, respectively). Evidence is presented that the lateral nucleus is also a permanent storage site for these associations. Consideration of the cellular mechanisms involved in fear conditioning builds on the discovery that long-term potentiation (LTP) occurs at the auditory inputs to the lateral nucleus during fear conditioning in awake, behaving animals. Thus, it is suggested that LTP and fear learning depend on similar cellular mechanisms and that LTP may be critical for storing associative memories during fear learning.

The fourth chapter ("On crucial roles of hippocampal NMDA receptors in acquisition and recall of associative memory") describes studies of the molecular basis of memory in mice. This chapter first describes the effects of deletion of the NR1 subunit of the NMDA receptor in CA1 pyramidal cells of adult mice (CA1-NR1 KO mice). Effects on the developing nervous system could be avoided because the deletion is not expressed until the animals are 1-month old. The mice were impaired at spatial learning (a task of declarative memory). Long-term potentiation and depression (LTP and LTD) were also deficient, and place fields recorded from CA1 cells exhibited abnormal properties.

The chapter then describes newer work with mice in which the NR1 subunit of the NMDA receptor was deleted in CA3 pyramidal cells beginning at about 5 weeks of age (CA3-NR1 KO mice). These mice were intact at spatial learning but were impaired when recall was tested under conditions of reduced spatial cues. In addition, in the reduced-cue condition, place cells recorded from the CA1 field were abnormal, and LTP was absent at synapses on CA3 cells where LTP depends on NMDA activation. It is suggested that the CA1 field is essential for forming and initially storing spatial memory, and that modifications in recurrent connections within the CA3 field during learning provide for subsequent pattern completion (and memory retrieval), as proposed by computational models of CA3 connectionist architecture. The pattern completion function becomes critical only under reduced-cue conditions. Pattern completion (and plasticity within CA3) is unnecessary when all the cues are present, and in that circumstance memory in CA1 is reactivated directly by the incoming cues. It will be interesting to extend these observations to other tasks, especially nonspatial memory tasks.

The era of the molecular genetics of behavioral memory has just begun. Such studies hold great promise for elucidating mechanisms of learning and memory, especially in the context of the conceptual framework and the information about brain systems that have become available from other techniques, as illustrated for example by the other chapters in this part.

9

Memory systems

LARRY R. SQUIRE AND CRAIG E. L. STARK

For all its diversity, one can view neuroscience as being concerned with two central issues – the hard wiring of the brain and the brain's capacity for plasticity. The former refers to how connections develop between cells, how cells function and communicate, and how an organism's inborn functions are organized (e.g., its sleep–wake cycles, hunger and thirst, and the ability to perceive the world). The nervous system has inherited such adaptations through evolution, because these are functions too important to be left to the vagaries of individual experience. In contrast, the capacity for plasticity refers to the fact that nervous systems can adapt or change as the result of experiences that occur during an individual lifetime. Experience can modify the nervous system, and as a result, organisms can learn and remember. Learning is the process by which new information is acquired about the world, and memory is the process by which this information can persist across time.

The scientific study of memory has reached a particularly fruitful stage. Memory is being studied at many levels of analysis – from questions about the cellular and molecular events that underlie synaptic change to questions about the organization of behavioral memory. This chapter considers memory from the perspective of brain systems and behavior and focuses on three topics (for recent reviews, see Squire & Bayley, 2007; Squire et al., 2004).

First, the hippocampus is part of an anatomically coherent system of structures in the medial temporal lobe that is essential for the formation of declarative memory. Declarative memory is what is meant by the term memory when it is used in everyday language. Declarative memory is memory for facts and events. A key feature of declarative memory is that the structures in the medial temporal lobe have only a time-limited role in memory. The system is needed for a lengthy period of time after learning to direct a process of reorganization in

Topics in Integrative Neuroscience: From Cells to Cognition, ed. James R. Pomerantz. Published by Cambridge University Press. © Cambridge University Press 2008.

neocortex (where long-term memory is ultimately stored). After this time it is not needed for storage or retrieval.

Second, the function of the hippocampus (and the medial temporal lobe system to which it belongs) is narrower than it was once thought to be. The medial temporal lobe memory system is involved only in declarative memory. In contrast, nondeclarative memory refers to a collection of learning and memory abilities that do not depend on the medial temporal lobe. Nondeclarative memory refers to a change in performance as a result of experience (and in that sense can be called "memory"), but the change in performance does not require access to any conscious memory content or even awareness that memory is being used. Examples of nondeclarative memory include the acquisition of skills and habits, the phenomenon of repetition priming, and simple forms of conditioning.

The third topic concerns the opportunities that exist for the use of animal models to study declarative memory in monkeys and in rodents. These opportunities can be illustrated with the phenomenon of recognition memory, an elemental form of declarative memory that underlies the capacity to detect familiarity. In the case of recognition memory, it is now possible to take the concepts that began in human studies and to follow them through the monkey and to the rat and mouse and to the promise of molecular analysis.

9.1   The medial temporal lobe and declarative memory

The modern era of the study of memory systems began in 1957 when Brenda Milner described the effects of bilateral medial temporal lobe surgery on human memory in the now famous patient HM. HM developed severe amnesia as the result of a medial temporal lobe resection that was carried out to relieve severe epilepsy. The hallmark of this amnesia is profound forgetfulness. Figure 9.1 shows the extent of HM's lesion in the medial temporal lobe. On the basis of MRI findings (Corkin et al., 1997), the resection is now understood to have included the hippocampus, the amygdala, the entorhinal cortex, and much of the perirhinal cortex (with some sparing of its ventro-caudal aspect). The more posterior parahippocampal cortex was largely spared. Although this case is often cited as evidence for the importance of the hippocampus in memory, HM's lesion extends well beyond the hippocampus to involve adjacent cortex. Accordingly, it is more accurate to say that this important case identified the importance of the medial temporal lobe for memory. It did not permit conclusions about the role of the hippocampus itself.

The landmark paper describing HM was clear on this point. Its final paragraph states: "It is concluded that the anterior hippocampus and the

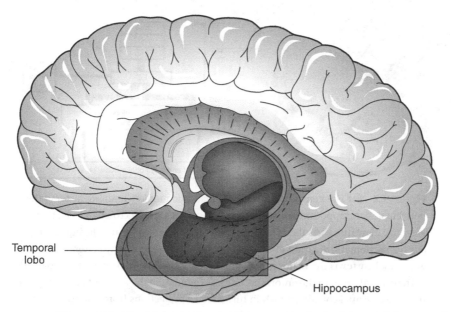

Figure 9.1   The hippocampus and adjacent structures of the medial temporal lobe were damaged bilaterally (i.e., in both hemispheres of the brain) in the amnesic patient HM (indicated by the darkly shaded area) (from Squire & Kandel, 1999).

hippocampal gyrus, either separately or together, are critically concerned in the retention of current experience" (Scoville & Milner, 1957). With respect to these three possibilities (that either the hippocampus, the hippocampal gyrus, or both are important for memory), it has turned out that the third possibility is the correct one. Both the hippocampus and the hippocampal gyrus are important. However, it took a number of years to decide this issue, that is, to determine which structures are responsible for HM's memory impairment. Indeed, these answers had to wait until the late 1970s and early 1980s and the development of an animal model of amnesia in the monkey (Mishkin, 1978; Mishkin *et al.*, 1982; Squire & Zola-Morgan, 1983). Once the animal model was developed, it was then possible over a period of years to identify the specific structures in the medial temporal lobe that are important for memory. Figure 9.2A shows the ventral surface of a monkey brain, highlighting the areas of the medial temporal lobe. Figure 9.2B illustrates schematically the structures now understood to be the constitutents of the medial temporal lobe memory system (Squire & Zola-Morgan, 1991). The hippocampus proper is located at the top of this information processing hierarchy. Together with the subiculum and the dentate gyrus, these areas constitute the hippocampal region. The adjacent entorhinal cortex originates the major cortical projections to the hippocampus. Finally, the perirhinal

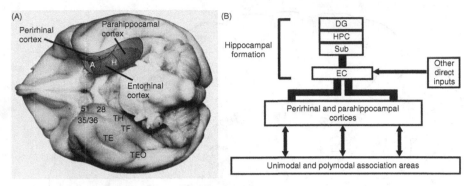

Figure 9.2   (A) The ventral surface of the macaque monkey brain identifying the perirhinal, parahippocampal, and entorhinal cortices. Using crosshatching, this view also identifies the subcortical location of the amygdala (A) and the hippocampus (H). (B) A schematic diagram of the medial temporal lobe memory system. The entorhinal cortex is the major source of projections to the hippocampus. Two-thirds of the cortical input to the entorhinal cortex originates in the adjacent perirhinal and parahippocampal cortices, which in turn receive projections from unimodal and polymodal areas in the frontal, temporal, and parietal lobes. The entorhinal cortex also receives other direct inputs from orbital frontal cortex, cingulate cortex, insular cortex, and superior temporal gyrus. All these projections are reciprocal (from Squire & Zola, 1991).

and parahippocampal cortices originate about two-thirds of the cortical projections to the entorhinal cortex (Suzuki & Amaral, 1994). The work with monkeys has shown that a large medial temporal lobe lesion is required to impair memory as severely as it is impaired in HM (Broadbent *et al.*, 2002; Squire & Zola-Morgan, 1991; Stefanacci *et al.*, 2000).

It is also now appreciated that damage limited to the hippocampus itself produces a more modest and quantitatively less severe memory impairment than is present in HM (Rempel-Clower *et al.*, 1996; Zola-Morgan & Squire, 1986). Figure 9.3 shows coronally oriented magnetic resonance images of the brain of a healthy volunteer (left panel) and the brain of amnesic patient LM (right panel). LM became amnesic in 1984 as a result of respiratory distress and then survived for 6 years during which time his memory impairment was documented repeatedly. When he died of lung carcinoma in 1990, we were able, with the consent and encouragement of his family, to obtain the brain shortly after death and to examine it in considerable detail. Structural abnormalities in the hippocampal region are readily apparent in the MRI (Figure 9.3), as it is reduced to about 55% of its normal area (Squire *et al.*, 1990). Neuropathological examination subsequently indicated that this abnormally small hippocampal region was the result of substantial cell loss (Rempel-Clower *et al.*, 1996). LM's lesion included most of

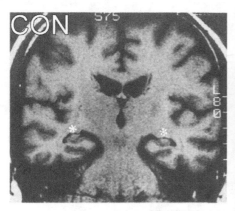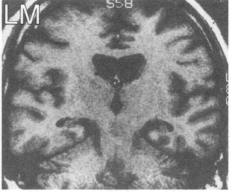

Figure 9.3   T1-weighted coronal MRI scans through the hippocampus from a
healthy control volunteer (CON) and from a patient (LM). Images are oriented
according to radiological convention (the right side of the brain is on the left side of
the image). The left and right hippocampus in the control volunteer lie immediately
below the white asterisk. Note the markedly shrunken appearance of the hippocampus in patient LM (from Squire *et al.*, 1990).

the CA1 region bilaterally, sparing only its most distal portion near the subicular
border. The CA2 field sustained some damage. In addition, there was essentially
complete loss of CA3 pyramidal cells bilaterally. In the dentate gyrus, there
was extensive loss of cells in the hilar region as well as a patchy loss of granule
cells. Finally, some cell loss was evident in layers II and III of the entorhinal
cortex.

   The memory loss associated with such a lesion is clinically significant and
easy to document. In one simple test of recognition memory (Wright *et al.*, 1985),
subjects see four floral patterns one at a time (1 second/pattern). After a variable
delay, subjects are asked to make a yes-or-no decision as to whether the probe
stimulus does or does not match one of the four that had been presented.
Figure 9.4 shows the performance of six patients with memory impairment
that resembled in severity the impairment exhibited by LM. When only 0–2
seconds elapsed between the presentation of the four study items and the probe
stimulus, performance was normal. However, after a delay of only 6–10 seconds,
the patients were distinctly impaired, and they were impaired as well at the
longer delays that were tested (Buffalo *et al.*, 1998).

   Figure 9.5 shows the performance of six amnesic patients (including patient
LM) on 11–25 different recognition memory tests that were administered over a
period of several years (Reed & Squire, 1997). All six patients were unequivocally
impaired. Of these six patients, detailed histological information is available for
three (GD, WH, and LM). All three of these patients had bilateral damage to the

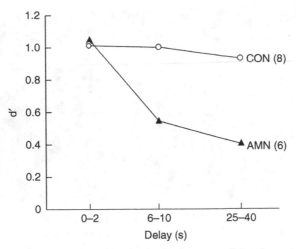

Figure 9.4   Discrimination accuracy (d′) as a function of retention delay for six amnesic patients with damage to the hippocampal region. Higher d′ scores reflect greater recognition accuracy. Amnesic patients performed normally with a 0–2 second delay between study and test, but were impaired when the delay exceeded 6 seconds (from Buffalo *et al.*, 1998).

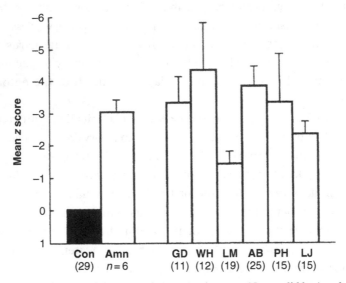

Figure 9.5   Performance of control volunteers (Con, solid bar) and six amnesic patients (Amn) with damage to the hippocampal region (as a group and individually, open bars) on 11–25 different tests of recognition memory. The raw performance scores from each test were converted to z scores based on the raw performance scores of control volunteers. By this method, control volunteers have a mean z score of zero on each test. The negative z scores indicate impaired performance, and higher negative z scores represent greater impairment (from Reed & Squire, 1997).

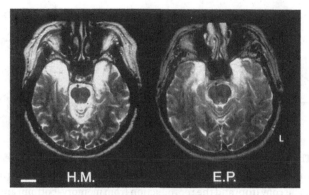

Figure 9.6   T2-weighted axial MRI scans of patients HM (left) and EP (right), through the level of the temporal lobes. Damaged tissue is indicated by bright signal. Images are oriented according to radiological convention (the right side of the brain is on the left side of the image) and the scale bar is 2 cm. Both patients sustained extensive damage to medial temporal lobe structures. HM's lesion was caused by surgery to relieve severe epilepsy. EP's lesion was caused by viral encephalitis (from Stefanacci *et al.*, 2000).

hippocampal region. In two of the cases (WH and LM), there was some damage to entorhinal cortex as well (Rempel-Clower *et al.*, 1996).

While it is easy to document the modest level of memory impairment when damage is restricted to the hippocampal region, it is also true that the impairment is much more severe in patients like HM, who have damage extending beyond the hippocampal region to involve large portions of adjacent cortex. Figure 9.6 shows horizontally oriented MRI brain scans of patient HM (left) and a second patient EP (right). Whereas HM's damage was caused by a surgical lesion, EP's damage was caused by viral encephalitis, which occurred in 1992 when he was 70 years old (Stefanacci *et al.*, 2000). The virus bilaterally damaged the amygdala, hippocampus, entorhinal cortex, perirhinal cortex, and much of the pararhippocampal cortex.

The severity of EP's memory impairment can be appreciated by comparing his performance on memory tests directly to the performance of patient LM. Figure 9.7 compares the ability of LM and EP to copy the Rey-Osterrieth figure and then to reproduce it from memory after a 10–15 minute delay. LM's reproduction was quite poor and resembled the original figure in only a general way. However, EP's performance was even worse. He stated that he could not remember having copied a figure earlier, and when encouraged to draw whatever came to mind he declined to try.

These examples illustrate the profound forgetfulness that characterize the memory impairment associated with extensive medial temporal lobe damage.

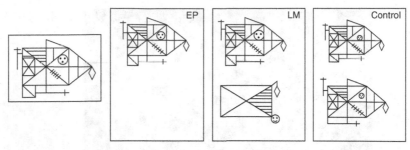

Figure 9.7   The Rey-Osterrieth figure. Subjects were first asked to copy the figure illustrated in the small box in the left panel and 10–15 minutes later to reproduce it from memory. The copy (top) and the reproduction from memory (bottom) are shown for EP, LM, and for a representative control in the larger panels at the right. EP did not recall copying the figure. Encouraged to draw whatever came to mind, he declined to try (from Stefanacci *et al.*, 2000).

Another important feature of this memory impairment is retrograde amnesia – the loss of memories that were acquired prior to the onset of amnesia. Clinical observers have long noted that when retrograde amnesia occurs, recent memory tends to be affected more than remote memory (Ribot, 1881; Russell & Nathan, 1946). However, it was only more recently that it was possible to identify patients with damage to the hippocampal formation who had become amnesic on a known calendar day and to test these patients formally with questions about past public events and questions about people who came into the news at different times in the past (Manns *et al.*, 2003). Studies of such patients suggested that retrograde amnesia can extend backwards in time, in a graded way, affecting several years of past memories (Bayley *et al.*, 2007; Manns *et al.*, 2003).

These observations suggest that the hippocampal function is needed for a limited period of time after learning and is not needed to retrieve remote memories. However, studies of humans encounter the difficulty that the methods for assessing retrograde manesia are almost always retrospective. Accordingly, it is difficult to assure that one is sampling past time periods in an equivalent way. Yet, to reach clear conclusions about the nature and extent of retrograde amnesia, one would want to be able to test material from different time periods that had been learned about to the same extent and was now in the course of being forgotten at the same rate.

While this standard is difficult to achieve in studies of human amnesia, one can meet all these conditions in studies of experimental animals. Experimental animals can be studied prospectively, and they can be given similar amounts of training at different times before surgery. Then one can ask how well animals remember what they have learned as a function of how long before surgery the training occurred.

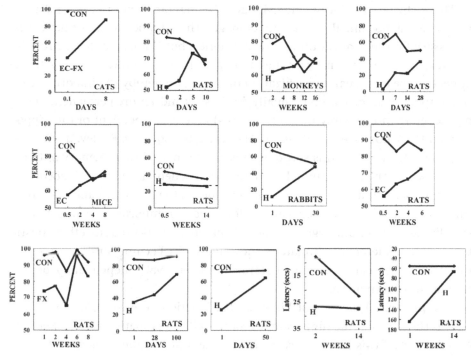

Figure 9.8 Summary of findings from 13 studies that examined retrograde amnesia prospectively (details available in Squire *et al.*, 2001). Data show performance of control (CON) and operated animals (H, hippocampus; EC, entorhinal cortex; FX, fornix) as a function of training–surgery interval. Performance scores are in percent (0–100 or 50–100) so that higher scores reflect better performance. In studies 12 and 13, the performance score is the latency to find a hidden goal, so that lower latencies (the upper end of the axis) reflect better performance. Temporally graded retrograde amnesia was observed in all but two of the studies (from Squire *et al.*, 2001).

Studies of retrograde amnesia following damage to the hippocampal formation or the fornix began in earnest in the 1990s. Figure 9.8 shows the results for 13 different studies in which equivalent training was given to animals on at least two different occasions before surgery (see Squire *et al.*, 2001 for details). The studies include a variety of different tasks and five different species (monkey, cat, rabbit, rat, and mouse). All but two of these studies (those illustrated in panels 6 and 12) found temporally graded retrograde amnesia. The amnesia extends across a time period that, depending on the study, covers as little as several days or as much as several weeks. In most of the studies, some forgetting is evident in the control animals across the time period being tested. Finally, in most of the studies the retrograde amnesia is not only temporally graded but remote memories are being recalled *better* than recent memories.

These studies provide strong evidence that remote memory can be spared following hippocampal formation damage. The hippocampal formation is necessary for the acquisition of new memories, but it appears that its role in the maintenance of memory is time-limited. As time passes after learning, there appears to be a gradual reorganization of memory whereby the importance of the hippocampal formation gradually diminishes and a more permanent memory develops (presumably in the neocortex) that is independent of the hippocampal formation (see also Squire & Alvarez, 1995; Squire & Bayley, 2007). It is important to note that this sort of idea is not a proposal that memory initially resides within the hippocampal formation and is then moved to the neocortex. The proposal is that the memory always resides in the neocortex and that, for a time after learning, the hippocampal formation is important for organizing, stabilizing, and binding together the distributed networks that together constitute a whole memory. Ultimately, these networks become sufficiently organized that they can function in storage and retrieval independently of the hippocampal formation.

One influential idea about hippocampal function derived from the rodent tests is the idea that the hippocampus forms and stores spatial maps (O'Keefe & Nadel, 1978). If this notion is correct, that the hippocampus is a repository of spatial maps, then it should be the case that no matter how long after learning hippocampal damage occurs, spatial maps should be lost.

We have had the opportunity to consider this issue in some detail in our studies of the severely amnesic patient EP (Teng & Squire, 1999). The work was inspired by initial impressions that EP seemed to know a good deal about the neighborhood in which he grew up. EP was born in 1922 and grew up in the East Bay area of San Francisco. He moved away as a young adult and has not lived there since. He moved to San Diego County in 1993, after he developed amnesia, and he currently resides there. We were able to obtain street maps of the Hayward-Castro Valley area of the East Bay – vintage 1940 – and to locate on the maps a number of landmarks that should be known to anyone who had lived in the area (Figure 9.9). Drawing from an area of about 50 square miles (a larger area than is illustrated in the figure), we identified about 20 such landmarks. In addition, we were also able to identify five individuals who attended EP's high school during the same period as EP, lived in the Hayward-Castro Valley area about as long as EP (26 years for the controls, 22 years for EP), subsequently moved away, and did not revisit the area.

These five individuals and EP were each given four tests that probed their spatial knowledge of the area. Three of the tasks were mental navigation tasks. In one task, they were asked to describe how they would navigate from their homes to different locations in the area (familiar navigation). In a second task,

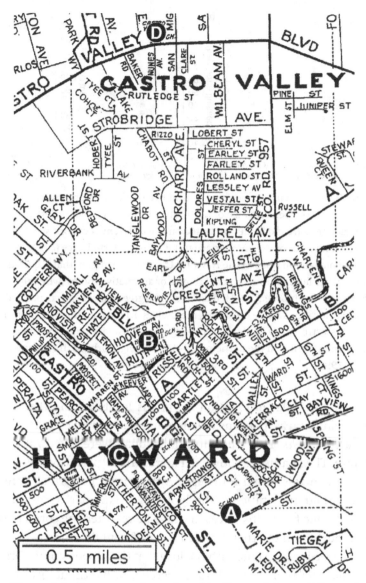

Figure 9.9   Street map of a portion of the Hayward-Castro Valley region from the 1940s (Thomas Bros. Map Co.). The locations of four representative landmarks used in the topographical memory tasks are shown (A–D). The locations used in the four spatial tasks encompassed an area of approximately 50 square miles, a larger area than is shown here (from Teng & Squire, 1999).

they were asked how they would navigate between two different locations (novel navigation). In the third, they were asked how they would navigate between these same two locations if a main street were blocked off (alternative routes). In addition to the navigation tasks, they were also asked to imagine

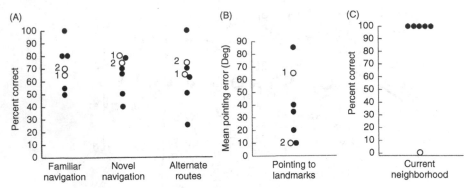

Figure 9.10 Patient EP's performance on five spatial memory tasks (open circles) together with the performance of five healthy controls (closed circles). For the four retrograde tests (A and B), EP was tested on two different occasions separated by 9 months (1 and 2). For the anterograde test (C), EP was tested once (A) Percent correct on three navigation tasks in the Hayward-Castro Valley region that required negotiating either familiar routes, novel routes, or alternative routes (when the most direct route was blocked). (B) Median error in degrees when subjects pointed to particular locations while imagining themselves oriented at other locations in the Hayward-Castro Valley region. (C) Percent correct on a task requiring the navigation of prominent routes in the participant's current neighborhood (from Teng & Squire, 1999).

themselves in a particular orientation at various locations and then to point toward specific landmarks (pointing to landmarks). EP was asked 8–10 questions for each of the four tests. The five control individuals were asked 7.8–9.8 questions on average. The results are shown in Figure 9.10. EP performed as well as or better than the controls on all four tests. Although EP performed somewhat poorly on the first administration of the "pointing to landmarks" test, this poor performance was due to two instances in which he reported the correct heading verbally (e.g., southwest) but then pointed in a different direction.

These results are inconsistent with the idea that the hippocampus forms and stores spatial maps (O'Keefe & Nadel, 1978), because EP has the ability to retrieve and utilize spatial maps that would have been stored long before the onset of his amnesia. One of the central tenets of the spatial hypothesis of hippocampal function is that the spatial maps stored in the hippocampus enable flexible navigation (O'Keefe & Nadel, 1978) by making it possible to find several routes to the same destination. EP's excellent performance on the "alternative routes" task indicates that even flexible navigation through environments learned long ago is possible despite virtually complete hippocampal damage.

In addition to testing the ability to mentally navigate in the environment learned long ago, we also asked all participants to describe how they would navigate from the homes where they currently reside to five locations in the neighborhood (e.g., post office, bank). All the controls were able to provide accurate directions in response to all five questions (100% correct). In contrast, EP, who moved to San Diego County in 1993 after he became amnesic, was unable to answer any of the questions (0% correct). Indeed, EP resides about 2 miles from the Pacific Ocean but is not able to point in the direction of the ocean when asked to do so.

These data provide strong evidence that the medial temporal lobe, including the hippocampus, is not essential for the long-term storage of spatial knowledge and does not maintain spatial layouts of learned environments that are necessary for successful navigation. These findings count against the so-called "spatial view" of the hippocampus and for the view that the hippocampus is a general purpose learner of new facts and events, both spatial and nonspatial. Further, the findings indicate that the hippocampus is not the final repository of long-term memory, either spatial or nonspatial.

Similar results were reported recently for patient KC, who developed memory impairment and hippocampal damage following a closed head injury (Rosenbaum *et al.*, 2000). KC was able to draw a detailed sketch of the neighborhood in which he grew up, he succeeded at finding novel routes from one location to another, and he succeeded at four other spatial tests. He performed poorly on one test that asked him to recognize buildings located in his neighborhood, and he also had difficulty locating cities on a map of Canada and on a map of the province of Ontario. Unfortunately, the anatomical substrates of KC's spared and impaired performance cannot be readily understood. According to MRI scans, his closed head injury produced asymmetric medial temporal lobe damage and involves only a small portion of the right medial temporal lobe. Moreover, the injury includes prominent damage to left frontal, left parietal, left retrosplenial, and left occipital cortices, and a smaller site of damage in the right parietal cortex (Tulving, 1991).

9.2   Nondeclarative memory

It is of considerable interest that the profound memory impairment in EP and other amnesic patients is narrow in the sense that many kinds of learning and memory abilities in these patients are spared (Squire, 2004). A particularly dramatic example of preserved learning and memory ability comes from the phenomenon of repetition priming. Repetition priming is a form of nondeclarative memory in which the ability to detect or identify stimuli is increased as a result of their recent exposure (Tulving & Schacter, 1990). Priming is a form of memory in the sense that behavior is modified by experience. However, studies of amnesic patients indicate that priming is quite a different kind of memory than what is studied when one queries individuals about their memory for past facts and events.

Consider a representative study in which 24 common English words were first presented to subjects one at a time (Hamann & Squire, 1997). After presentation of the words, one can test for memory of these words in a number of different ways. For example, one can test declarative memory by giving tests of recognition memory. In this case, participants can be shown two words (one from the list and one new word) and then asked to decide which of the two words was from the list (forced-choice recognition). Alternatively, participants can be shown words one at a time (either from the studied list or not) and asked to make a yes or no judgment as to whether each word was or was not on the list.

In contrast, one can ask whether the word list has had any effect on behavior without making explicit reference to the study episode. Consider the following two different ways of testing the effects of past experience on present performance. In the case of word–stem completion, one sees word beginnings or word stems such as MOT__ and is asked to complete each word stem to form the first word that comes to mind. If one has not recently seen a particular word that begins with this stem (e.g., motel), there is a 10–20% chance that participants will complete the stem to form this word. However, if participants have recently seen the word "motel", there is an increased probability (30–40%) of generating "motel" when asked to complete MOT__ with the first word that comes to mind. Thus, the recent presentation of a word creates a bias so that later one tends to complete the word stem to form the presented word. A similar repetition priming effect can be observed with a task called perceptual identification. In this task, words are flashed on a computer screen one at a time and at a duration of approximately 30 ms, which is too brief to read the words successfully. The finding of interest is that recent experience with a word increases the probability that it can be read (from 30%–35% to about 50%). Thus, experience with the words improves the perceptual fluency of the words, and they can be identified more readily.

Figure 9.11 shows the results with control subjects and amnesic patients, including EP. As measured by the two conventional recognition memory tests (forced-choice and yes or no), control subjects performed very well. For example, in the forced-choice test, controls recognized on average about 90% of the 24 words that had been presented. Three moderately-impaired amnesic patients performed poorly on the two recognition tests but had some residual memory capacity. In contrast, the severely amnesic patient EP performed at chance on both tests. That is, he performed on these simple recognition tests no better than if he had flipped a coin to decide his answer.

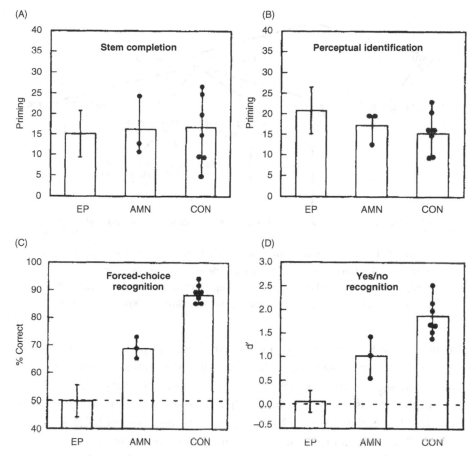

Figure 9.11 Performance on two tests of repetition priming (A,B) and two tests of recognition memory (C,D) for patient EP, three other amnesic patients (AMN), and seven healthy control volunteers (CON). (A) Stem-completion priming scores. Priming scores reflect the increased probability of completing a word stem to the studied word. (B) Perceptual identification priming scores. Priming scores reflect the increased probability of accurately identifying a briefly presented word. (C) Percent correct in a two-alternative, forced-choice recognition task. Higher scores reflect better recognition memory. (D) Discriminability (d') scores in a yes/no recognition memory task. Higher d' scores reflect better recognition memory (from Hamann & Squire, 1997).

The findings were strikingly different on the word–stem completion task and the perceptual identification task. On both these tests, the three moderately-impaired amnesic patients and EP performed entirely normally. On the word completion test the patients had the same tendency as normal individuals to complete word stems to form words that were on the study list. Additionally, on the perceptual identification task, the patients were (like normal subjects) able to read a briefly presented word more easily if they had just seen the word on the list.

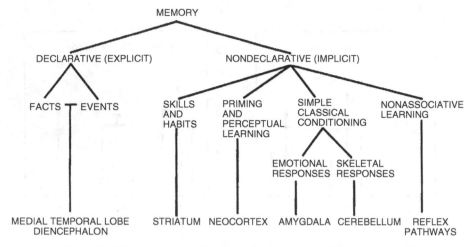

Figure 9.12   A taxonomy of memory. Declarative (explicit) memory refers to conscious recollection of facts and events and depends on the integrity of the medial temporal lobe. Nondeclarative memory (implicit) refers to a collection of abilities and is independent of the medial temporal lobe (from Squire & Knowlton, 1999).

In further studies of this type, EP has continued to perform at chance on recognition tests and appears unable to use the information available to him through priming to inform his recognition judgements (Conroy *et al.*, 2005). In one example, EP was given a test in which, a word–stem completion probe was administered on each trial immediately prior to a recognition probe. Despite the fact that EP often generated the studied item in response to the word–stem completion probe (e.g., he said "motel" in response to MOT__), when immediately given a forced-choice recognition task (e.g., was "motel" or "motor" on the study list?), he scored at chance (Stark & Squire, 2000). These findings show that the phenomenon of priming is independent of the medial temporal lobe.

Priming is an example of a large category of memory phenomena which are intact in amnesia and are supported by brain systems other than the medial temporal lobe system. Figure 9.12 illustrates several different kinds of memory, as they are currently understood. Here memory has been divided into declarative memory (memory for facts and events) and a number of forms of nondeclarative memory. Declarative memory is representational. It provides a way of modeling the external world and is available as conscious recollection. Nondeclarative memory is dispositional and is expressed through performance rather than recollection. Nondeclarative memory refers to a collection of nonconscious learning abilities that depend on brain systems other than the medial temporal lobe. Priming and perceptual learning are thought to be intrinsic to the perceptual machinery of the cortex (Gilbert, this volume; Schacter & Buckner,

1998). Emotional memory requires the amygdala, as when one acquires a phobia through some aversive experience (LeDoux, this volume). Skill and habit learning require the neostriatum. Skill learning includes perceptual skills like learning to read upside down, motor skills as expressed in a good tennis backhand, as well as cognitive skills such as can be acquired in solving puzzles or programming computers. Habit learning involves gradual changes in behavior, as when one comes to wash one's hands before dinner or to say "please" and "thank you." Such behaviors develop without reference to particular events and in the absence of conscious efforts to memorize.

Simple forms of classical conditioning, such as eyeblink conditioning in vertebrates (Thompson & Krupa, 1994), depend on the cerebellum. Other forms of classical conditioning can also be demonstrated in invertebrate animals such as *Aplysia* and *Drosophila*. Classical conditioning, as well as nonassociative forms of memory (habituation and sensitization), have been preserved through evolutionary history and they are present in all animals with a sufficiently developed nervous system.

In vertebrates, these categories of memory can be related to the operation of several different brain systems, which operate in parallel. Although one can debate which terms are the most appropriate for labeling these forms of memory, it is evident that psychology has matured to the point that it can draw on biology to identify categories of memory. Thus, during this century the problem of memory moved beyond philosophical discussion, psychological intuition, and behavioral observation to a point where biological findings provide the clearest and most unambiguous evidence about the organization of memory.

9.3   Animal models of declarative memory

The final topic of this chapter concerns how animal models can be used to illuminate the anatomy and organization of declarative memory. The promise of this approach can be illustrated by the capacity of recognition memory. Recognition memory can be studied with an elementary task that takes advantage of the natural tendency of mammals to seek novelty. This task, known as the visual paired-comparison task (or novel object recognition), can be studied in humans, monkeys, and rodents in a rather similar fashion. In the case of humans, one first presents two identical pictures, placed side by side, and then after a variable delay the original picture is presented together with a new picture. The finding of interest is that during a 5-second viewing period, participants tend to look at the new picture longer than the old picture. For example, an individual might spend 3.5 seconds viewing the new picture and only 1.5 seconds viewing the old picture.

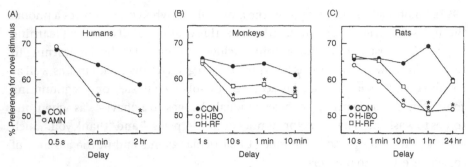

Figure 9.13 Performance of humans, monkeys, and rats on the visual paired-comparison task, a task of recognition memory. Asterisks indicate impaired performance of the lesion group relative to the control (CON) group. Chance performance is 50%. (A) Performance of human amnesic patients (AMN) with damage to the hippocampal formation or diencephalon and control volunteers (CON). Data from 9 to 11 individuals contribute to each delay point. (B) Performance of five monkeys with radio frequency (H-RF) lesions of the hippocampal region, four monkeys with ibotenic acid (H-IBO) lesions of the hippocampal region, and five control animals. (C) Performance of eight rats with H-RF lesions, eight rats with H-IBO lesions, and sixteen controls (from Broadbent et al., in press).

Figure 9.13A shows the findings when this task was given to amnesic patients. When there was no delay between the original presentation of two pictures and the subsequent presentation of two different pictures, both control subjects and amnesic patients, like controls, exhibited the normal tendency to look at the novel picture; that is, amnesic patients spent about two-thirds of the time (65% of the time) looking at the novel picture. When the delay was increased to 2 minutes, control subjects continued to express a strong preference for the novel picture. However, amnesic patients began to divide their time more equally between the new and old picture. Finally, when the delay was increased to one hour, the looking preference of the amnesic patients no longer discriminated between the two pictures.

This same task was adapted for the monkey by Jocelyne Bachevalier (Bachevalier, 1990). Figure 9.13B shows the results with this task for normal monkeys and monkeys with radio frequency or ibotenate lesions of the hippocampal region (Zola et al., 2000). The monkeys with lesions performed normally when the delay was only one second, indicating that the hippocampal lesion has not affected perception or the appreciation of novelty per se. However, at delays of 10 seconds, 1 minute, and 10 minutes, the monkeys with lesions did not effectively discriminate between the novel picture and the old picture.

This same task has also been adapted for the rodent (Ennaceur & Delacour, 1988). In the case of rodents, one takes advantage of the readiness with which rodents explore large spaces. A rat is first introduced to an arena where it encounters two identical objects. The animal is allowed to explore until it accumulates 30 seconds of contact time with the objects. Then the animal is removed from the arena for a variable interval. When the animal is later reintroduced to the arena, it again encounters two objects – a copy of the original object and a new object – and it again explores until it accumulates 30 seconds of contact time with the objects. The finding of interest is that the animal tends to spend most of its time with the novel object. Figure 9.13C shows the effects of radio frequency or ibotenic acid lesions of the hippocampus on this task (Clark et al., 2000). Control animals showed a preference for the novel object across all the delays tested, from 10 seconds to 24 hours. In contrast, the rats with hippocampal lesions preferred to explore the novel object only when the delay was 10 seconds. Thereafter this preference weakened. In the ibotenate group, no preference was evident after one minute. The radio frequency group's performance was more variable. Nevertheless, averaging across the longer delays (10 minutes, 1 hour and 24 hours), performance was significantly impaired relative to the control group.

Taken together, the results are quite similar across humans, monkeys, and rats. This finding is encouraging because it suggests that one can take tasks and concepts that began in cognitive science, in the clinic, and in the human neuropsychological laboratory, and take these to the monkey and ultimately to the rodent. Indeed, this particular task has been extended successfully to the mouse (Mansuy et al., 1998; Tang et al., 1999). In such a case, one can have some confidence that one is studying memory operations in the rat and in the mouse that have relevance to the human condition. One thus has the promise that molecular analysis of this task may be feasible and, if so, the results should reveal information relevant to the molecular basis of human memory.

9.4   Conclusion

This chapter summarizes recent findings concerning the medial temporal lobe memory system, the distinction between declarative and nondeclarative memory, and the use of animal models to illuminate the anatomy and organization of declarative memory. The study of memory has been advantaged by the possibility of extending the concepts and findings from human memory to simpler animals, including rat and mouse.

Acknowledgments

The research summarized here was supported by the Medical Research Service of the Department of Veterans Affairs, the National Institute of Mental Health, and the Metropolitan Life Foundation.

References

Bachevalier, J. (1990). Ontogenetic development of habit and memory formation in primates. *Annals of the New York Academy of Sciences*, **608**, 457–74.

Bayley, P. J., Hopkins, R. O., and Squire, L. R. (2007). The fate of old memories following medial temporal lobe damage. *Journal of Neuroscience*, **26**, 13311–17.

Broadbent, N., Clark, R. E., Zola, S., and Squire, L. R. (2002). The medial temporal lobe and memory. In L. R. Squire and D. Schacter, eds., *The Neuropsychology of Memory*, 3rd edn. New York: Guilford Press, pp. 3–23.

Buffalo, E. A., Reber, P. J., and Squire, L. R. (1998). The human perirhinal cortex and recognition memory. *Hippocampus*, **8**, 330–9.

Clark, R. E., Zola, S. M., and Squire, L. R. (2000). Impaired recognition memory in rats after damage to the hippocampus. *Journal of Neuroscience*, **20**, 8853–60.

Conroy, M. A., Hopkins, R. O., and Squire, L. R. (2005). Contribution of perceptual fluency and priming to recognition memory. *Cognitive, Affective, and Behavioral Neuroscience*, **5**, 14–20.

Corkin, S., Amaral, D. G., Gonzalez, R. G., Johnson, K. A., and Hyman, B. T. (1997). H.M.'s medial temporal lobe lesion: findings from magnetic resonance imaging. *Journal of Neuroscience*, **17**, 3964–80.

Ennaceur, A. and Delacour, J. (1988). A new one-trial test for neurobiological studies of memory in rats: 1. Behavioural data. *Behavioral Brain Research*, **31**, 47–59.

Hamann, S. B. and Squire, L. R. (1997). Intact perceptual memory in the absence of conscious memory. *Behavioral Neuroscience*, **111**, 850–4.

Manns, J. R., Hopkins, R. O., and Squire, L. R. (2003). Semantic memory and the human hippocampus. *Neuron*, **37**, 127–33.

Mansuy, I. M., Mayford, M., Jacob, B., Kandel, E. R., and Bach, M. E. (1998). Restricted and regulated overexpression reveals calcineurin as a key component in the transition from short-term to long-term memory. *Cell*, **92**, 39–49.

Mishkin, M. (1978). Memory in monkeys severely impaired by combined but not by separate removal of amygdala and hippocampus. *Nature*, **273**, 297–8.

Mishkin, M., Spiegler, B. J., Saunders, R. C., and Malamut, B. J. (1982). An animal model of global amnesia. In S. Corkin, K. L. Davis, J. H. Growdon, E. Usdin, and R. J. Wurtman, eds., *Toward a Treatment of Alzheimer's Disease*. New York: Raven, pp. 235–47.

O'Keefe, J. and Nadel, L. (1978). *The Hippocampus as a Cognitive Map*. London: Oxford University Press.

Reed, J. M. and Squire, L. R. (1997). Impaired recognition memory in patients with lesions limited to the hippocampal formation. *Behavioral Neuroscience*, **111**, 667–75.

Rempel-Clower, N., Zola, S. M., Squire, L. R., and Amaral, D. G. (1996). Three cases of enduring memory impairment following bilateral damage limited to the hippocampal formation. *Journal of Neuroscience*, **16**, 5233–55.

Ribot, T. (1881). *Les Maladies de la Memoire*. English translation: Diseases of Memory. New York: Appleton-Century-Crofts.

Rosenbaum, D. L., Priselac, S., Kohler, S., et al. (2000). Remote spatial memory in an amnesic person with extensive bilateral hippocampal lesions. *Nature Neuroscience*, **3**, 1044–8.

Russell, W. R. and Nathan, P. W. (1946). Traumatic amnesia. *Brain*, **69**, 280–300.

Schacter, D. L. and Buckner, R. L. (1998). Priming and the brain. *Neuron*, **20**, 185–95.

Scoville, W. B. and Milner, B. (1957). Loss of recent memory after bilateral hippocampal lesions. *Journal of Neurology, Neurosurgery, and Psychiatry*, **20**, 11–21.

Squire, L. R. (2004). Memory systems of the brain. A brief history and current perspective. *Neurobiology of Learning and Memory*, **82**, 171–4.

Squire, L. R. and Alvarez, P. (1995). Retrograde amnesia and memory consolidation: a neurobiological perspective. *Current Opinion in Neurobiology*, **5**, 169–77.

Squire, L. R., Amaral, D. G., and Press, G. A. (1990). Magnetic resonance measurements of hippocampal formation and mammillary nuclei distinguish medial temporal lobe and diencephalic amnesia. *Journal of Neuroscience*, **10**, 3106–17.

Squire, L. R., and Bayley, P. J. (2007). The neuroscience of remote memory. *Current Opinion in Neurobiology*, **17**, 185–96.

Squire, L. R., Clark, R. E., and Knowlton, B. J. (2001). Retrograde amnesia. *Hippocampus*, **11**, 50–5.

Squire, L. R., Stark, C. E. L., and Clark, R. E. (2004). The medial temporal lobe. *Annual Review of Neuroscience*, **27**, 279–306.

Squire, L. R. and Zola-Morgan, S. (1983). The neurology of memory: the case for correspondence between the findings for human and nonhuman primate. In J. A. Deutsch, ed., *The Physiological Basis of Memory*. New York: Academic Press, pp. 199–268.

Squire, L. R. and Zola-Morgan, S. (1991). The medial temporal lobe memory system. *Science*, **253**, 1380–6.

Stark, C. E. L. and Squire, L. R. (2000). Chance recognition memory performance in severe amnesia: no evidence for the use of repetition priming in familiarity judgments. *Behavioral Neuroscience*, **114**, 459–67.

Stefanacci, L., Buffalo, E. A., Schmolck, H., and Squire, L. R. (2000). Profound amnesia after damage to the medial temporal lobe: a neuroanatomical and neuropsychological profile of E.P. *Society for Neuroscience*, **20**, 7024–36.

Suzuki, W. A. and Amaral, D. G. (1994). Perirhinal and parahippocampal cortices of the macaque monkey: cortical afferents. *Journal of Comparative Neurology*, **350**, 497–533.

Tang, Y. P., Shimizu, E., Dube, G. R., et al. (1999). Genetic enhancement of learning and memory in mice. *Nature*, **401**, 63–9.

Teng, E. and Squire, L. R. (1999). Memory for places learned long ago is intact after hippocampal damage. *Nature*, **400**, 675–7.

Thompson, R. F. and Krupa, D. J. (1994). Organization of memory traces in the mammalian brain. *Annual Review of Neuroscience*, **17**, 519–50.

Tulving, E. (1991). Concepts in human memory. In L. R. Squire, N. M. Weinberger, G. Lynch, and J. L. McGaugh, eds., *Memory: Organization and Locus of Change X*. New York: Oxford University Press, pp. 3–32.

Tulving, E. and Schacter, D. L. (1990). Priming and human memory systems. *Science*, **247**, 301–6.

Wright, A. A., Santiago, H. C., Sands, S. F., Kendrick, D. F., and Cook, R. G. (1985). Memory processing of serial lists by pigeons, monkeys and people. *Science*, **229**, 287–9.

Zola, S. M., Squire, L. R., Teng, E., *et al.* (2000). Impaired recognition memory in monkeys after damage limited to the hippocampal region. *Journal of Neuroscience*, **20**, 451–63.

Zola-Morgan, S. and Squire, L. R. (1986). Memory impairment in monkeys following lesions limited to the hippocampus. *Behavioral Neuroscience*, **100**, 155–60.

10

A brain system for declarative memory

SETH J. RAMUS AND HOWARD B. EICHENBAUM

Our understanding about the brain system that mediates memory began in the 1950s with the landmark case study of patient HM (Scoville & Milner, 1957). To relieve epilepsy that was intractable to pharmacological intervention, surgeons removed a large part of this patient's temporal lobes, including the amygdala, part of the hippocampus, and the cortex immediately surrounding the hippocampus and amygdala. Following surgery, HM exhibited a severe amnesia, leaving nonmemory aspects of intelligence and cognition intact. This observation demonstrated that memory could be separated from other cognitive functions and that structures of the medial temporal lobe are critical to memory.

While the early neuropsychological reports clearly pointed to the importance of the temporal lobes in memory, there was debate over precisely *which* temporal structures were important. Because the available clinical cases did not provide highly specific anatomical resolution, efforts were made to develop animal models in which experimental brain lesions could be performed with the necessary anatomical specificity. However, the early efforts to model amnesia in monkeys and rats did not yield a consistent pattern of severe and selective amnesia, precluding useful insights into the anatomical identification of the memory system. With hindsight, it is now clear that the difficulty in characterizing the brain system responsible for memory arose for two reasons (Eichenbaum et al., 2000). First, while the memory deficit following medial temporal damage was initially thought to be global in nature, it is now understood that damage to the medial temporal region causes amnesia that is limited to a specific domain of memory, and that other brain systems mediate other types of memory. Second, a valid animal model of amnesia had to wait for the development of behavioral tests that emphasized the specific functions of the

Topics in Integrative Neuroscience: From Cells to Cognition, ed. James R. Pomerantz. Published by Cambridge University Press. © Cambridge University Press 2008.

medial temporal lobe in animals. Only when this model was established, some 20 years after Scoville and Milner's original report, were researchers able to begin elaborating which structures damaged in patient HM were critical for normal memory function. In this chapter, we briefly discuss the history of these developments, and then outline our current understanding of the brain system that mediates memory.

10.1   The hippocampal memory system and declarative memory

The first major breakthrough in characterizing the domain of human memory dependent on the medial temporal lobe region came when Cohen and Squire (1980) reported that the amnesia associated with medial temporal damage is selective for "declarative memory," the ability to form new long-term memories about facts and everyday events – information that can be verbally "declared" in a statement. This type of memory has also been described as "episodic" (Tulving, 1993), in referring to one's ability to recollect specific experiences, or "explicit" in that declarative memories are subject to conscious expression (Graf & Schacter, 1985). Despite the variety of terminology used to characterize this form of memory, there is consensus that the medial temporal lobes are important for the rapid formation and representation of episodes within a general semantic framework. These memories are available to conscious recollection, and are able to be expressed "flexibly", that is, in a variety of contexts outside repetition of the learning event (Cohen & Eichenbaum, 1993; Schacter & Tulving, 1994). By contrast, the medial temporal lobes are not necessary for a heterogeneous collection of other memory processes that depend on brain systems not involving the hippocampus. These "nondeclarative" abilities include the acquisition of skills and biases that are expressed unconsciously through alterations in performance on a variety of tasks. Examples of nondeclarative memory are habit and motor skill learning, which depend on the neostriatum and cerebellum (Bechara *et al.*, 1995; Gabrieli, 1995; Hallet *et al.*, 1996; Knowlton *et al.*, 1996; Salmon & Butters, 1995; Woodruff-Pak *et al.*, 1996), emotional memory dependent on the amygdala (LeDoux, 1994), short-term or working memory (Vallar & Shallice, 1990) and perceptual priming (Tulving & Schacter, 1990) that are dependent on neocortical structures.

The second major breakthrough came with the establishment of a valid animal model of human amnesia. Since the degenerative processes and cerebral insults that typically result in human memory disorders rarely respect anatomical boundaries, the development of an animal model of human amnesia and the development of surgical procedures that could target specific anatomical structures were critical to characterizing the pathways that mediate declarative memory. The problem can be illustrated by considering the damage to patient HM's brain. The parts of his brain that were removed included many structures in the temporal lobes, including the amygdala, part of the hippocampus, and the cortical areas (parts of the perirhinal, parahippocampal, and entorhinal cortices) immediately adjacent to these regions. Further, each of these structures is comprised of several subdivisions. Because several anatomically distinct areas were damaged in HM as well as in other cases of amnesia, the early clinical studies could not provide sufficient anatomical resolution to identify which structures and nuclei within the medial temporal lobe are critical for memory. It was clear that this question would best be addressed by the use of experimental animals in which the precise locus and extent of the brain damage could be controlled with precision.

Almost immediately after the initial reports of HM and other amnesic patients, efforts began to reproduce the syndrome in monkeys by damaging the same structures as were damaged in HM. However, the early animal studies failed to demonstrate consistent, severe, and selective deficits in learning and memory, as was observed in human patients after large lesions of the temporal lobes (see Eichenbaum *et al.*, 2000 for a discussion of these early attempts). A major breakthrough occurred with the development of new procedures for testing memory in animals. In parallel efforts, Gaffan (1974) and Mishkin and Delacour (1975) developed a novel variant of the delayed nonmatching to sample (DNMS) task that tested recognition of items that had been previously encountered only once. In these studies, animals were initially presented with a novel memory cue, then, following a variable memory delay, were tested for memory of the cue vs. a different novel stimulus. This version of the DNMS test emphasizes episodic learning and flexible expression of memory, properties characteristic of declarative memory in humans. This new version of the DNMS task would be instrumental in the development of the nonhuman primate model of human amnesia, and ultimately for delineating the structures in the temporal lobe important for memory.

Initially, human neuropsychological studies pointed to the hippocampus as the crucial structure within the medial temporal lobe for memory, because the extent of hippocampal damage correlated with severity of amnesia (Milner, 1974). However, on the basis of the initial findings from the newly established monkey model, Mishkin (1978) suggested that it was a combination of damage to *both* the hippocampus and the amygdala that was required to produce amnesia. Apparently, the human and animal work were once again at odds. However, cortical structures surrounding the hippocampus and amygdala were incidentally damaged during the surgical approach both in the human amnesic patients and in the experimental monkeys. These structures are now known to be critical for memory. But the resolution of this discrepancy had to wait another decade as animal researchers carefully worked out the anatomical connectivity and individual contributions of the various medial temporal lobe structures.

A more complete and accurate story began to unfold after anatomical studies revealed that the cortex immediately surrounding the hippocampus is highly interconnected with the hippocampus itself (Insausti et al., 1987). This parahippocampal region, including the perirhinal, entorhinal, and parahippocampal cortices, was typically damaged during the surgeries in which the amygdala or hippocampus was destroyed. Furthermore, the parahippocampal region was damaged to a greater extent when both the hippocampus and amygdala were lesioned together. Thus, a potential confound in the early behavioral studies was that the severity of the deficit might be due to the extent of parahippocampal region damage, as much as, or more so, than damage to the amygdala or hippocampus per se. Recognizing this problem, Murray, Mishkin and colleagues, and Zola-Morgan, Squire and their colleagues, examined the separate roles in memory of the amygdala, and the overlying parahippocampal region. Damage limited to the amygdala that spared the overlying cortex did not produce deficits in declarative memory. Furthermore, circumscribed lesions of the amygdala did not exacerbate the memory deficits seen after large lesions including the hippocampus (Zola-Morgan et al., 1989a). By contrast, damage to the overlying cortex that spared the hippocampus and amygdala, was sufficient in itself to produce severe declarative memory deficits in monkeys (Murray & Mishkin, 1986; Zola-Morgan et al., 1989b). Although many of the subtleties of function, and much of the connectivity, had yet to be fully characterized (see Section 10.2.1), the medial temporal lobe structures that are important for declarative memory had been identified (Squire & Zola-Morgan, 1991). By this view, the structures of the medial temporal lobe that are critical for memory include the hippocampus, and the parahippocampal region (including the perirhinal, entorhinal, and parahippocampal cortices). Together, these structures form a module for declarative memory that has been termed the "hippocampal memory system."

But before we move on to describe this system in detail, the initial behavioral findings, as well as more recent behavioral, anatomical, and neurophysiological studies, suggest the importance of a further component of the hippocampal memory system, namely the association neocortex. This region has received particular attention in recent human neuroimaging studies, which have suggested that the neocortex may normally interact with medial temporal lobe structures in memory storage and retrieval (e.g., Nyberg et al., 2000; Wheeler et al., 2000; for reviews see Buckner & Wheeler, 2001; Fletcher et al., 1997). The importance of the association neocortex is best illustrated by a consideration of the temporal specificity of memories dependent on the hippocampal system. Damage to the medial temporal lobe prevents the ability to form new long-term memories (anterograde amnesia), but spares short-term or immediate memory. It is generally believed that the neocortical areas that send inputs to the medial temporal lobe mediate this capacity for short-term memory and provide the gateway to the hippocampal system. Second, damage to the medial temporal lobe also results in a retrograde memory loss, characterized by impaired memory for information acquired recently before the brain damage, but spared memory for information acquired remotely before the damage. This observation indicates that the medial temporal lobe is not the final repository of memories. Rather, it is generally believed that the final repository for declarative memories is also in the association cortex. These two lines of evidence suggesting a critical role for the association cortex in declarative memory will be considered in turn.

A spared capacity for short-term memory can be dissociated from the deficit in long-term memory that is characteristic of human amnesia (Corkin, 1984; Squire et al., 1993). Human amnesic patients can acquire and immediately repeat a brief story or a short series of digits or words, even though their capacity to recall or recognize the items following a brief distraction is severely impaired (Drachman & Arbit, 1966). The same pattern of spared short-term or immediate memory and impaired long-term memory is also observed across a broad range of nonverbal materials (Milner, 1971). Furthermore, the same dissociation is observed in the performance of animals with medial temporal lobe damage on the DNMS task. Monkeys and rats with damage to medial temporal lobe structures are typically able to learn the task at a normal rate when trained with very short memory delays, but are impaired on the task when the memory delay interval is lengthened. This observation indicates that, like human amnesic patients, animals with medial temporal lobe damage have selective deficits in long-term memory, sparing of short-term memory as well as the perceptual and cognitive capacities and the motivation necessary for learning the task (Eichenbaum et al., 2000).

Conversely, evidence from a broad range of neuropsychological studies implicate the association neocortex in short-term and working memory in humans (Vallar & Shallice, 1990). Similarly, in animals, lesions of association cortex impair learning of the DNMS task even when trained with the briefest possible delay, suggesting an impairment in perception or in acquiring the task rules (Buffalo et al., 2000; Otto & Eichenbaum, 1992a; the role of specific structures in DNMS performance is discussed in more detail in later sections). Also, electrophysiological studies in monkeys have pointed to the role of association neocortex in forming and maintaining short-term representations of relevant stimuli during performance of a variety of short-term or working memory tasks (for reviews, see: Fuster, 1995; Goldman-Rakic, 1995; Miller, 2000). In these studies, neurons in the inferotemporal and prefrontal cortex often demonstrate stimulus-selective activation that is sustained after the offset of a memory cue and that is maintained until a delayed behavioral response is made. For example, Funahashi *et al.* (1989) found cells in prefrontal cortex that showed target-selective firing during the interval between the offset of a spatial memory target and the corresponding delayed oculomotor response. The combination of these studies suggest that one role of association neocortex in declarative memory is to briefly maintain sensory representations until they enter the domain of long-term memory.

In addition, neocortical association areas may be the ultimate site for storage of declarative memories. In addition to anterograde amnesia, damage to the medial temporal lobe results in a loss of memories acquired before the onset of amnesia. However, the retrograde memory loss in human amnesia is time-limited. It is characterized by a severe loss of memories that were acquired recently prior to the brain damage, and a relative sparing of childhood memories and general world knowledge that were acquired in early life (Corkin, 1984; Squire *et al.*, 1993). This pattern of temporally limited retrograde memory loss has also been successfully modeled in animals with medial temporal damage (see Squire & Alvarez, 1995 for a review). While the scope of memories involved in temporally graded retrograde amnesia remains controversial (e.g., Nadel & Moscovitch, 1997), recent work has indicated that the time-limited involvement of the hippocampal region is broad, extending to spatial as well as nonspatial memories (Teng & Squire, 1999). Moreover, the observation of a time-limited involvement of the medial temporal area indicates that this region cannot be the ultimate site of memory storage. Rather, the medial temporal region must be considered as critical for the formation of long-term memories, but not as the final storage site. By this view, the role of the medial temporal lobe is to facilitate the gradual establishment of long term memories elsewhere in the brain – a process called memory consolidation. The proposed ultimate storage site for long-term memory is the neocortical association areas that initially processed the to-be-learned information (Alvarez & Squire, 1994; Squire & Alvarez, 1995).

The findings outlined above suggest that functions of association neocortex are critical for normal declarative memory. Neocortex is likely involved in the short-term representation of sensory stimuli, and neocortex also serves as the ultimate storage site for declarative memories. These ideas are consistent with the interconnectivity of the cortex and temporal lobes outlined in Section 10.2.1. The interactions between the cortex and medial temporal areas subserving short-term memory and memory consolidation remain poorly understood. However, it is clear that components of the cerebral cortex are intimately involved in the hippocampal memory system, and understanding their role will be critical to understanding the operation of the full system. Some preliminary insights into the complementary roles of the cortex and hippocampal region will be discussed below.

In sum then, the work on animal models has been successful in replicating the hallmark features of human amnesia, including both the selective patterns of anterograde amnesia and temporally graded retrograde amnesia in the absence of other cognitive deficits (Eichenbaum, 1997; Squire, 1992). Also, the animal work has been critical to identifying the key structures for declarative memory, and to improving our understanding about the nature of memory processing by medial temporal structures. In the late 1980s, this work showed that the cortical structures adjacent to the hippocampus were critical for long-term memory. This led to a broader anatomical definition of the system that mediates declarative memory, expanding beyond a focus on hippocampus itself to include the parahippocampal region. Additionally, recent findings have focused attention on the role of association neocortex. Again, we need to broaden the anatomical definition of the hippocampal memory system to include critical contributions of these regions to normal declarative memory. Our goal in this chapter is to outline recent progress in characterizing the operation of the broader hippocampal memory system.

10.2   The organization of this chapter

Over the last several decades, substantial research has focused on iden-tifying the structures of the medial temporal lobe that are important for declarative memory, and to identify their separate contributions to memory. More recently, it is becoming clear that structures within the medial temporal region participate in a broader network that includes association neocortex. The purpose of this chapter is to discuss the functional contributions of major components of this system, and their interaction within this larger network. Each major component of this system – the hippocampus, the parahippocampal region, and the association neocortex – makes separate contributions to the formation and storage of declarative memories. We will discuss recent behavioral and neurophysiological findings, and relate them both to the anatomy of the hippocampal system and to current thinking about how the system may accomplish its mnemonic function.

The remainder of this chapter is divided into four sections. The first section will begin with a description of the anatomical connectivity of the broader hippocampal memory system. In the next three sections, we will discuss the individual contributions to memory of each of the three major components of this system. The second section of this chapter discusses the function of the hippocampus proper. The third section discusses the distinct contribution of the parahippocampal region, including the perirhinal and entorhinal cortices. This section will deal primarily with direct comparisons between the functional roles of the hippocampus and the parahippocampal region. The fourth section will discuss the contribution of association neocortex in the ultimate storage of declarative memories. While the chapter will focus primarily on findings from rats and monkeys, we will also consider some recent important findings from human subjects.

10.2.1   Anatomical pathways

The three components of the broader hippocampal memory system include the hippocampus, the parahippocampal region (including the entorhinal, perirhinal, and parahippocampal/postrhinal cortex), and neocortical association areas. The anatomy of this system is illustrated in Figure 10.1. It turns out that the anatomical connectivity of these regions has been extremely helpful in making sense of how the individual components of the system contribute to memory, and how they interact with one another.

Using animals, a large body of neuroanatomical tracer studies has outlined the neural pathways through the hippocampal memory system (Burwell & Amaral, 1998; Deacon *et al.*, 1983; Martin-Elkins & Horel, 1992; Suzuki & Amaral, 1994; Van Hoesen & Pandya, 1975a,b; Van Hoesen *et al.*, 1972, 1975). The pathways through this system are largely similar in rats and primates. Broadly outlined, information flow through the hippocampal memory system is marked by hierarchical stages of processing, involving convergence of information from neocortex to the parahippocampal region, then to the hippocampus. A corresponding set of back projections involves divergent projections from the hippocampus, returning to the parahippocampal region, which, in turn, sends major projections back to several areas of the neocortex (Suzuki & Eichenbaum, 2000). The projections to the parahippocampal region arise from virtually every neocortical association area (Burwell & Amaral, 1998; Suzuki & Amaral, 1994). Each of these cortical outputs projects to one or more subdivisions of the parahippocampal region (Burwell *et al.*, 1995; Suzuki, 1996). All of the areas of the parahippocampal region in turn project to multiple subdivisions of the hippocampus itself, including the dentate gyrus, CA3, CA1, as well as the adjacent subiculum. Thus, the parahippocampal region serves as a convergence site for cortical input and distributes these inputs within the hippocampus. The hippocampus supports mechanisms of plasticity that could mediate the rapid coding of new conjunctions of information (Bliss & Collingridge, 1993) within its broadly convergent and divergent intrinsic connections (Amaral & Witter,

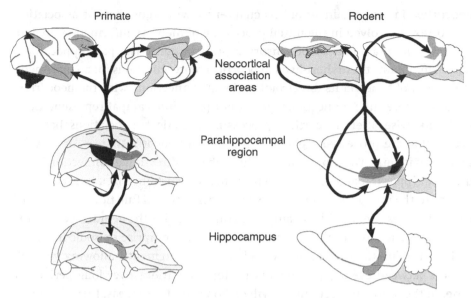

Figure 10.1 Anatomy of the hippocampal memory system. The connectivity of the hippocampal memory system is similar in rats and monkeys. The parahippocampal region (middle) receives projections from all neocortical association areas (top). The parahippocampal region, including the perirhinal cortex (*medium grey*) entorhinal cortex (*light grey*), and parahippocampal/postrhinal cortex (*dark grey*), in turn provide the majority of the cortical input to the hippocampus (bottom). Therefore, the parahippocampal region is a site of convergence for cortical afferent input and distributes these inputs to the hippocampus. The hippocampus itself, through a wide network of convergent and divergent intrinsic connections, could support a large network of associations or conjunctions of information. Hippocampal processing is directed back to the parahippocampal cortex through its reciprocal connections with this region. Likewise, the output of the parahippocampal region is distributed through reciprocal connections to the cortical areas that originally processed the information (adapted from Eichenbaum, 2000).

1989). The output from the hippocampus is directed back to the entire parahippocampal region, and then to the same neocortical association areas from which the input originated (Burwell & Amaral, 1998; Suzuki & Amaral, 1994). This pattern of neuroanatomical pathways is consistent with the idea that there is a broad convergence of sensory information onto the hippocampal system. Furthermore, through backprojections, the hippocampus and parahippocampal region are positioned to alter the nature, persistence and organization of memory representations within neocortex.

The anatomical connectivity of these regions suggests a functional organization for the broader hippocampal system, with three distinct but related levels of processing, specifically in the hippocampus, parahippocampal region, and neocortex. In the remainder of this chapter we will argue that the association neocortex is involved in the initial processing of memory information, including the brief maintenance of sensory representations. The parahippocampal region maintains these short-lived neocortical representations for an intermediate period of time via its direct bidirectional connections with the neocortex. Through these interconnections, persistent parahippocampal representations could likewise alter neocortical processing to reflect associations between events that are processed separately in different neocortical areas, or that are separated in time. The hippocampus, through its bidirectional connections with the parahippocampal region, is also privy to these sustained representations, as well as to the integration of information across time and functional domains of cortical processing. The hippocampus, in turn, contains the neural mechanisms for rapidly encoding the sequences of events that comprise episodic memory, and for linking these episodes by their common elements, allowing generalization between events, and for linking representations over long periods of time. In the following sections we will elaborate on these ideas, first describing the role of the hippocampus in declarative memory, then the role of the parahippocampal region, and finally the role of the association neocortex.

10.2.2   *The role of the hippocampus in memory*

Reports of human patients with damage limited to the hippocampus are relatively rare in the literature (Rempel-Clower *et al.*, 1996; Vargha-Khadem *et al.*, 1997; Victor & Agamanolis, 1990; Zola-Morgan, *et al.*, 1986), so it is particularly important that carefully controlled lesion studies in animals have been successful in producing many of the central aspects of human amnesia. Some of the properties of declarative memory in humans, in particular, the access to conscious recollection, cannot be examined directly in animal models. However, other aspects of declarative memory can be studied in animals. Declarative memories are acquired through the record of everyday personal experience. In humans, hippocampal damage disrupts "episodic memory" (Vargha-Khadem *et al.*, 1997), as well as the development of the general semantic network in which episodic memories reside (Squire & Zola, 1998). For example, a typical episodic memory might include memory of where one parked a car on the streets of Boston and memory for the subsequent path taken in walking to one's workplace. This representation would include the sequence of events, places passed, and the route taken while walking from the car to work. This memory is not in isolation but is integrated within general knowledge of the streets in the vicinity of one's workplace, which, in turn, has been developed in large part from a synthesis of many episodic memories from other days of parking one's car and walking via different paths to work.

In humans, the declarative memory for this episodic and semantic information is expressed through conscious, effortful recollection. Furthermore, the contents of memory for episodic and semantic information can be accessed flexibly. In the case of the example above, one might be able to recollect several intersecting paths and describe alternative routes to and from the car and work. In this way, declarative memories can be used to solve new problems by recovering several related memories and then making inferences from relations among the stored information from each memory. In the example above, this use of declarative memory would be reflected in a capacity for novel route-finding. This is an example of a 'memory space,' a network of memories whose development and use is mediated by hippocampal function (Eichenbaum *et al.*, 1999). By this view, declarative memory is comprised of a wide range of these networks organized by episodic memories that are linked via common events and places.

10.3   Animal models of hippocampal function

Animal research has sought to relate the properties of declarative memory to memory performance. One way to assess declarative memory capacity is to study the creation of memory spaces from overlapping experiences. Animals can be trained on distinct episodes that share common elements and then asked to solve new problems using inferences from their acquired knowledge. This approach has been applied in a large number of domains, including learning about spatial relationships between items in the environment, categorizing of foods, organizing odor and visual stimuli, and learning social relationships.

Probably the best known experimental protocol for assessing hippocampal function is spatial learning, similar to the route-finding example described above. In this case, simply requiring animals to synthesize several overlapping experiences (routes) is sufficient to require hippocampal function. For example, in the Morris water maze task, rats learn to escape from cloudy water in a swimming pool by climbing onto a platform submerged just below the surface of the water. The platform is always in the same position relative to several distant, fixed spatial cues. In the conventional version of this task, rats must learn the position of the escape platform in relation to four separate starting points, and therefore must learn four separate routes to the common goal. Importantly, rats with hippocampal damage fail to learn the position of the platform in relation to the distal cues (Morris *et al.*, 1982). But when the demand for integrating across episodes is removed, by always starting the rat in the same position relative to the escape platform, rats with damage to this system (specifically, fornix damage) learn the task quickly (Eichenbaum *et al.*, 1990). Although rats with fornix damage learned this version of the task, further probe testing revealed that they did not learn the task in the same way as normal animals. In probe tests, rats with fornix damage that had already learned the position of the escape platform relative to one start position were now started at a new position. From this new position they were unable to find the escape platform readily, even though they had successfully navigated to it from the original position. By contrast, normal rats located the platform quickly on probe trials (Eichenbaum *et al.*, 1990). This finding demonstrates that the hippocampal system is required for new problem solving even in familiar environments.

Another task with the same formal demand of flexibly using familiar knowledge to solve a new problem is the social transmission of food preferences task. In this task, a rat is allowed to interact socially with a "demonstrator" rat that has recently eaten a novel food. During this interaction, the subject sniffs the breath of the demonstrator and acquires an association between the novel food odor and a particular constituent of the demonstrator's breath, carbon disulfide (Galef *et al.*, 1988). The test of the flexible expression of this association is that rats will now preferentially eat the demonstrated food, even in the absence of the social context present during learning. The normal memory for this association, expressed as a food preference in a choice between the demonstrated and another food, may last days or even weeks. Rats with selective lesions of the hippocampus show a preference for the demonstrated food when tested immediately after the social encounter, but no memory when tested 24 hours later (Bunsey & Eichenbaum, 1995; Winocur, 1990). This pattern of spared short-term memory and impaired long-term memory is, of course, a hallmark feature of human amnesia. These findings also show that the hippocampus is not essential for the perceptual or motivational components of learning, for the social interaction, or for expression of the food preference. The hippocampus *is* critical, however, for the flexible representation of a long-term memory for a single social episode.

Tests of transitive inference have also been used to demonstrate that flexible expression of memory depends on the hippocampus. In this line of experiments, animals with selective damage to the hippocampus are able to learn a set of distinct, overlapping experiences, but are unable to express their memories when asked to make inferences based upon the linkage of these experiences. In one protocol, rats were trained on a series of odor–odor associations (Bunsey & Eichenbaum, 1996). On each trial, one of two odors was presented, followed by a choice between that odor's "associate" which was baited, and a foil odor which was not baited (A goes with B, not X; X goes with Y, not B). Following training on the first set of two paired associates, rats were trained on a second, overlapping set (B goes with C; Y goes with Z). Rats were then given probe tests to assess their ability to infer indirect relationships among the odors, specifically the indirect association between odors A and C and between X and Z. Both normal rats and rats with hippocampal damage rapidly learned the original odor–odor associations. Normal rats were then able to show in two ways that they could link these overlapping experiences to make inferences. First, intact rats were able to make transitive inferences about indirect relations among the odor pairings that contained a shared item. Having learned that A goes with B, and that B goes with C, they inferred that A goes with C. Second, intact rats demonstrated symmetry within paired-associates. Having learned that B goes with C, they inferred that C goes with B. Rats with selective hippocampal lesions, despite the fact that they could learn the odor–odor associations, were unable to demonstrate either transitivity or symmetry.

In a second protocol, rats were trained on the classic transitive inference task (Dusek & Eichenbaum, 1997), in which rats had to make inferences about the hierarchical organization of a set of odors that were presented as overlapping pairwise discriminations. Rats sequentially learned the premise pairs: A > B, B > C, C > D, and D > E, in which the ">" indicates that the first item in the pair is to be selected (i.e., is rewarded) over the second item (i.e., is not rewarded). Once the rats learned the premise pairs, they were then tested on the four premise pairs in random order, together with occasional probe trials for the critical test of transitivity, B vs. D. Normal rats acquired each of the initial premise pairs and showed robust transitivity by choosing odor B over odor D. In this way, they demonstrated that they were able to link information acquired about the odors in separate experiences and were able to infer the hierarchical structure of the series. Rats with hippocampal damage were able to learn the premise pairs as well as normal rats, but they showed no ability to make the transitive judgment. These last two studies indicate that the hippocampus itself is not necessary for the acquisition of some forms of stimulus–stimulus associations. However, in the absence of a hippocampus, representations of these associations are "hyperspecific" and can be expressed only within the context of the original learning (Schacter, 1985). The hippocampus is necessary if separate experiences are to be linked in such a way to support flexible or inferential expression of the memories.

10.4   Neurophysiology of hippocampal function

Observations from electrophysiological recordings from neurons in the hippocampal region are largely consistent with the ideas presented in the preceding section. These findings support the notion that hippocampal networks represent the sequences of places and events that compose episodic memories. The firing patterns of hippocampal neurons reflect both conjunctions of events and places that define specific episodes, as well as features common to related episodes.

O'Keefe and Dostrovsky (1971) first reported that principal cells of the hippocampus fired when a rat was in a particular location in its environment. These "place" cells have been used as evidence for the selective role of the hippocampus in spatial mapping (O'Keefe & Nadel, 1978). But hippocampal cells do not simply fire in response to spatial stimuli and locations, they also show changes in firing patterns related to conditioned behavioral responses in eyeblink classical conditioning (Berger et al., 1976), related to olfactory cues (Wood et al., 1999; Wiebe & Stäubli, 1999, 2001), and in human neurosurgical patients, related to categories of visual stimuli (Fried et al., 1997). Furthermore, the pattern of activity of place cells is not determined entirely by an animal's location. Activity can also be strongly affected by the direction and speed of movement of the rat (McNaughton et al., 1983; Muller et al., 1994), by the position of the movement goal (Gothard et al., 1996), and by the behavioral demands of the task (Markus et al., 1995; Wiener et al., 1989).

As mentioned in the previous section, one way to conceptualize episodic memory is that it is comprised of stored sequences of events and places where these events occurred. Some of the most illuminating studies on the nature of the information represented by hippocampal cells are studies in which animals learn behavioral sequences. In each of several such studies, the firing of hippocampal neurons has been related to a broad range of events (Eichenbaum et al., 1999). For example, in tasks where rats were required to shuttle back and forth between a common start position and one or more goal positions, different place cells fire when the rat is in different positions along the path between the start and the goal. These cells fire sequentially, each cell firing when the rat reaches the cell's preferred position along the pathway. On the return trip, a largely different set of place cells fires as the animal passes through the same positions (Gothard et al., 1996; McNaughton et al., 1983; Muller et al., 1994; Wiener et al., 1989). Thus, each cell could be characterized as being a part of a hippocampal network representing the episode of either the outbound or inbound journey, as if the network maintains a 'videoclip' of the trial episode in which each cell represents where the rat was and what it was doing in a particular "frame" of the clip (Eichenbaum, 2000).

Similarly, hippocampal principal cells fire in relation to specific task events as rats perform a variety of simple and complex learning tasks (Berger et al., 1976; Wiener et al., 1989). For example, during odor discrimination learning, different hippocampal cells fire sequentially as a rat approaches an odor port, samples the odor stimuli, executes the appropriate behavioral responses, and consumes the reward (Wiener et al., 1989). As in the spatial memory tasks described above, the findings from odor discrimination learning are consistent with the notion that hippocampal networks represent sequences of events in each trial, with each cell encoding one specific behavioral event together with the place where that behavior occurred.

A key observation is that some hippocampal cells fire only during particular kinds of episodes, such as when the odor stimuli are presented in a particular configuration. The location of the animal in space is sometimes irrelevant. In addition, other cells fire during events or in places common to every trial, such as during the approach to the stimulus sampling location in each trial. This pattern of findings was apparent in the results from a recent recording study of rats performing an odor recognition memory task. Hippocampal neurons were monitored while rats performed the same DNMS task at different places in an open field. The activity of some hippocampal cells was associated with specific combinations of events and places that were unique to a given trial, whereas the activity of other cells was associated with events or places that were common across many related trials (Wood et al., 1999). As in the previous studies, different cells fired during distinct and sequential trial events. Some fired in relation to almost unique events, such as when a particular odor was presented in a particular place. Other cells fired in relation to features that were common across trials. Some cells fired when the rat approached an odor stimulus, or when the rat sampled a particular odor, regardless of where the odor was presented on the open field. Conversely, other cells always fired when the rat was in a particular position, regardless of the odor that was presented there (Figure 10.2).

There is also evidence that hippocampal cells can code for information about specific *types* of episodes, even when the animal's behavior, and the locations of the behavioral episodes, are identical. In one study involving a spatially cued variant of the DNMS task, Hampson et al. (1999) described hippocampal cells that fired when a rat pressed one of two levers, specifically during the sample or the test phase of the task. These cells can be characterized as encoding the conjunction of sample or test event, and the place where it was performed, each of which is a single event (defined temporally, spatially, and behaviorally) within a broader framework of particular types of trial episodes. Other cells fired when the rat pressed one of the two levers, regardless of the phase of the task, and other cells fired during one phase of the task, regardless of the position of the rat in space. Thus, as in other experiments described above, some hippocampal cells seem to code for the highly specific conjunctions of events within particular types of episodes, while other cells code for elements of these events

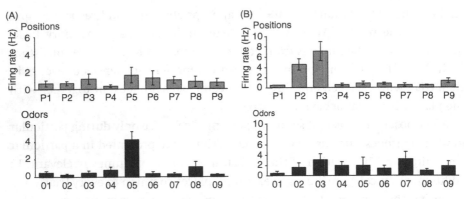

Figure 10.2 Patterns of neuronal activity in the hippocampus of rats performing a version of the DNMS task in which the stimuli were nine different odors, and trials were performed in nine different locations. Some cells in the hippocampus fire when the rat approaches a particular odor regardless of its position. Other cells code particular positions, regardless of the odor presented there. Panel (A) illustrates a cell that fires selectively to odor 5 (O5), but does not fire differentially among positions (P1–P9) in which the task was performed. The cell in panel (B) fires preferentially in positions 2 and 3 (P2 & P3), but does not have a selective odor response (adapted from Wood *et al.*, 1999).

that are common across different types of episodes. The latter cells could link representations of the different types of trials. Most interestingly, the functional anatomy of the hippocampus may lend itself to this sort of organization, because Hampson *et al.* found cells responsive to spatial position and cells responsive to phase of the trial to be topographically clustered within the dorsal hippocampus.

More direct evidence of episodic-like representation by hippocampal networks comes from another report by Wood *et al.* (2000). In this study, hippocampal cells were recorded in rats performing a spatial alternation task in a T-maze. On each trial, a rat had to traverse the stem of the maze, and then make a left or a right turn into one of the two choice arms of the maze. At the choice point, the rat had to remember which direction it turned on the previous trial and then make the opposite choice. Importantly, the behavior of the rat was identical as it traversed the stem of the maze on every trial, until it arrived at the locus where it made its behavioral choice. As expected, Wood *et al.* found that different hippocampal cells fired sequentially as the rat passed through the various locations on the maze. In addition, the future path of the rat strongly modulated the firing of these cells. Despite the similarity in overt behavior and in the set of locations traversed on the stem of the maze, some cells fired selectively on trials when the rat was *going* to make a left turn at the choice

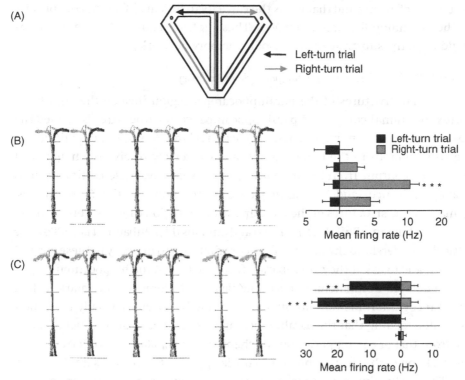

Figure 10.3   Patterns of neuronal activity in the hippocampus of rats performing a continuous T-maze alternation task. (A) Schematic view of the T-maze in which rats traversed the stem of the maze on each trial and alternated between left and right turns at the T-junction. Water rewards were provided at water ports (small circles) for each correct alternation. (B & C) The firing patterns of two hippocampal cells. (B) This cell fired almost exclusively on right-turn trials. (C) This cell fired almost exclusively on left-turn trials. For each cell, the paths taken by the rat are shown in the left panel. The second and third panels indicate the location of the rat when individual spikes occurred separately for left-turn and right-turn trials, respectively. For each cell the right panel shows the mean firing rate of the cell for each of the four sectors of the maze stem, with the firing rate adjusted to eliminate variability associated with the animal's head direction and speed (adapted from Wood et al., 2000).

point, and other cells fired selectively when the rat was *going* to make a right turn (Figure 10.3). Many of these cells fired to some extent when the rat was at a common location on all trials. Thus, the hippocampus distinctly encoded the left-turn and right-turn episodes as distinct representations within a broader network that also included common elements by which the distinct representations could be linked. This evidence, consistent with the findings from the other studies described above, indicates that the hippocampus encodes specific sequences of events and that it has the capacity to link distinct types of episodes by their common features and places. These linked, sequential representations could form the substrate of an episodic memory network.

10.4.1   *The role of the parahippocampal region in memory*

The structures of the parahippocampal region include the entorhinal cortex, perirhinal cortex, and parahippocampal cortex (the latter is termed the postrhinal cortex in rats). These cortical regions provide the majority of the cortical input to the hippocampus, and conversely receive the majority of the cortical output from the hippocampus. Presumably, these cortical regions heavily influence (and are influenced by) processing in the hippocampus. Damage to the structures of the parahippocampal region causes severe memory deficits in humans (Buffalo *et al.*, 1998) and animals (Eichenbaum *et al.*, 2000). It is critical to understand the nature of the contributions to memory of these cortical regions, and to ask if they are separate from the role of the hippocampus.

The delayed nonmatching to sample task has become a benchmark task of visual recognition memory in the monkey, and has been especially important for understanding that the parahippocampal region has a role distinct in memory from that of the hippocampus (Eichenbaum *et al.*, 2000). During training in this task, on each trial the monkey is initially presented with a 'sample' stimulus. Then following a minimal (5–8 seconds) memory delay, the monkey is presented in the test phase with a choice between the sample and another novel stimulus. Reward is given for selecting the novel (nonmatching) stimulus and not the stimulus identical to the sample (the matching choice stimulus). Once monkeys have learned the nonmatching rule, they are tested at progressively longer delay intervals. Typically, monkeys with damage to all or part of the parahippocampal region do well remembering the sample when the memory delay interval is relatively short. However, when the delay is lengthened to increase memory demands, severe deficits emerge (Figure 10.4, *left*; Meunier *et al.*, 1993; Zola-Morgan *et al.*, 1989b). However, in these reports, monkeys with parahippocampal region damage require more trials than normal monkeys to learn the nonmatching rule. This finding leaves open the question of whether the parahippocampal region may be important for perception or short-term memory. Recent studies have addressed this issue using an automated testing apparatus that allows training with very brief memory delays. These studies have demonstrated that monkeys with damage including the parahippocampal region are able to learn the nonmatching rule normally with very short (0.5 second) delays between the sample and choice (Alvarez *et al.*, 1994; Buffalo *et al.*, 2000), indicating that poor performance on the delay portion of the task is not due to perceptual or motivational problems.

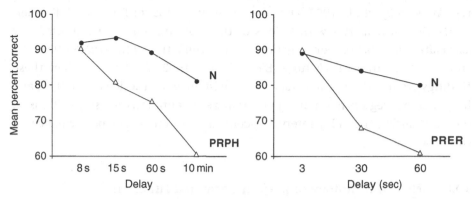

Figure 10.4 Performance of monkeys (left) and rats (right) on the delayed non-matching to sample task. Normal animals (N) of both species perform correctly on approximately 90% of the trials when the memory delay is brief, and show very most forgetting when the delay is lengthened. In both species, animals with lesions of the parahippocampal region perform as well as normal animals when the memory delay interval is relatively short, but demonstrate impaired memory when the interval is lengthened. N – normal control animals; PRPH – monkeys with lesions of the para-hippocampal region (including the perirhinal and the parahippocampal cortex; Zola-Morgan *et al.*, 1989b); PRER – rats with lesions of the perirhinal and entorhinal cortices (Otto & Eichenbaum, 1992a).

Importantly, the pattern of deficits in DNMS is different following lesions of the parahippocampal region, the hippocampus, or the neocortex. Deficits on DNMS performance following parahippocampal damage are more severe than those following damage limited to the hippocampus (Murray & Mishkin, 1998; Zola *et al.*, 2000) or its primary subcortical input, the fornix (Gaffan, 1994). By contrast, damage to visual association cortex (area TE) impairs learning of the task even at the briefest of delays (Buffalo *et al.*, 2000). This latter finding suggests that area TE is involved in perceptual processes or short-term memory that are important for the performance of the DNMS rather than in long-term memory *per se*.

A similar pattern of results has been observed in parallel studies in rats (Figure 10.4, *right*). One of these studies examined the effects of damage to different brain areas on performance of an odor-guided version of the DNMS task. In this study, rats with lesions of the parahippocampal region were able to learn the task at the normal rate, and continued to perform well at the briefest delay intervals. However, these rats were impaired when the delay between sample and choice was lengthened beyond a few seconds, indicating a deficit in their ability to maintain the memory for the sample stimulus. Also, in rats, as in monkeys, damage to the hippocampal region produces less severe impairment on nonspatial versions of the DNMS than does damage to the parahippocampal region (Mumby *et al.*, 1992; Otto & Eichenbaum, 1992b; Rothblat & Kromer, 1991). By contrast, rats with lesions of the orbitofrontal cortex (an olfactory association neocortex) were impaired on the acquisition of the DNMS rule at the shortest delay intervals (Otto & Eichenbaum, 1992a). Taken together, these findings from monkeys and rats are consistent with the idea that the parahippocampal region maintains persistent representations for single items in memory during the delay interval, a central requirement for performance on the DNMS task.

10.5   Neurophysiology of parahippocampal function

Electrophysiological studies of single unit activity have supported the view of parahippocampal function described in the previous section. These recordings, from the parahippocampal region in both rats and monkeys, have provided clues about the neural coding mechanisms that underlie DNMS performance. In general, three kinds of responses have been observed (Suzuki & Eichenbaum, 2000; Young *et al.*, 1997). First, some cells show enhanced firing in relation to one or a few stimuli, and not to others. Therefore, these cells demonstrate coding of the identity of individual stimuli while the stimuli were present. Second, some cells maintain stimulus-specific firing during the delay interval when the sample cue is no longer present. These cells demonstrate a persistent memory representation of the sample stimulus (Figure 10.5). Third, many cells show an increase or a decrease in firing rate to familiar stimuli when they reappear during the choice phase of the task. Interestingly, a recent study examining unit activity in the human entorhinal cortex and hippocampus also found changes in firing rate related to the familiarity of stimuli (Fried *et al.*, 1997). In particular, the stimulus-specific suppression of neuronal firing to repeated stimuli can be long-lasting (Fahy *et al.*, 1993; Xiang & Brown, 1998).

Each of these three types of responses has been observed in the perirhinal and entorhinal cortex of monkeys performing a visual delayed matching to sample task (Miller *et al.*, 1991, 1993; Suzuki *et al.*, 1997). However, differences between the specific tasks used in rat and monkey studies (especially visual vs. olfactory modality) make direct comparisons difficult (Suzuki & Eichenbaum, 2000). Nevertheless, it is likely that the perirhinal and entorhinal cortex, because of their different patterns of input, may contribute to memory in different ways. For instance, the perirhinal cortex receives a prominant input from unimodal visual areas, while the entorhinal cortex receives strong inputs from olfactory areas (Deacon *et al.*, 1983; Suzuki & Amaral, 1994). So the perirhinal cortex may be more important for visual recognition memory, while the entorhinal cortex is more important for olfactory memory. Consistent with this

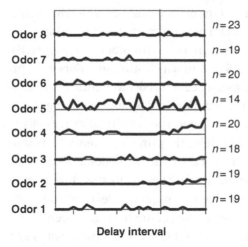

Figure 10.5 Example of an entorhinal cortex neuron with a persistent representation of an odor stimulus. This cell was recorded from the entorhinal cortex of a rat performing an odor version of the DNMS. Sustained firing is apparent during the delay interval after the presentation of odor 5, but not following the presentation of any of the other seven odors (adapted from Young *et al.*, 1992).

idea is that in the monkey there was found to be a preponderance of visually stimulus-selective cells in the perirhinal cortex (Suzuki *et al.*, 1997), while in the rat a preponderance of olfactory selective cells was found in the entorhinal cortex (Young *et al.*, 1997).

10.6   Comparison of coding mechanisms in the hippocampus and parahippocampal region

The studies that have used the DNMS task indicate that the parahippocampal region and hippocampus encode information differently. Cells in the parahippocampal region provide two types of memory signals that could guide performance in the task (Young *et al.*, 1997). Some cells show sustained stimulus-selective firing during the memory delay in the absence of the sample stimulus. Other cells show differential responses to the memory test stimuli depending on whether the stimulus is a match or a nonmatch. In contrast with the stimulus-selective activity of neurons in the parahippocampal region, cells in the hippocampus convey more abstract recognition memory signals. In one study (Otto & Eichenbaum, 1992b), no cells with sustained, stimulus-selective firing were found in the hippocampus. Instead, some cells recorded in the rat hippocampus during the DNMS task fire differently on match and nonmatch trials, and this firing is similar for *all* match and nonmatch stimuli. These observations suggest that the outcome of the match or nonmatch judgment is being encoded.

While early reports failed to demonstrate stimulus-selective firing in the hippocampus, more recent reports have shown that stimulus identity may be encoded by the hippocampus in conjunction with other task events. For example, in a novel version of the DNMS task in which stimulus odors were presented in several places, some hippocampal cells fired differentially on match and nonmatch trials, irrespective of odor identity (an abstract recognition signal, similar to that described above). However, the activity of other cells reflected more specific information. For example, they fired differentially when a given odor was presented in a particular place, or when an odor appeared as a match or nonmatch stimulus (Wood *et al.*, 1999). These cells therefore demonstrated the 'episode-specific' coding described in sequence learning tasks discussed above. Similar patterns of episode-specific coding have also been found in rats performing a spatial delayed match to sample task (Hampson *et al.*, 1993) and in rats performing an olfactory delayed nonmatching to sample task (Wiebe & Stäubli, 1999). Hippocampal cells may represent stimulus-specific information particularly when task demands require distinguishing and linking different types of related trials, as was the case in each of the studies discussed above.

The differences between the representations encoded by cells in the parahippocampal region and the hippocampus may be understood in terms of the connectivity of these regions. The parahippocampal region receives a convergence of inputs from neocortical regions that process information within distinct functional domains. Accordingly, the parahippocampal region is in an ideal position to have access to and to maintain information about stimulus identity. By contrast, the hippocampus receives convergent cortical input primarily from the parahippocampal region. The hippocampus is therefore in a position to combine information about a broad variety of events and places, and to abstract common information from these signals. Via backprojections, these representations could be used to establish selective representations in neocortex.

10.6.1   *The role of association neocortex in memory*

According to the view developed in this chapter, the association neocortex is the source of the sensory signals sent via the parahippocampal region to the hippocampus. Conversely, the neocortex receives memory signals from the hippocampal region via reciprocal backprojections through the parahippocampal region. One would therefore predict that lesions of association cortex would affect performance on memory tasks, and that neurons in association cortex represent both sensory information and memory information. Further, one would predict that memory representations in association neocortex are dependent on the integrity of the hippocampus and the parahippocampal region.

Emerging evidence suggests that neocortical association areas play a critical role in declarative memory that is distinct and complementary to the role of the parahippocampal region. Lesions of orbitofrontal cortex (an olfactory association area) in the rat impair learning of the nonmatching rule in an odor-guided version of the DNMS. Because the rule is learned at a delay that is brief enough to involve only the most minimal memory demands, this finding suggests that the orbitofrontal cortex is important either for perceptual processing or for learning the nonmatching rule. By contrast, rats with lesions of the parahippocampal region learn the task at a normal rate, but are impaired when the memory demand is increased by lengthening the delay interval between sample and choice (Otto & Eichenbaum, 1992a). Findings from monkeys parallel the findings from rats. In monkeys, lesions of a visual association cortex (area TE) impair learning of the nonmatching rule on a visual version of the DNMS, while lesions of the perirhinal cortex impair performance on the delay portion of the task (Buffalo et al., 1999, 2000). There is a dissociation based on anatomical boundaries between a role in perceptual processes for association cortex function and a distinct role in memory for the parahippocampal region.

A recent study in our laboratory with rats directly compared the firing of neurons in the orbitofrontal cortex with those in the parahippocampal region (Ramus & Eichenbaum, 2000). Cells in the orbitofrontal cortex demonstrated all of the characteristics of cells recorded in the parahippocampal region: namely, in orbitofrontal cells, we found stimulus-specific firing, sustained stimulus-specific firing during the delay interval, and differential firing on match and nonmatch trials (Figure 10.6), the same three properties observed in the parahippocampal region. This suggests that the orbitofrontal cortex shares much information with parahippocampal region, an observation consistent with the interconnectivity of these regions.

However, there were two key differences between the firing of neurons in these two regions (Figure 10.7). First, we found more cells in the parahippocampal region than in orbitofrontal cortex that demonstrated sustained delay firing, whereas we found more cells in the orbitofrontal cortex that demonstrated stimulus-selective match suppression or match enhancement. The proportion of cells in orbitofrontal cortex that displayed match suppression or match enhancement increased with performance of the rat on the DNMS task (Figure 10.8). Together with the finding that orbitofrontal lesions impair acquisition of the DNMS task (Otto & Eichenbaum, 1992a), the finding that orbitofrontal neurons prominently code the critical match or nonmatch judgment suggests that the orbitofrontal cortex may play a key role in the abstraction and representation of the nonmatching rule.

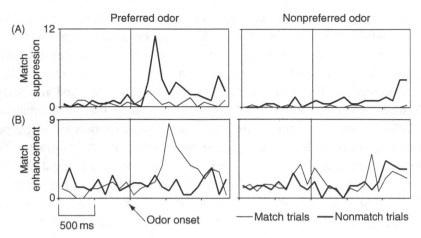

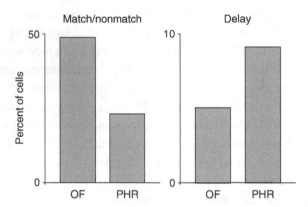

Figure 10.6   Examples of two association neocortex neurons with odor-selective enhancement or suppression of firing responses to a match stimulus. These cells were recorded in the orbitofrontal cortex of rats performing an odor-guided version of the DNMS. *Dark lines* indicate average firing rates on nonmatch trials; *light lines* indicate average firing rates on match trials. (A) Example of a match suppression cell. (B) Example of a match enhancement cell (from Ramus & Eichenbaum, 2000).

Figure 10.7   Differences in the distribution of firing patterns of cells in association neocortex and the parahippocampal region. These cells were recorded in the orbito-frontal cortex (OF; Ramus & Eichenbaum, 2000) and the parahippocampal region (PHR; Young *et al.*, 1992) of rats, performing an odor version of the DNMS. A greater proportion of cells in the OF demonstrated stimulus-selective match enhancement or suppression, while a greater proportion of cells in the PHR demonstrated sustained stimulus-selective firing during the delay interval.

Second, the firing of cells in the orbitofrontal cortex was more complex than the firing of cells recorded in the parahippocampal region – cells fired in relation to more task events or to complex behavioral states of the rat. Together, these findings from orbitofrontal neurons are consistent with the

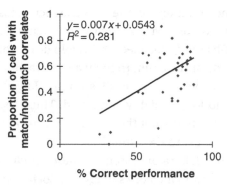

Figure 10.8 The proportion of cells in association neocortex that demonstrate stimulus-selective match enhancement or suppression varies with performance. This figure represents the proportion of odor-selective match/nonmatch cells recorded in orbitofrontal cortex of the rat as a function of performance on the odor-guided version of the DNMS task. The number of match/nonmatch cells recorded in the orbitofrontal cortex during a given session increased as the performance of the rat improved (adapted from Ramus & Eichenbaum, 2000).

idea that the orbitofrontal cortex is a "mixing pot" for sensory signals originating from piriform cortex and memory signals arising in the parahippocampal region. They also suggest that the orbitofrontal cortex participates both in the memory representations for specific stimuli and in the acquisition and application of task rules. Similar findings have been reported in the monkey lateral prefrontal cortex (Miller et al., 1996). Although task and species differences make direct comparison to the rodent work difficult, Miller and coworkers have come to similar conclusions about the role of prefrontal cortex in recognition memory performance (Miller, 2000).

Several studies in monkeys have examined the origin of the sensory and memory signals in association cortex. In these studies, monkeys were implanted with electrodes in either area TE, or in both TE and the perirhinal cortex. Sakai and Miyashita (1991) found stimulus-selective cells in anterior inferotemporal cortex with two memory properties. The first type of cell, "pair-coding" neurons, fired maximally to presentations of either of two previously learned paired-associates, but not to other stimuli involved in other pairings (i.e., the firing of cells became highly correlated for the items in each paired-associate). The second type of cell, "pair-recall" neurons, showed sustained firing during the delay when the paired-associate of the cell's optimal stimulus was used as the sample. These two types of cells were found in both the parahippocampal region *and* in area TE. Neuronal representations of paired-associates in area TE develop during learning and with a time-course that parallel behavioral learning (Messinger et al., 2001). To examine the origin of these memory signals,

Higuchi and Miyashita (1996) trained monkeys on the paired-associate task, and then recorded from TE neurons in monkeys with and without unilateral lesions of the parahippocampal region. Observing the electrophysiological properties of the cells in TE on the lesioned side of the brain, Higuchi and Miyashita found that cells maintained their responsiveness to visual stimuli. However, the responses to paired-stimuli were no longer highly correlated. Thus, lesions of the parahippocampal region appeared to disrupt the associative code in area TE without impairing visual responsiveness to the stimuli.

A more recent study from the same laboratory extended these conclusions by examining the time-course of sensory and memory signals in association cortex and the parahippocampal region. Simultaneous recordings in TE and in perirhinal cortex revealed that the latency of the visual response was shorter in TE than in the perirhinal cortex, consistent with the forward propagation of these sensory signals. Conversely, pair-recall cells showed increases in firing rate with a shorter latency in perirhinal cortex than in area TE, consistent with the backward propagation of the memory signal from the parahippocampal region to association neocortex (Naya et al., 2001). These findings support the view developed here that sensory signals arising in neocortex propagate through the hippocampal memory system, where they are attached with mnemonic information. These mnemonic signals then propagate backwards through the network to the association areas that originally processed the information. This view is consistent with the expectation that both sensory and memory information should be represented by cells in the association neocortex. In addition, the findings are consistent with the idea that association cortex, the parahippocampal region, and the hippocampus, all contribute to memory in different, but complementary ways.

10.7   Conclusions

The studies described here support a model of declarative memory based on the known anatomical connectivity of three separate regions of the "broader" hippocampal memory system – the hippocampus, the parahippocampal region, and association neocortex. By this view, association neocortex initially processes sensory and behavioral information, and can maintain this information for at least a few seconds and longer if attention is sustained. The information is propagated via convergent projections to the parahippocampal region. The parahippocampal cortex appears to sustain these otherwise relatively short-lived representations of single items. In order to link representations that are separated by long periods of time, or to form generalizations, these signals must be passed into the hippocampus. The hippocampus represents organized sequences of events that compose coherent episodic memories, and abstracts information that is common between episodes items, binding episodic representations by their common elements. This mnemonic information is then passed back to the neocortex via divergent backprojections through the parahippocampal region.

Because damage to the hippocampal system does not abolish remote memories, the associations and episodic representations laid down by the hippocampal system must ultimately reside elsewhere in the brain, likely the neocortical areas that originally processed the information. By this view, hippocampal neurons do not store detailed information, but rather may serve to coordinate the establishment of detailed representations in association neocortex. The divergent connections between the hippocampus and neocortex (via the parahippocampal region) could serve to coactivate representations in widespread cortical areas. Ultimately, through iterative activation of this network, linkages between elements of detailed memories could be built that would be independent of hippocampal function. Thus, hippocampal processing could underlie the consolidation of cortical memories (McClelland *et al.*, 1995; Squire & Alvarez, 1995). In addition, association neocortex (especially prefrontal cortex) is in the privileged position to receive and integrate sensory-specific information, memory information from the parahippocampal region and hippocampus, information about the motivational and emotional significance of stimuli, as well as information about the behavioral state of the animal. This integration of information is critical to behavioral decision-making and to the abstraction of task rules.

Each component of the memory system – association neocortex, the parahippocampal region, and the hippocampus – contributes to memory in different, but complementary ways. However, this is a brain "system" in the proper sense of the term, a system in which distinct functions are not completely segregated but require the integrated activity of the individual parts of the system.

References

Alvarez, P. and Squire, L. R. (1994). Memory consolidation and the medial temporal lobe: a simple network model. *Proceedings of the National Academy of Sciences USA*, **91**, 7041–5.

Alvarez, P., Zola-Morgan, S., and Squire, L. R. (1994). The animal model of human amnesia: long-term memory impaired and short-term memory intact. *Proceedings of the National Academy of Sciences USA*, **91**, 5637–41.

Amaral, D. G. and Witter, M. P. (1989). The three-dimensional organization of the hippocampal formation: a review of anatomical data. *Neuroscience*, **31**, 571–91.

Bechara, A., Tranel, D., Damasio, H. D., *et al.* (1995). Double dissociation of conditioning and declarative knowledge relative to the amygdala and hippocampus in humans. *Science*, **269**, 1115-18.

Berger, T. W., Alger, B. E., and Thompson, R. F. (1976). Neuronal substrates of classical conditioning in the hippocampus. *Science*, **192**, 483-5.

Bliss, T. V. P. and Collingridge, G. L. (1993). A synaptic model of memory: long-term potentiation in the hippocampus. *Nature*, **361**, 31-9.

Buckner, R. L. and Wheeler, M. E. (2001). The cognitive neuroscience of remembering. *Nature Reviews, Neuroscience*, **2**, 624-34.

Buffalo, E. A., Ramus, S. J., Clark, R. E., *et al.* (1999). Dissociation between the effects of damage to perirhinal cortex and area TE. *Learning and Memory*, **6**, 572-99.

Buffalo, E. A., Ramus, S. J., Squire, L. R., and Zola, S. M. (2000). Perception and recognition memory in monkeys following lesions of area TE and perirhinal cortex. *Learning and Memory*, **7**, 375-82.

Buffalo, E. A., Reber, P. J., and Squire, L. R. (1998). The human perirhinal cortex and recognition memory. *Hippocampus*, **8**, 330-9.

Bunsey, M. and Eichenbaum, H. (1995). Selective damage to the hippocampal region blocks long-term retention of a natural and nonspatial stimulus-stimulus association. *Hippocampus*, **5**, 546-56.

Bunsey, M. and Eichenbaum, H. (1996). Conservation of hippocampal memory function in rats and humans. *Nature*, **379**, 255-7.

Burwell, R. D. and Amaral, D. G. (1998). Cortical afferents of the perirhinal, postrhinal and entorhinal cortices. *Journal of Comparative Neurology*, **398**, 179-205.

Burwell, R. D., Witter, M. P., and Amaral, D. G. (1995). Perirhinal and postrhinal cortices in the rat: a review of the neuroanatomical literature and comparison with findings from the monkey brain. *Hippocampus*, **5**, 390-408.

Cohen, N. J. and Eichenbaum, H. (1993). *Memory, Amnesia, and the Hippocampal System*. Cambridge, MA: MIT Press.

Cohen, N. J. and Squire, L. R. (1980). Preserved learning and retention of a pattern-analyzing skill in amnesia: dissociation of knowing how and knowing that. *Science*, **210**, 207-10.

Corkin, S. (1984). Lasting consequences of bilateral medial temporal lobectomy: clinical course and experimental findings in H. M. *Seminars in Neurology*, **4**, 249-59.

Deacon, T. W., Eichenbaum, H., Rosenberg, P., and Eckman, K. W. (1983). Afferent connections of the perirhinal cortex in the rat. *Journal of Comparative Neurology*, **220**, 168-290.

Drachman, D. A. and Arbit, J. (1966). Memory and the hippocampal complex. II. Is memory a multiple process? *Archives of Neurology*, **15**, 52-61.

Dusek, J. A. and Eichenbaum, H. (1997). The hippocampus and memory for orderly stimulus relations. *Proceedings of the National Academy of Science (United States of America)*, **94**, 7109-14.

Eichenbaum, H. (1997). Declarative memory: insights from cognitive neurobiology. *Annual Review of Psychology*, **48**, 547-72.

Eichenbaum, H. (2000). A cortical-hippocampal system for declarative memory. *Nature Reviews, Neuroscience*, **1**, 41–50.

Eichenbaum, H., Alvarez, P., and Ramus, S. J. (2000). Animal models of amnesia. In L. S. Cermak, ed., *Memory and its Disorders*. Vol. 2 of *Handbook of Neuropsychology*, 2nd edn. Amsterdam: Elsevier, pp. 1–24.

Eichenbaum, H., Dudchenko, P., Wood, E., Shapiro, M., and Tanila, H. (1999). The hippocampus, memory, and place cells: is it spatial memory or memory space? *Neuron*, **23**, 1–20.

Eichenbaum, H., Stewart, C., and Morris, R. G. M. (1990). Hippocampal representation in spatial learning. *The Journal of Neuroscience*, **10**, 331–9.

Fahy, F. L., Riches, I. P., and Brown, M. W. (1993). Neuronal activity related to visual recognition memory: long-term memory and encoding of recency and familiarity information in the primate anterior and medial inferior temporal and rhinal cortex. *Experimental Brain Research*, **96**, 457–72.

Fletcher, P. C., Frith, C. D., and Rugg, M. D. (1997). The functional neuroanatomy of episodic memory. *Trends in Neuroscience*, **20**, 213–18.

Fried, I., MacDonald, K. A., and Wilson, C. L. (1997). Single neuron activity in human hippocampus and amygdala during recognition of faces and objects. *Neuron*, **18**, 753–65.

Funahashi, S., Bruce, C. J., and Goldman-Rakic, P. S. (1989). Mnemonic coding of visual space in the primate dorsolateral prefrontal cortex. *Journal of Neurophysiology*, **61**, 331–49.

Fuster, J. (1995). *Memory in the Cerebral Cortex*. Cambridge, MA: MIT Press.

Gabrieli, J. (1995). Contributions of the basal ganglia to skill learning and working memory in humans. In J. C. Houk, J. L. Davis, and D. G. Beiser, eds., *Models of Information Processing in the Basal Ganglia*. Cambridge, MA: MIT Press, pp. 227–94.

Galef, B. G., Mason, J. R., Preti, G., and Bean, N. J. (1988). Carbon disulfide: a semiochemical mediating socially-induced diet choice in rats. *Physiology and Behavior*, **42**, 119–24.

Gaffan, D. (1974). Recognition impaired and association intact in the memory of monkeys after transection of the fornix. *Journal of Comparative and Physiological Psychology*, **86**, 1100–9.

Gaffan, D. (1994). Scene-specific memory of objects: a model of episodic memory impairment in monkeys with fornix transection. *Journal of Cognitive Neuroscience*, **6**, 305–20.

Goldman-Rakic, P. S. (1995). Cellular basis of working memory. *Neuron*, **14**, 477–85.

Gothard, K. M., Skaggs, W. E., and McNaughton, B. L. (1996). Dynamics of mismatch correction in the hippocampal ensemble code for space: interaction between path integration and environmental cues. *The Journal of Neuroscience*, **16**, 8027–40.

Graf, P. and Schacter, D. L. (1985). Implicit and explicit memory for new association in normal and amnesic subjects. *Journal of Experimental Psychology: Learning, Memory and Cognition*, **11**, 501–18.

Hallet, M., Pascual-Leone, A., and Topka, H. (1996). Adaptation and skill learning: evidence for different neural substrates. In J. R. Bloedel, T. J. Ebner, and S. P. Wise, eds., *The Acquisition of Motor Behavior in Vertebrates*. Cambridge, MA: MIT Press, pp. 289–302.

Hampson, R. E., Heyser, C. J., and Deadwyler, A. (1993). Hippocampal cell firing correlates of delayed-match-to-sample performance in the rat. *Behavioral Neuroscience*, **107**, 715–39.

Hampson, R. E., Simeral, J. D., and Deadwyler, A. (1999). Distribution of spatial and nonspatial information in dorsal hippocampus. *Nature*, **402**, 610–14.

Higuchi, S. and Miyashita, Y. (1996). Formation of mnemonic neural responses to visual paired associations in inferotemporal cortex is impaired by perirhinal and entorhinal lesions. *Proceedings of the National Academy of Sciences USA*, **93**, 739–43.

Insausti, R., Amaral, D. G., and Cowan, W. M. (1987). The entorhinal cortex of the monkey: II. Cortical afferents. *Journal of Comparative Neurology*, **264**, 356–95.

Knowlton, B. J., Mangels, J. A., and Squire, L. R. (1996). A neostriatal habit learning system in humans. *Science*, **273**, 1399–401.

LeDoux, J. E. (1994). Emotion, memory and the brain. *Scientific American*, **270**, 32–9.

Markus, E. J., Qin, Y.-L., Leonard, B., *et al.* (1995). Interactions between location and task affect the spatial and directional firing of hippocampal neurons. *The Journal of Neuroscience*, **15**, 7079–94.

Martin-Elkins, C. L. and Horel, J. A. (1992). Cortical afferents to behaviorally defined regions of the inferior temporal and parahippocampal gyri as demonstrated by WGA-HRP. *Journal of Comparative Neurology*, **321**, 177–92.

McClelland, J. L., McNaughton, B. L., and O'Reilly, R. C. (1995). Why there are complementary learning systems in the hippocampus and neocortex: insights from the successes and failures of connectionist models of learning and memory. *Psychological Review*, **102**, 419–57.

McNaughton, B. L., Barnes, C. A., and O'Keefe, J. (1983). The contributions of position, direction, and velocity to single unit activity in the hippocampus of freely-moving rats. *Experimental Brain Research*, **52**, 41–9.

Messinger, A., Squire, L. R., Zola, S. M., and Albright, T. D. (2001). Neuronal representations of stimulus associations develop in the temporal lobe during learning. *Proceedings of the National Academy of Science USA*, **98**, 12239–44.

Meunier, M., Bachevalier, J., Mishkin, M., and Murray, E. A. (1993). Effects on visual recognition of combined and separate ablations of the entorhinal and perirhinal cortex in rhesus monkeys. *The Journal of Neuroscience*, **13**, 5418–32.

Miller, E. K. (2000). The prefrontal cortex and cognitive control. *Nature Reviews, Neuroscience*, **1**, 9–65.

Miller, E. K., Erickson, C. A., and Desimone, R. (1996). Neural mechanism of visual working memory in prefrontal cortex of the macaque. *The Journal of Neuroscience*, **16**, 5154–67.

Miller, E. K., Li, L., and Desimone, R. (1991). A neural mechanism for working and recognition memory in inferior temporal cortex. *Science*, **254**, 1377–9.

Miller, E. K., Li, L., and Desimone, R. (1993). Activity of neurons in anterior inferior temporal cortex during a short-term memory task. *The Journal of Neuroscience*, **13**, 1460–78.

Milner, B. (1971). Interhemispheric differences in the localization of psychological process in man. *British Medical Bulletin*, **27**, 272–7.

Milner, B. (1974). Hemispheric specialization: scope and limits. In F. O. Schmitt and F. G. Worden, eds., *The Neurosciences: Third Research Program*. Cambridge, MA: MIT Press.

Mishkin, M. (1978). Memory in monkeys severely impaired by combined but not separate removal of the amygdala and hippocampus. *Nature*, **273**, 297–8.

Mishkin, M. and Delacour, J. (1975). An analysis of short-term visual memory in the monkey. *Journal of Experimental Psychology: Animal Behavior Processes*, **1**, 326–34.

Morris, R. G. M., Garrud, P., Rawlins, J. P., and O'Keefe, J. (1982). Place navigation impaired in rats with hippocampal lesions. *Nature*, **297**, 681–3.

Muller, R. U., Bostock, E., Taube, J. S., and Kubie, J. L. (1994). On the directional firing properties of hippocampal place cells. *The Journal of Neuroscience*, **14**, 7235–51.

Mumby, D. G., Wood, E. R., and Pinel, J. P. J. (1992). Object-recognition memory is only mildly impaired in rats with lesions of the hippocampus and amygdala. *Psychobiology*, **20**, 18–27.

Murray, E. A. and Mishkin, M. (1986). Visual recognition in monkeys following rhinal cortical ablations combined with either amygdalectomy or hippocampectomy. *The Journal of Neuroscience*, **6**, 1991–2003.

Murray, E. A. and Mishkin, M. (1998). Object recognition and location memory in monkeys with excitotoxic lesions of the amygdala and hippocampus. *The Journal of Neuroscience*, **18**, 6568–82.

Nadel, L. and Moscovitch, M. (1997). Memory consolidation, retrograde amnesia and the hippocampal complex. *Current Opinion in Neurobiology*, **7**, 217–27.

Naya, Y., Yoshida, M., and Miyashita, Y. (2001). Backward spreading of memory-retrieval signal in the primate temporal cortex. *Science*, **291**, 661–4.

Nyberg, L., Habib, R., McIntosh, A. R., and Tulving, E. (2000). Reactivation of encoding-related brain activity during memory retrieval. *Proceedings of the National Academy of Sciences USA*, **97**, 11120–4.

O'Keefe, J. A. and Dostrovsky, J. (1971). The hippocampus as a spatial map. Preliminary evidence from single unit activity in the freely-moving rat. *Brain Research*, **34**, 71–175.

O'Keefe, J. A. and Nadel, L. (1978). *The Hippocampus as a Cognitive Map*. New York: Oxford University Press.

Otto, T. and Eichenbaum, H. (1992a). Complementary roles of orbital prefrontal cortex and the perirhinal-entorhinal cortices in an odor-guided delayed non-matching to sample task. *Behavioral Neuroscience*, **106**, 763–76.

Otto, T. and Eichenbaum, H. (1992b). Neuronal activity in the hippocampus during delayed non-match to sample performance in rats: evidence for hippocampal processing in recognition memory. *Hippocampus*, **2**, 323–34.

Ramus, S. J. and Eichenbaum, H. (2000). Neural correlates of olfactory recognition memory in the rat orbitofrontal cortex. *The Journal of Neuroscience*, **20**, 8199–208.

Rempel-Clower, N. L., Zola, S. M., Squire, L. R., and Amaral, D. G. (1996). Three cases of enduring memory impairment following bilateral damage limited to the hippocampal formation. *The Journal of Neuroscience*, **16**, 5233–55.

Rothblat, L. A. and Kromer, L. F. (1991). Object recognition memory in the rat: the role of the hippocampus. *Behavioural Brain Research*, **42**, 25–32.

Sakai, K. and Miyashita, Y. (1991). Neural organization for the long-term memory of paired associates. *Nature*, **354**, 152–5.

Salmon, D. P. and Butters, N. (1995). Neurobiology of skill and habit learning. *Current Opinion in Neurobiology*, **5**, 184–90.

Schacter, D. L. (1985). Multiple forms of memory in humans and animals. In N. M. Weinberger, J. L. McGaugh, and G. Lynch, eds., *Memory Systems of the Brain*. New York: Guilford Press, pp. 351–80.

Schacter, D. L. and Tulving, E. (1994). What are the memory systems of 1994? In D. L. Schacter and E. Tulving, eds., *Memory Systems*. Cambridge: MIT Press, pp. 1–38.

Scoville, W. B. and Milner, B. (1957). Loss of recent memory after bilateral hippocampal lesions. *Journal of Neurology, Neurosurgery and Psychiatry*, **20**, 11–12.

Squire, L. R. (1992). Memory and the hippocampus: a synthesis of findings with rats, monkeys, and humans. *Psychological Review*, **99**, 195–231.

Squire, L. R. and Alvarez, P. (1995). Retrograde amnesia and memory consolidation: a neurobiological perspective. *Current Opinion in Neurobiology*, **5**, 169–77.

Squire, L. R., Knowlton, B., and Musen, G. (1993). The structure and organization of memory. *Annual Review of Psychology*, **44**, 453–95.

Squire, L. R. and Zola, S. M. (1998). Episodic memory, semantic memory and amnesia. *Hippocampus*, **8**, 205–11.

Squire, L. R. and Zola-Morgan, S. M. (1991). The medial temporal lobe memory system. *Science*, **253**, 1380–6.

Suzuki, W. A. (1996). Neuroanatomy of the monkey entorhinal, perirhinal, and parahippocampal cortices: organization of cortical inputs and interconnections with amygdala and striatum. *Neuroscience*, **8**, 3–12.

Suzuki, W. A. and Amaral, D. G. (1994). The perirhinal and parahippocampal cortices of the macaque monkey: cortical afferents. *Journal of Comparative Neurology*, **350**, 497–533.

Suzuki, W. A. and Eichenbaum, H. (2000). The neurophysiology of memory. *Annals of the New York Academy of Sciences*, **911**, 175–91.

Suzuki, W. A., Miller, E. K., and Desimone, R. (1997). Object and place memory in the macaque entorhinal cortex. *Journal of Neurophysiology*, **78**, 1062–81.

Teng, E. and Squire, L. R. (1999). Memory for places learned long ago is intact after hippocampal damage. *Nature*, **400**, 675–7.

Tulving, E. (1993). What is episodic memory? *Current Directions in Psychological Science*, **2**, 67–70.

Tulving, E. and Schacter, D. L. (1990). Priming and human memory systems. *Science*, **247**, 301–6.

Vallar, G. and Shallice, T. (eds.) (1990). *Neuropsychological Impairments of Short-Term Memory*. Cambridge: Cambridge University Press.

Van Hoesen, G. W. and Pandya, D. N. (1975a). Some connections of the entorhinal (area 28) and perirhinal (area 35) cortices of the rhesus monkey. I. Temporal lobe afferents. *Brain Research*, **95**, 1–24.

Van Hoesen, G. W. and Pandya, D. N. (1975b). Some connections of the entorhinal (area 28) and perirhinal (area 35) cortices of the rhesus monkey. III. Efferent connection, *Brain Research*, **95**, 48–67.

Van Hoesen, G. W., Pandya, D. N., and Butters, N. (1972). Cortical afferents to the entorhinal cortex of the rhesus monkey. *Science*, **175**, 1471–3.

Van Hoesen, G. W., Pandya, D. N., and Butters, N. (1975). Some connections of the entorhinal (area 28) and perirhinal (area 35) cortices of the rhesus monkey. II. Frontal lobe afferents. *Brain Research*, **95**, 25–38.

Vargha-Khadem, F., Gadin, D. G., Watkins, K. E., *et al.* (1997). Differential effects of early hippocampal pathology on episodic and semantic memory. *Science*, **277**, 376–80.

Victor, M. and Agamanolis, D. (1990). Amnesia due to lesions confined to the hippocampus: a clinical-pathological study. *Journal of Cognitive Neuroscience*, **2**, 246–57.

Wheeler, M. E., Petersen, S. E., and Buckner, R. L. (2000). Memory's echo: vivid remembering reactivates sensory-specific cortex. *Proceedings of the National Academy of Sciences USA*, **97**, 11125–9.

Wiebe, S. P. and Stäubli, U. V. (1999). Dynamic filtering of recognition memory codes in the hippocampus. *The Journal of Neuroscience*, **19**, 10562–74.

Wiebe, S. P. and Stäubli, U. V. (2001). Recognition memory correlates of hippocampal theta cells. *The Journal of Neuroscience*, **21**, 3955–67.

Wiener, S. I., Paul, C. A., and Eichenbaum, H. (1989). Spatial and behavioral correlates of hippocampal neuronal activity. *The Journal of Neuroscience*, **9**, 2737–63.

Winocur, G. (1990). Anterograde and retrograde amnesia in rats with dorsal hippocampal or dorsomedial thalamic lesions. *Behavioural Brain Research*, **38**, 145–54.

Wood, E., Dudchenko, P. A., and Eichenbaum, H. (1999). The global record of memory in hippocampal neuronal activity. *Nature*, **397**, 613–16.

Wood, E., Dudchenko, P. A., Robitsek, R. J., and Eichenbaum, H. (2000). Hippocampal neurons encode information about different types of memory episodes occurring in the same location. *Neuron*, **27**, 623–33.

Woodruff-Pak, D. S., Papka, M., and Ivry, R. B. (1996). Cerebellar involvement in eyeblink classical conditioning in humans. *Neuropsychology*, **10**, 443–58.

Xiang, J. Z. and Brown, M. W. (1998). Differential neuronal encoding of novelty, familiarity and recency in regions of the anterior temporal lobe. *Neuropharmacology*, **37**, 657–76.

Young, B. J., Otto, T., Fox, G. D., and Eichenbaum, H. (1997). Memory representation within the parahippocampal region. *The Journal of Neuroscience*, **17**, 5183–95.

Zola, S. M., Squire, L. R., Teng, E., *et al.* (2000). Impaired recognition memory in monkeys after damage limited to the hippocampal region. *The Journal of Neuroscience*, **20**, 451–63.

Zola-Morgan, S., Squire, L. R., and Amaral, D. G. (1986). Human amnesia and the medial temporal region: enduring memory impairment following a bilateral lesion limited to field CA1 of the hippocampus. *The Journal of Neuroscience*, **6**, 2950–67.

Zola-Morgan, S., Squire, L. R., and Amaral, D. G. (1989a). Lesions of the amygdala that spare adjacent cortical regions do not impair memory or exacerbate the impairment following lesions of the hippocampal formation. *The Journal of Neuroscience*, **9**, 1922–36.

Zola-Morgan, S., Squire, L. R., Amaral, D. G., and Suzuki, W. A. (1989b). Lesions of perirhinal and parahippocampal cortex that spare the amygdala and hippocampal formation produce severe memory impairment. *The Journal of Neuroscience*, **9**, 4355–70.

The role of the lateral nucleus of the amygdala in auditory fear conditioning

HUGH T. BLAIR, KARIM NADER, GLENN E. SCHAFE, ELIZABETH P. BAUER, SARINA M. RODRIGUES, AND JOSEPH E. LEDOUX

11.1 Introduction

Classical fear conditioning is a form of associative learning in which subjects are trained to express fear responses to a neutral conditioned stimulus (CS) that is paired with an aversive unconditioned stimulus (US). As a result of such pairing, the CS comes to elicit behavioral, autonomic, and endocrine responses that are characteristically expressed in the presence of danger (Blanchard & Blanchard, 1969; Bolles & Fanselow, 1980; Smith *et al.*, 1980). Fear conditioning has emerged as an especially useful behavioral model for investigating the neurobiological mechanisms of learning and memory, because fear memories are rapidly acquired and long-lasting, involve well-defined stimuli and responses, and depend upon similar neural circuits in different vertebrate species (see Davis & Lee, 1998; LeDoux, 2000; Maren, 1999; Rogan *et al.*, 2001).

In this chapter, we review studies that have investigated the role of the amygdala in fear learning. We argue that neural plasticity in the lateral amygdala is critical for storing memories of the association between the CS and US during fear conditioning, and discuss how learning and memory are achieved at the cellular or molecular level. Alternative views of amygdala contributions to fear conditioning are also considered.

11.2 The amygdala and fear conditioning

Fear learning depends critically upon the amygdala (Davis & Shi, 2000; Fendt & Fanselow, 1999; LeDoux, 1996, 2000), a cluster of nuclei in the brain's temporal lobe that plays a key role in regulating emotions (Kluver & Bucy, 1939; LeDoux, 1996). Numerous studies have shown that damage to the amygdala

Topics in Integrative Neuroscience: From Cells to Cognition, ed. James R. Pomerantz. Published by Cambridge University Press. © Cambridge University Press 2008.

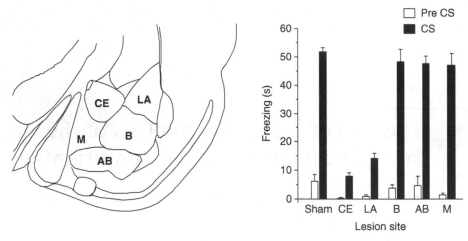

Figure 11.1 The amygdala consists of several distinct subnuclei (anatomical diagram at left adapted from the atlas of Paxinos & Watson, 1997). After the auditory CS is paired with the US, unlesioned (Sham) rats freeze much more during the CS (black bars) than during the period immediately prior to CS presentation (white bars), indicating that these rats have learned to fear the CS. Lesions of the LA or CE nucleus impair auditory fear conditioning, whereas lesions of the B, AB, or M nucleus do not (data from Nader *et al.*, 2001; see text for abbreviations).

impairs a broad variety of fear learning tasks in rodents (Amorapanth *et al.*, 2000; Campeau & Davis, 1995; Goosens & Maren, 2001; Kapp *et al.*, 1979; LeDoux *et al.*, 1988; Nader *et al.*, 2001; Poremba & Gabriel, 1997; Roozendaal *et al.*, 1991; Sananes & Davis, 1992; Walker & Davis, 1997).

Much of what is currently known about the amygdala's role in fear learning has come from studies of *auditory fear conditioning*, a simple task in which rats learn to fear a neutral auditory tone (the CS) that is paired with an electric shock (the US). Prior to such pairing, the tone elicits very little response from the rat. However, after the tone has been paired with electric shock, subsequent presentations of the tone can elicit a variety of fearful responses from the rat, such as freezing (defensive crouching and immobility), elevated startle reflex, and autonomic responses such as changes in heart rate and blood pressure. The emergence of these defensive responses indicates that the rat has learned to fear the tone CS after it has been paired with the shock US.

Auditory fear conditioning depends upon the amygdala, and is severely impaired by amygdala damage (Kapp *et al.*, 1992; LeDoux, 1996; Maren & Fanselow, 1996). However, the amygdala is a heterogeneous structure consisting of many different subnuclei (Figure 11.1), which differ in their contributions to emotional learning processes. Lesions restricted to the lateral (LA) or central (CE) amygdaloid nucleus prevent the acquisition of conditioned freezing responses to an auditory CS, but lesions of the basal (B), accessory basal (AB), or medial (M) nucleus do not (Nader *et al.*, 2001; see Figure 11.1). These findings indicate that, among the major subnuclei of the amygdala, only LA and CE are essential for classical auditory fear conditioning. Although other subnuclei are not essential for this task, they may be critical for other types of fear learning and emotional processing. For example, the B nucleus is important for instrumental fear learning tasks (Amorapanth *et al.*, 2000; Killcross *et al.*, 1997), even though it does not seem to be necessary for classical fear conditioning to an auditory CS (although there is evidence that the anterior portion of the B nucleus may contribute to auditory fear conditioning [Goosens & Maren, 2001]). In the present chapter, we shall focus specifically on the role of the amygdala, and especially the LA nucleus, in classical auditory fear conditioning.

11.3 A cellular hypothesis of associative fear learning

Why are LA and CE so critical for auditory fear conditioning? LA receives direct auditory sensory inputs from the thalamus and cortex, and serves as the main sensory interface of the amygdala (Figure 11.2A; Doron & LeDoux, 1999; McDonald, 1998; Pitkänen *et al.*, 1997). LA sends direct and indirect projections to CE (Pare *et al.*, 1995; Pitkänen *et al.*, 1997), which, in turn, projects to the brain stem and the hypothalamic regions that govern defensive behaviors and accompanying autonomic and endocrine responses. Thus, the amygdala, and specifically the LA–CE circuitry, is well-positioned to provide an anatomical channel through which the CS, after pairing with the US, may gain access to defense response systems in the brainstem and elsewhere (Davis & Lee, 1998; Fendt & Fanselow, 1999; LeDoux, 2000; Maren & Fanselow, 1996). There is considerable evidence that synaptic plasticity in the amygdala's LA nucleus is critical for allowing the CS to gain access to defense response circuits during associative fear learning.

It has long been believed that synaptic plasticity (i.e., alterations in synaptic transmission) is a critical component of the cellular changes that underlie associative learning (Cajal, 1909; Eccles, 1965; Hebb, 1949; Kandel & Spencer, 1968). The most influential statement of this synaptic hypothesis was proposed by Donald Hebb (1949), who theorized that when two interconnected neurons fire at the same time, the synapses between them become stronger, and remain stronger for a long time afterward. This form of synaptic strengthening has come to be called *Hebbian synaptic plasticity*. Hebbian plasticity could provide a neural mechanism for long-term memory storage during classical conditioning (see Hawkins *et al.*, 1983; Kandel & Spencer, 1968; Kelso *et al.*, 1986; Levy & Steward, 1979; McNaughton *et al.*, 1978). When a neutral CS is paired with a US,

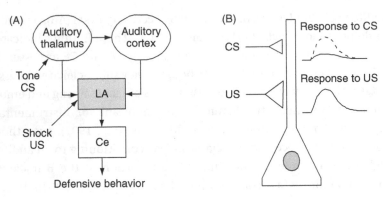

Figure 11.2 LA neurons provide a pathway by which auditory signals can gain access to circuits controlling defensive responses. (A) During auditory fear conditioning, sensory information about the tone CS reaches LA via a thalamic pathway and a cortical pathway. (B) Auditory CS inputs to individual LA neurons may be weak prior to conditioning, but become strengthened by Hebbian plasticity following CS–US pairing (dashed line indicates enhanced CS response after conditioning).

neurons that respond to the CS become activated simultaneously with neurons that respond to the US. According to Hebb's theory, synaptic connections between these neural populations should become stronger, and remain stronger for a long time afterwards, thereby storing a long-term memory for the association between the CS and US.

Figure 11.2B shows how Hebbian synaptic plasticity in LA could store long-term memories of the CS–US association during auditory fear conditioning. Prior to auditory fear conditioning, the synapses formed by auditory thalamic and cortical projections onto LA neurons are believed to be weak, so that the tone CS cannot strongly stimulate the amygdala, and thus does not elicit large postsynaptic responses. In contrast, synapses formed by nociceptive (US) projections to LA may be stronger, and may generate larger postsynaptic responses, since electric shock is an innately aversive stimulus. During auditory fear conditioning, when a tone CS is presented simultaneously with a shock US, weak auditory CS inputs are activated concurrently with strong nociceptive US inputs to LA. This simultaneous activation of CS and US inputs may cause the CS inputs to become strengthened by a Hebbian process of synaptic plasticity. After CS–US pairing, the CS inputs may become sufficiently strengthened to stimulate the amygdala by themselves, and activate amygdala-driven defensive responses in the absence of the US. These strengthened synapses would provide a long-term memory for the association between CS and US, which is stored in LA.

If Hebbian plasticity in LA is essential for storing associative memories during fear conditioning, then this could explain why damage restricted to the LA prevents the acquisition (Figure 11.1) and expression of fear responses to an auditory CS (Amorapanth *et al.*, 2000; Goosens & Maren, 2001; LeDoux *et al.*, 1990; Nader *et al.*, 2001). It could also explain why functional inactivation of LA (and adjacent areas) with the GABA agonist muscimol during conditioning impairs the acquisition of auditory CS-elicited fear responses (Helmstetter & Bellgowan, 1994; Muller *et al.*, 1997; Wilensky *et al.*, 1999, 2000), since plasticity probably cannot occur in LA while it is inactivated by muscimol. Further evidence for Hebbian plasticity in LA comes from physiological studies of neural activity in the amygdala, as reviewed below.

11.4   Synaptic plasticity in LA

At the time Hebb (1949) proposed his influential theory, there was little evidence available to support the view that the connection between two neurons increases when those neurons are simultaneously active. However, later studies of the rodent hippocampus showed that high frequency stimulation of hippocampal afferents leads to long-term enhancement of synaptic transmission, called *long-term potentiation (LTP)* (Bliss & Lomo, 1973). It has also been shown that LTP can exhibit two key properties that are predicted by Hebb's theory. First, LTP at certain synapses is *associative*, in that coactivation of weak inputs and strong inputs onto the same neuron can lead to strengthening of the weak inputs (Levy & Steward, 1979; McNaughton *et al.*, 1978). Second, such LTP is *synapse-specific*, in that synaptic strengthening occurs only at synapses of active, but not inactive, presynaptic afferents to the postsynaptic cell (Andersen *et al.*, 1977; Lynch *et al.*, 1977). The LTP that exhibits these two properties – associativity and synapse specificity – is commonly referred to as *associative* or *Hebbian* LTP. Hebbian LTP has gained prominence as the leading biological model of associative memory formation (see Bliss & Collingridge, 1993; Brown *et al.*, 1988; Hölscher, 2001; Martin *et al.*, 2000; Rogan *et al.*, 2001).

Since the initial discovery of LTP in the hippocampus, it has subsequently been shown that LTP can occur in many structures throughout the brain, including the amygdala (Bauer *et al.*, 2001; Chapman *et al.*, 1990; Clugnet & LeDoux, 1990; Gean *et al.*, 1993; Huang & Kandel, 1998; Huang *et al.*, 2000; Humeau *et al.*, 2003, 2005; Rogan & LeDoux, 1995; Weisskopf *et al.*, 1999). Most importantly for the present discussion, LTP has been demonstrated at thalamic and cortical inputs to LA, the same synapses where Hebbian plasticity is thought to support memory storage during auditory fear conditioning (Bauer *et al.*, 2001, 2002; Huang & Kandel, 1998; Huang *et al*, 2000; Humeau *et al.*, 2003, 2005; Rogan & LeDoux, 1995; Weisskopf *et al.*, 1999).

The principle excitatory neurons in LA are spiny, glutamatergic pyramidal cells (McDonald, 1984; Rainnie *et al.*, 1993; Washburn & Moises, 1992), which receive glutamatergic inputs onto their dendritic spines from presynaptic neurons in the auditory thalamus and cortex (LeDoux & Farb, 1991). Cellular mechanisms of LTP have been investigated at these synaptic inputs to LA in vitro using whole-cell recordings of intracellular excitatory postsynaptic potentials (EPSPs) or extracellular recordings of field EPSPs in amygdala brain slices (Bauer *et al.*, 2002; Huang & Kandel, 1998; Huang *et al.*, 2000; Weisskopf *et al.*, 1999). Such studies have shown that Hebbian LTP can be induced experimentally at LA synapses by artificial stimulation, and that, as in other brain structures (such as the hippocampus and neocortex), some forms of LTP in LA depend on the influx of calcium into the postsynaptic cell. This rise in postsynaptic calcium then triggers a cascade of other intracellular processes that ultimately induce synaptic enhancement (Carew, 1996; Elgersma & Silva, 1999; Frank & Greenberg, 1994; Kandel, 1997; Lisman, 1994; Malenka, 1991; Sweatt, 1999, 2000).

There are two major mechanisms known for calcium influx into the postsynaptic cell during associative LTP. The first involves the N-methyl-D-aspartate class of glutamate receptors (NMDARs; Bliss & Collingridge, 1993; Hollmann & Heinemann, 1994; Malenka & Nicoll, 1999; Monyer *et al.*, 1992; Muller *et al.*, 1988; Nakanishi, 1992; Regehr & Tank, 1990; Watkins & Olverman, 1987), and the second involves voltage-gated calcium channels (VGCCs; Aniksztejn & Ben-Ari, 1991; Grover & Teyler, 1990; Miyakawa *et al.*, 1992; Sabatini & Svoboda, 2000). Both of these mechanisms may be important for mediating Hebbian synaptic plasticity in LA. Hebbian LTP can be induced experimentally at LA synapses in two different ways – by either *tetanic* or *paired* stimulation – and evidence indicates that the role of NMDARs vs. VGCCs for inducing LTP differs, depending on which type of stimulation is used to induce LTP.

During tetanic stimulation, a high-frequency train of pulses, or *tetanus*, is delivered to presynaptic fibers. This tetanic stimulation is so intense that it causes strong depolarization of postsynaptic cells, and thus, pre- and postsynaptic neurons are simultaneously activated to induce Hebbian LTP. In amygdala brain slices, LTP induced by tetanic stimulation of the cortical or thalamic inputs to LA is abolished by bath application of the NMDAR antagonist APV during the tetanus (Bauer *et al.*, 2002; Huang & Kandel, 1998; Huang *et al.*, 2000), or by the selective NR2B antagonist ifenprodil (Bauer *et al.*, 2002). The synaptic changes are also abolished by loading the postsynaptic cell with the calcium chelator BAPTA, indicating that induction of LTP requires calcium entry into the postsynaptic cell (Huang & Kandel, 1998). Thus, tetanus-induced Hebbian LTP in LA probably involves calcium entry into the postsynaptic cell through NMDARs.

During the tetanus protocol, concurrent pre- and postsynaptic activity is achieved by strong stimulation of a single presynaptic input pathway to LA. By contrast, associative learning that occurs during fear conditioning is thought to require the conjunctive activation of weak presynaptic CS inputs to LA during strong depolarization of these same neurons by the US (Figure 11.2B). Hence, natural activity patterns that occur in LA during behavioral fear learning may be very different from activity that occurs during tetanic stimulation. For this reason, another in vitro method of LTP induction – paired-stimulation – may more closely approximate natural activity patterns that occur in LA during fear conditioning.

During paired-stimulation, the presynaptic pathway is weakly stimulated while the postsynaptic neuron is concurrently depolarized by current injection (Bi & Poo, 1998; Kelso et al., 1986; Magee & Johnston, 1997; Malinow & Miller, 1986; Markram et al., 1997; Wigström & Gustafsson, 1986). Again, combined pre- and postsynaptic activity occurs to produce Hebbian LTP. Such a pairing protocol may better approximate the stimulus conditions that occur during associative learning, because the presynaptic stimulation is like a weak CS that activates the postsynaptic neuron, and the postsynaptic depolarization is like a strong activation of the same cell by the US (Kelso & Brown, 1986; Kelso et al., 1986).

Huang and Kandel (1998) induced LTP in the cortico-LA pathway by pairing low-frequency (0.2 Hz) presynaptic stimulation pulses with prolonged (50 ms) injection of current (2–4 nA) into the postsynaptic LA neuron (Huang & Kandel, 1998). This LTP was attenuated, but not completely blocked, by NMDA antagonists. Huang and Kandel (1998) speculated that the NMDA-independent component of this pairing-induced LTP might depend on postsynaptic VGCCs, but they did not experimentally test this hypothesis. Later findings by Humeau et al. (2003) suggest that the NMDA-independent component of cortico-thalamic LTP may be presynaptic, and thus completely independent of postsynaptic mechanisms (see further discussion below).

Weisskopf et al. (1999) used a pairing protocol to explore the role of NMDARs and VGCCs in LTP in the thalamo-LA pathway. In their repeated pairing protocol, trains of 10 presynaptic pulses at 30 Hz were paired with brief postsynaptic depolarizations (1 nA for 5 ms) delivered 5–10 ms after the onset of each EPSP in the train. Pairing-induced LTP of the thalamo-LA pathway did not affect the EPSP elicited by cortical stimulation, demonstrating that this form of LTP is synapse-specific, as required for Hebbian plasticity. Further, the LTP was not at all affected by the NMDA antagonists APV and MK-801 (Weisskopf et al., 1999), indicating that NMDARs are not involved. The LTP was, instead, abolished by bath application of the L-type VGCC antagonist nifedipine, as well as by loading the postsynaptic cell with BAPTA (Weisskopf *et al.*, 1999). Subsequent studies showed that this form of LTP could also be blocked by the L-type VGCC antagonist verapamil (Bauer *et al.*, 2002). Similarly, Humeau *et al.* (2005) showed that pairing-induced LTP at thalamo-amygdala synapses depends upon R-type VGCCs located in dendritic spines that receive inputs from thalamic afferents. These findings indicate that pairing-induced LTP in the thalamo-LA pathway requires high-threshold VGCCs (such as R-type and L-type channels), but not NMDARs.

Together, the above findings suggest that Hebbian LTP in LA can involve either NMDARs or VGCCs, depending on the stimulation conditions. Tetanization of presynaptic inputs to LA produces LTP that depends on NMDARs but not VGCCs, whereas pairing weak presynaptic stimulation with strong postsynaptic depolarization produces LTP that requires VGCCs but not NMDARs. Although these experiments show that it is possible to artificially induce LTP in LA that requires VGCCs but not NMDARs, or vice versa, this does not mean that LTP must always depend on only one of these mechanisms, and not the other. In the hippocampus, some stimulation protocols produce LTP that requires both NMDARs and VGCCs (Huber *et al.*, 1995; Magee & Johnston, 1997; Nishiyama *et al.*, 2000).

Recently it has been shown that convergent activation of cortical and thalamic inputs to LA can induce LTP of the cortical input pathway, and this LTP does not depend upon postsynaptic calcium influx, but instead depends upon presynaptic mechanisms (Humeau *et al.*, 2003). Hence, this novel form of LTP does not require postsynaptic NMDA receptors or VGCCs. This intriguing form of LTP may be considered 'associative' since it is induced by convergent activation of thalamic and cortical inputs to LA, but it is not 'Hebbian' since it does not require activation of the postsynaptic target neuron as originally postulated by Hebb. This raises the intriguing possibility that CS and US inputs might converge upon LA neurons to induce a nonHebbian form of associative plasticity. For example, if CS information is conveyed to LA through cortical inputs and US information is conveyed via thalamic inputs, then nonHebbian associative LTP could occur when these inputs are activated simultaneously, thereby strengthening the CS inputs to LA in a manner that does not require activation of the targeted LA neuron. This alternative to the Hebbian hypothesis is somewhat speculative, but further study is warranted to investigate whether it is a viable alternative to the Hebbian view. In the remainder of this chapter, we shall focus upon the Hebbian hypothesis outlined in Figure 11.2.

In summary, Hebbian LTP that depends on NMDARs or VGCCs (or both) may be induced in LA by artificial stimulation in amygdala brain slices. Can a similar LTP-like process be engaged by natural patterns of neural activity that occur in response to the CS and US during fear conditioning? In the following section, we review evidence that LTP does indeed occur at auditory inputs to LA in awake, behaving animals during auditory fear conditioning. We next discuss findings which indicate that this LTP depends upon both NMDARs and VGCCs, as suggested by in vitro physiology studies.

11.5   Plasticity of neural responses in LA

The Hebbian theory of fear learning reviewed above (Figure 11.2B) predicts that CS and US signals converge upon single neurons in LA, and that CS inputs to these neurons become strengthened by Hebbian plasticity during CS–US pairing. Supporting this view, neurons in LA are known to fire action potentials in response to both an auditory CS and an electric shock US (Blair & LeDoux, 2000; Romanski *et al.*, 1993), indicating that sensory information about the CS and US converges onto LA neurons. Furthermore, following fear conditioning, responses of single LA neurons evoked by an auditory CS are enhanced in LA, implying that auditory inputs to these LA neurons are strengthened by an LTP-like process when the CS is paired with the US (Collins & Pare, 2000; Goosens *et al.*, 2003; Maren, 2000; Quirk *et al.*, 1995, 1997; Repa *et al.*, 2001). In addition, auditory stimuli elicit field potentials in the LA of awake, freely behaving rats (Rogan & LeDoux, 1995), and fear conditioning results in a potentiation of these field potentials recorded from LA (Rogan *et al.*, 1997). Thus, several studies have shown that auditory fear conditioning is accompanied by an enhancement of auditory-evoked responses in LA, providing evidence that LTP occurs in LA of behaving animals during fear conditioning.

However, it must be noted that CS-evoked responses of neurons in the auditory thalamus are also enhanced after an auditory CS has been paired with an aversive US (Maren *et al.*, 2001; Poremba & Gabriel, 2001). Since the auditory thalamus provides much of the auditory input to LA, the possibility must be considered that enhancement of CS-evoked auditory responses in LA is due primarily to upstream neural plasticity in the thalamus, rather than LTP occurring at synapses within LA itself. Contradicting this alternative explanation is the fact that conditioned neural responses in the auditory thalamus depend on the integrity of the amygdala (Poremba & Gabriel, 2001). Further, fear conditioning potentiates synaptic inputs to LA, as recorded in postmortem brain slices from rats that are sacrificed after conditioning (McKernan & Shinnick-Gallagher, 1997), suggesting that LTP does indeed occur at auditory inputs to LA during fear learning. Recent studies have shown that potentiation of thalamo-LA synapses during fear conditioning involves molecular signaling cascades in the thalamic projection neurons (Apergis-Schoute *et al.*, 2005), supporting the view that thalamic plasticity is not an amygdala-independent mechanism for fear memory storage, but rather that the thalamic plasticity that occurs during fear conditioning is specifically related to potentiation of the thalamo-LA pathway. Further evidence that LTP occurs in LA during fear learning comes from pharmacological studies showing that drugs that interfere with Hebbian LTP can disrupt fear learning when they are infused into the amygdala, as described next.

11.6   Role of NMDARs and VGCCs in fear conditioning

Hebbian synaptic plasticity in vitro typically requires activation of either NMDARs or VGCCs (or both) in LA (see above). Thus, if fear conditioning depends upon Hebbian LTP in LA, then it should also depend upon the function of NMDARs and VGCCs in LA. To determine whether this is the case, several studies have investigated the role of amygdala NMDARs and VGCCs in associative fear learning.

If NMDARs in the amygdala are required for memory storage, then fear learning should be impaired if NMDARs are blocked during the acquisition phase of fear conditioning (i.e., when the task is initially learned). Supporting this prediction, infusion of the selective NMDAR antagonist APV into the amygdala impairs acquisition of fear learning in a variety of tasks, including auditory fear conditioning (Lee & Kim, 1998), contextual fear conditioning (Fanselow & Kim, 1994; Maren *et al.*, 1996), fear-potentiated startle (Campeau *et al.*, 1992; Gewirtz & Davis, 1997; Miserendino *et al.*, 1990), and inhibitory avoidance (Kim & McGaugh, 1992; Liang *et al.*, 1994). In each of these studies, APV was administered into the amygdala immediately before the training procedure, and animals showed learning deficits when they were later tested drug-free. This suggests that NMDARs may participate in the induction of synaptic plasticity that underlies memory storage in the amygdala during fear learning.

However, interpretation of these results is complicated by the finding that APV can block synaptic transmission in LA (Bauer *et al.*, 2002; Li *et al.*, 1995, 1996; Weisskopf & LeDoux, 1999). Thus, instead of specifically impairing plasticity in LA, APV may functionally inactivate LA by impairing synaptic activity. If APV selectively blocks the induction of synaptic plasticity in LA (without impairing synaptic transmission), then infusing APV into LA should not interfere with previously learned fear tasks. However, contrary to this prediction, pretesting infusion of APV into the amygdala impairs performance of previously learned auditory fear conditioning (Lee & Kim, 1998; Lee *et al.*, 2001b), contextual fear conditioning (Maren *et al.*, 1996), and inhibitory avoidance (Kim & McGaugh, 1992). Some studies have reported that intra-amygdala infusions of APV do not impair performance of previously learned fear-potentiated startle to a visual CS

(Campeau *et al.*, 1992; Gewirtz & Davis, 1997; Miserendino *et al.*, 1990; Walker & Davis, 2000), but other studies report that performance of fear-potentiated startle is impaired by APV (Fendt, 2001), much like other fear learning tasks.

It is difficult to interpret the effects of APV infusions on synaptic plasticity in behaving rats, since the behavioral studies reviewed above have produced conflicting evidence that does not consistently and unequivocally distinguish effects on synaptic transmission from effects on plasticity. However, recent experiments using an alternative method provide a means for more clearly distinguishing the role of NMDARs in synaptic plasticity and transmission in LA during fear conditioning.

APV is a nonselective antagonist that blocks all NMDARs, regardless of their molecular composition. However, NMDARs are heteromeric molecules, consisting of two NR1 subunits plus some combination of subunits from the NR2 class: the NR2A, NR2B, NR2C, or NR2D subunits (Behe *et al.*, 1995; Schoepfer *et al.*, 1994). NMDARs that incorporate the NR2B subunit can be selectively blocked using the NR2B-specific antagonist ifenprodil.

It has been shown that hippocampal LTP is accompanied by increased tyrosine phosphorylation of NMDARs at the NR2B subunit (Rosenblum *et al.*, 1996; Rostas *et al.*, 1996), suggesting a link between the NR2B subunit and synaptic plasticity that may underlie memory storage. Supporting this, the NR2B subunit in the insular cortex has been implicated in memory for novel tastes (Rosenblum *et al.*, 1997), and genetic overexpression of the NR2B subunit in hippocampus leads to increased LTP and enhanced learning of hippocampal-dependent tasks (Tang *et al.*, 1999). Recent in vivo experiments from our laboratory have shown that ifenprodil, unlike APV, is effective at blocking tetanus-induced LTP in LA at concentrations that do not interfere with synaptic transmission (Bauer *et al.*, 2002). Thus, by selectively blocking NMDARs that incorporate the NR2B subunit, ifenprodil seems to disrupt NMDAR-dependent synaptic plasticity without impairing synaptic transmission.

Rodrigues *et al.* (2001) infused ifenprodil into LA during the acquisition phase of auditory fear conditioning to a tone CS. As with APV, conditioning was impaired when rats were tested drug-free after training. However, unlike the effects of APV, infusion of ifenprodil into LA prior to testing did not block the expression of previously learned tone conditioning. This suggests that ifenprodil selectively blocks synaptic plasticity in LA, without disrupting normal synaptic transmission. Hence, NMDARs in LA that incorporate the NR2B subunit may be particularly important for synaptic plasticity that occurs during fear learning, while other classes of NMDARs may be more important for normal synaptic transmission. It thus appears that NMDARs do indeed contribute significantly to fear conditioning in LA, and that the NR2B subunit plays an important role.

In addition to NMDARs, LTP in LA can also depend upon VGCCs (Bauer *et al.*, 2002; Weisskopf *et al.*, 1999). Bauer *et al.* (2002) found that infusion of the L-type VGCC blocker verapamil into LA during training blocked the acquisiton of fear conditioning, but did not impair the expression of previously learned conditioned fear responses. They also examined the effects of verapamil on synaptic transmission and LTP induction in amygdala brain slices, and found that verapamil had no effect on synaptic transmission but prevented LTP induction, in agreement with previous studies in which LTP was impaired by applying nifedipine to block VGCCs (Weisskopf *et al.*, 1999). L-type VGCCs in LA thus appear to play a parallel role in behavioral fear conditioning and pairing-induced associative LTP.

In summary, both NMDARs and VGCCs in LA appear to be necessary at the time of learning for fear conditioning to occur, but they are not necessary for the expression of previously learned fear. A likely explanation for these findings is that NMDARs and VGCCs are required for Hebbian LTP to occur in LA at the time of learning. This interpretation is further supported by evidence that molecular process in the amygdala are necessary for forming stable long-term memories of the CS–US association.

11.7   Memory consolidation in the amygdala

As each of us knows from personal experience, some memories last longer than others. *Memory consolidation* is the process by which short-term memories are transformed, over time, into stable long-term memories. The nervous system cannot store permanent memories of everything that happens to us, so the brain must select which experiences to consolidate into long-term memory storage, and which to forget after they have expired from short-term memory.

Synaptic plasticity is widely thought to underly memory storage (Cajal, 1909; Eccles, 1965; Hebb, 1949; Kandel & Spencer, 1968). In a straightforward extension of this view, it is believed that short-term memories may involve short-term changes in synaptic strength, whereas long-term memories are implemented by more permanent modifications of synaptic strength (see Bailey *et al.*, 1996; Davis & Squire, 1984; Dudai, 1989; Goelet *et al.*, 1986; Kandel, 1997; Schafe *et al.*, 2001). A large body of evidence indicates that, at the level of a single synapse, the cellular mechanisms for short-term synaptic plasticity are distinct from the mechanisms for long-term plasticity. Broadly, short-term synaptic plasticity is thought to involve regulatory modifications of existing proteins at the synapse, without requiring protein or RNA synthesis, whereas long-term plasticity is believed to depend upon more permanent structural modifications of the synapse that depend on synthesis of protein and RNA.

Fearful experiences are easily consolidated to long-term memory, probably because they convey vital information about danger in the environment, which is important for survival. However, this long-term persistence of fear memories can be selectively impaired (without affecting short-term fear memories) by infusion of drugs into LA that block molecular processes that are essential for long-term synaptic modification. For example, blockade of protein synthesis in LA does not disrupt short-term fear memory, but prevents the consolidation of the short-term changes into long-lasting memories (Schafe & LeDoux, 2000). Long-term fear memories are also inhibited by intra-amygdala infusion of RNA synthesis inhibitors (Bailey et al., 1999). Long- and short-term memory of fear conditioning can also be dissociated by blockade of several second messenger pathways in LA, including the mitogen-activated protein kinase (MAPK) and protein kinase A (PKA) pathways (Bourtchouladze et al., 1998; Schafe & LeDoux, 2000; Schafe et al., 1999, 2000). In the amygdala, as in other neural systems, PKA and MAPK may support LTP by helping to activate CRE-dependent transcription (Impey et al., 1996, 1998), a conclusion that is supported by the finding that overexpression of CREB in the amygdala using viral transfection methods facilitates LTM, but not STM, of fear-potentiated startle (Josselyn et al., 2001). Finally, EGR-1 (Zif-268) mRNA is upregulated in the amygdala following contextual fear conditioning, and blockade of EGR-1 protein translation by antisense oligonucleotides impairs contextual fear memory consolidation (Hall et al., 2000; Malkani & Rosen, 2000).

The above findings suggest that short-term fear memories are stored by immediate synaptic changes that occur in LA when the CS is paired with the US, and these changes do not involve gene transcription or synthesis of RNA or proteins. However, in order for these changes to persist as long-term memories, macromolecular synthesis is necessary to consolidate the immediate short-term synaptic enhancements into permanent synaptic modifications. Interestingly, the same signaling pathways that are required for consolidating long-term fear memories in LA of behaving animals are also required for inducing long-lasting enhancement of synaptic transmission at LA synapses in amygdala slice experiments. Huang et al. (2000) investigated synaptic correlates of short- and long-term fear memory by inducing two different forms of LTP in LA. The first form, called early LTP (E-LTP), produces synaptic enhancement which lasts only 60–90 minutes, and is induced by stimulating the input pathway with a single high-frequency tetanus. The second form, called late LTP (L-LTP), produces enhancement lasting many hours, and is induced by applying tetanic stimulation five times to the input pathway. They showed that selective impairment of L-LTP (and sparing of E-LTP) can be obtained by applying inhibitors of MAPK, PKA, and protein synthesis, the same treatments that selectively impair long-term memory (but not short-term memory) of fear conditioning when they are infused into LA.

Memory consolidation has been traditionally regarded as a unidirectional process, in which labile short-term memories are transformed over time into stable long-term memories that are resistant to erasure or forgetting. In the last several decades, however, a number of studies have suggested that memories that have already been consolidated into stable, long-term memories can once again become unstable, or labile, when they are retrieved. For example, if electroconvulsive shock is delivered near the time when a stable long-term memory is retrieved, then subsequent retrieval of this memory may be impaired in future recall tests (Mactutus *et al.*, 1979; Misanin *et al.*, 1968; Sara, 2000). Such findings have been interpreted as evidence that stable long-term memories return to a labile state during retrieval, and that following retrieval, such memories can be lost unless they are *reconsolidated* back into a stable form.

Recently, our laboratory has used the auditory fear conditioning paradigm to investigate memory reconsolidation processes in the amygdala (Nader *et al.*, 2000a,b). In these reconsolidation experiments, rats were given intra-amygdala infusions of the protein synthesis inhibitor anisomycin not at the time of training (as in the standard consolidation experiments reviewed above), but rather 24 hours later, in conjunction with a retrieval test in which the CS was presented to the rat. Rats treated with anisomycin at the time of retrieval showed marked impairment of fear, relative to vehicle controls, on subsequent recall tests conducted 24 hours later (but not on recall test conducted 4 hours later, suggesting that reconsolidation, like standard memory consolidation, is a slow process). This effect was dependent on retrieval of the previously learned CS–US association, because anisomycin did not cause a memory deficit when administered without reexposure to the CS. Further, this effect was observed not only when the initial recall test and drug infusion were given 24 hours after training, but also if given 14 days later. Thus, fear memories appear to return to a labile state after retrieval. In order to become stable again, these memories must be put back into long-term storage via a protein synthesis-dependent mechanism in the amygdala.

In recent years, much work has been done to investigate the phenomenon of memory reconsolidation. The basic reconsolidation effect, in which memories become vulnerable to disruption after they are recalled, has been reported in a variety of different memory systems in diverse species (for review see Alberini, 2005; Dudai & Eisenberg, 2004; Nader *et al.*, 2000b). While there are still many unanswered questions about the nature of reconsolidation and the mechanisms involved, the fast pace of research is producing significant advances and these questions may soon be answered.

11.8   Alternative theories

As we have shown, available evidence strongly suggests that Hebbian neural changes occur in LA during fear conditioning, and that these changes are critical for the conditioning of fear responses to an auditory CS. However, several alternative theories have been proposed to explain the amygdala's role in fear learning.

In principle, there are a variety of possible explanations for why the amygdala – especially LA and CE – are necessary for fear conditioning to an auditory CS. A trivial explanation could be that the amygdala is required for CS processing, so that damage to LA or CE would render the animal unable to detect the auditory CS. However, there is no evidence that amygdala lesions cause hearing impairment, so this explanation seems highly unlikely. Alternatively, amygdala lesions could impair US processing, rendering the animal insensitive to the electric shock US. This explanation is contradicted by studies showing that amygdala damage or inactivation does not affect rats' behavioral reactivity to electric shock (Cahill & McGaugh, 1990; Helmstetter & Bellgowan, 1994; Miserendino et al., 1990). Finally, amygdala lesions could impair an animal's ability to perform certain defensive responses, such as the freezing response that is typically used to assess conditioned fear, without impairing the animal's ability to learn an association between the CS and US. Contradicting this explanation, amygdala damage or inactivation does not always impair the unconditioned performance of defensive responses elicited by the US (LeDoux et al., 1990; Wallace & Rosen, 2001), although performance of defensive responses is sometimes impaired by amygdala damage (Davis, 1997; Walker & Davis, 1997).

Given the overwhelming amount of evidence that the amygdala is involved in learning, there is broad agreement that the amygdala plays a key role in storing memories for the CS–US association during fear conditioning. However, there remains some controversy about whether such memories are stored within the amygdala itself, or elsewhere in the brain (Cahill et al., 1999; Fanselow & LeDoux, 1999). In contrast to the theory that synaptic modification in LA provides a substrate for storing memories of the CS–US association, a competing theory argues that fear memories are not stored anywhere within the amygdala, but instead, the amygdala merely modulates the storage of such memories in other brain structures during and briefly after learning (Cahill & McGaugh, 1998; Cahill et al., 1999). Key to this argument is the fact that immediate post-training manipulations of the amygdala (especially the LA and the adjacent B nucleus) influence the strength of memory in a variety of different appetitive and aversive instrumental learning tasks. However, evidence shows that classical Pavlovian fear conditioning is *not* affected by these types of immediate posttraining manipulations of the amygdala in the same manner as instrumental tasks (Lee *et al.*, 2001a; Wilensky *et al.*, 2000). This indicates that modulation of memory storage in other brain regions is not essential for the amygdala-dependent aspects of Pavlovian fear conditioning. Instead, Pavlovian fear conditioning appears to depend chiefly upon memories stored by synaptic plasticity occuring in the amygdala itself.

11.9   Summary and conclusions

Hebbian LTP has gained prominence as the leading biological model of associative memory formation (see Bliss & Collingridge, 1993; Brown *et al.*, 1988; Hölscher, 2001; Martin *et al.*, 2000; Rogan *et al.*, 2001). But in order for LTP to account for memory formation, it would be necessary to show that the same mechanisms engaged by artificial stimulation in LTP experiments are also triggered by natural activity patterns during learning. Indirect support for this notion comes from studies showing that hippocampal-dependent memory can be impaired or enhanced in behaving animals by pharmacological and genetic manipulations that alter hippocampal LTP (Bach *et al.*, 1996; Davis *et al.*, 1992; Mayford *et al.*, 1996; Tang *et al.*, 1999; Tsien *et al.*, 1996). But despite advances such as these, it has been difficult to clarify the contribution of specific hippocampal circuits to memory, and thus to relate LTP at specific synapses to memory (see Barnes, 1995; Eichenbaum, 1997; Martin *et al.*, 2000; Stevens, 1998).

In this chapter, we have argued that Hebbian LTP occurs in LA, both in vivo and in vitro, and that fear conditioning and Hebbian LTP in LA depend on similar cellular mechanisms. We have reviewed several lines of evidence that support this view. First, damage restricted to the LA prevents the acquisition and expression of fear responses to an auditory CS (Amorapanth *et al.*, 2000; Goosens & Maren, 2001; LeDoux *et al.*, 1990; Nader *et al.*, 2001) showing that the LA is a necessary component of the circuitry through which the CS–US association is formed. Second, functional inactivation of LA (and adjacent areas) with the GABA agonist muscimol during conditioning impairs the acquisition of auditory CS-elicited fear responses (Helmstetter & Bellgowan, 1994; Muller *et al.*, 1997; Wilensky *et al.*, 1999, 2000), demonstrating that neural activity in LA during conditioning is required for this type of fear learning to take place. Third, the auditory CS and nociceptive US converge on single neurons in LA (Blair & LeDoux, 2000; Romanski *et al.*, 1993), providing a substrate through which the US might modify the processing of the CS. Fourth, neural responses evoked in LA by the auditory CS are enhanced when the CS is paired with US (Collins & Pare, 2000; Goosens *et al.*, 2003; McKernan & Shinnick-Gallagher, 1997; Quirk *et al.*, 1995, 1997; Repa *et al.*, 2001; Rogan *et al.*, 1997), supporting the Hebbian prediction that temporal overlap of the CS and US leads to the strengthening of the synaptic connections activated by the CS. Fifth, disruption of macromolecular synthesis in LA and surrounding areas prevents the consolidation of long-term memory for associative auditory fear conditioning (Bailey *et al.*, 1999; Nader *et al.*, 2000a; Schafe *et al.*, 2000), consistent with the fact that macromolecular synthesis is essential for the conversion of short to long-term memory in neurons that store associative memories (Bailey *et al.*, 1996; Davis & Squire, 1984; Dudai, 1989; Goelet *et al.*, 1986; Kandel, 1997). From this evidence we conclude that, although LA may not be the only site of neural plasticity during fear learning (e.g., Maren *et al.*, 2001; Poremba & Gabriel, 2001; Weinberger, 1995), it is very likely a site where neural changes relevant to behavioral fear learning occur.

In conclusion, we believe that by advancing our knowledge of how synaptic plasticity in LA contributes to fear learning, it is possible to gain novel insights into how LTP participates in memory storage.

References

Alberini, C. M. (2005). Mechanisms of memory stabilization: are consolidation and reconsolidation similar or distinct processes? *Trends Neuroscience*, **28**, 51–6.

Amorapanth, P., LeDoux, J. E., and Nader, K. (2000). Different lateral amygdala outputs mediate reactions and actions elicited by a fear-arousing stimulus. *Nature Neuroscience*, **3**, 74–9.

Andersen, P., Sundberg, S. H., Sveen, O., and Wigstrom, H. (1977). Specific long-lasting potentiation of synaptic transmission in hippocampal slices. *Nature*, **266**, 736–7.

Aniksztejn, L. and Ben-Ari, Y. (1991). Novel form of long-term potentiation produced by a K$^+$ channel blocker in the hippocampus, *Nature*, **349**, 67–9.

Apergis-Schoute, A. M., Debiec, J., Doyere, V., LeDoux, J. E., and Schafe, G. E. (2005). Auditory fear conditioning and long-term potentiation in the lateral amygdala require ERK/MAP kinase signaling in the auditory thalamus: a role for presynaptic plasticity in the fear system. *Journal of Neuroscience*, **25**, 5730–9.

Bach, M. E., Hawkins, R. D., Osman, M., Kandel, E. R., and Mayford, M. (1996). Impairment of spatial but not contextual memory in CaMKII mutant mice with a selective loss of hippocampal LTP in the range of the theta frequency. *Cell*, **81**, 905–15.

Bailey, C. H., Bartsch, D., and Kandel, E. R. (1996). Toward a molecular definition of long-term memory storage. *Proceedings of the National Academy of Sciences USA*, **93**, 13445–52.

Bailey, D. J., Sun, W., Thompson, R. F., Kim, J. J., and Helmstetter, F. J. (1999). Acquisition of fear conditioning in rats requires the synthesis of mRNA in the amygdala. *Behavioral Neuroscience*, **113**, 276–82.

Barnes, C. A. (1995). Involvement of LTP in memory: are we "searching under the street light"? *Neuron*, **15**, 751–4.

Bauer, E. P., LeDoux, J. E., and Nader, K. (2001). Fear conditioning and LTP in the lateral amygdala are sensitive to the same stimulus contingencies. *Nature Neuroscience*, **4**, 687–8.

Bauer, E. P., Schafe, G. E., and LeDoux, J. E. (2002). NMDA receptors and L-type voltage-gated calcium channels contribute to long-term potentiation and different components of fear memory formation in the lateral amygdala. *Journal of Neuroscience*, **22**, 5239–49.

Behe, P., Stern, P., Wyllie, D. J., *et al.* (1995). Determination of NMDA NR1 subunit copy number in recombinant NMDA receptors. *Proceedings of the Royal Society of London [Biol]*, **262**, 205–13.

Bi, G. Q. and Poo, M. M. (1998). Synaptic modifications in cultured hippocampal neurons: dependence on spike timing, synaptic strength, and postsynaptic cell type. *Journal of Neuroscience*, **18**, 10464–72.

Blair, H. T. and LeDoux, J. E. (2000). Single-unit recording of auditory and nociceptive responses from lateral amygdala neurons during auditory fear conditioning in freely behaving rats. *Society for Neuroscience Abstracts*, **26**, 1254.

Blanchard, D. C. and Blanchard, R. J. (1969). Crouching as an index of fear. *Journal of Comparative Physiology Psychology*, **67**, 370–5.

Bliss, T. V. P. and Collingridge, G. L. (1993). A synaptic model of memory: long-term potentiation in the hippocampus. *Nature*, **361**, 31–9.

Bliss, T. V. P. and Lomo, T. (1973). Long-lasting potentiation of synaptic transmission in the dentate area of the anaesthetized rabbit following stimulation of the perforant path. *Journal of Physiology*, **232**, 331–56.

Bolles, R. C. and Fanselow, M. S. (1980). A perceptual-defensive-recuperative model of fear and pain. *Behavioral and Brain Sciences*, **3**, 291–323.

Bourtchouladze, R., Abel, T., Berman, N., *et al.* (1998). Different training procedures recruit either one or two critical periods for contextual memory consolidation, each of which requires protein synthesis and PKA. *Learning and Memory*, **5**, 365–74.

Brown, T. H., Chapman, P. F., Kairiss, E. W., and Keenan, C. L. (1988). Long-term synaptic potentiation. *Science*, **242**, 724–8.

Cahill, L. and McGaugh, J. L. (1990). Amygdaloid complex lesions differentially affect retention of tasks using appetitive and aversive reinforcement. *Behavioral Neuroscience*, **104**, 532–43.

Cahill, L. and McGaugh, J. L., (1998). Mechanisms of emotional arousal and lasting declarative memory. *Trends in Neurosciences*, **21**, 294–9.

Cahill, L., Weinberger, N. M., Roozendaal, B., and McGaugh, J. L. (1999). Is the amygdala a locus of 'conditioned fear'? Some questions and caveats. *Neuron*, **23**, 227–8.

Cajal, S. R. Y. (1909). *Histologie du systeme nerveux de l'homme et des vertebres*. Paris: A. Maloine.

Campeau, S. and Davis, M. (1995). Involvement of subcortical and cortical afferents to the lateral nucleus of the amygdala in fear conditioning measured with fear-potentiated startle in rats trained concurrently with auditory and visual conditioned stimuli. *Journal of Neuroscience*, **15**, 2312–27.

Campeau, S., Miserendino, M. J. D., and Davis, M. (1992). Intra-amygdala infusion of the N-Methyl-D-Aspartate receptor antagonist AP5 blocks acquisition but not expression of fear-potentiated startle to an auditory conditioned stimulus. *Behavioral Neuroscience*, **106**, 569–74.

Carew, T. J. (1996). Molecular enhancement of memory formation. *Neuron*, **16**, 5–8.

Chapman, P. F., Kairiss, E. W., Keenan, C. L., and Brown T. H. (1990). Long-term synaptic potentiation in the amygdala. *Synapse*, **6**, 271–8.

Clugnet, M. C. and LeDoux, J. E. (1990). Synaptic plasticity in fear conditioning circuits: induction of LTP in the lateral nucleus of the amygdala by stimulation of the medial geniculate body. *Journal of Neuroscience*, **10**, 2818–24.

Collins, D. R. and Pare, D. (2000). Differential fear conditioning induces reciprocal changes in the sensory responses of lateral amygdala neurons to the CS(+) and CS(−). *Learning and Memory*, **7**, 97–103.

Davis, H. P. and Squire, L. R. (1984). Protein synthesis and memory. A review. *Psychology Bulletin*, **96**, 518–59.

Davis, M. (1997). Neurobiology of fear responses: the role of the amygdala. *Journal of Neuropsychology and Clinical Neuroscience*, **9**, 382–402.

Davis, M. and Lee, Y. (1998). Fear and anxiety: possible roles of the amygdala and bed nucleus of the stria terminalis. *Cognition and Emotion*, **12**, 277–305.

Davis, M. and Shi, C. (2000). The amygdala. *Current Biology*, **10**, R131.

Davis, S., Butcher, S. P., and Morris, R. G. (1992). The NMDA receptor antagonist D-2-amino-5-phosphonopentanoate (D-AP5) impairs spatial learning and LTP in vivo at intracerebral concentrations comparable to those that block LTP in vitro. *Journal of Neuroscience*, **12**, 21–34.

Doron N. N. and LeDoux, J. E. (1999). Organization of projections to the lateral amygdala from auditory and visual areas of the thalamus in the rat. *Journal of Comparative Neurology*, **412**, 383–409.

Dudai, Y. (1989). *The Neurobiology of Memory*. New York: Oxford University Press.

Dudai, Y. and Eisenberg, M. (2004). Rites of passage of the engram: reconsolidation and the lingering consolidation hypothesis. *Neuron*. Sep. 30, **44**(1), 93–100.

Eccles, J. C. (1965). Conscious experience and memory. Academic address. *Recent Advances in Biological Psychiatry*, **8**, 235–56.

Eichenbaum, H. (1997). To cortex: thanks for the memories. *Neuron*, **19**, 481–4.

Elgersma, Y. and Silva, A. J. (1999). Molecular mechanisms of synaptic plasticity and memory. *Current Opinion in Neurobiology*, **9**, 209–13.

Fanselow, M. S. and Kim, J. J. (1994). Acquisition of contextual Pavlovian fear conditioning is blocked by application of an NMDA receptor antagonist

D,L-2-amino-5-phosphonovaleric acid to the basolateral amygdala. *Behavioral Neuroscience*, **108**, 210–12.

Fanselow, M. S. and LeDoux, J. E. (1999). Why we think plasticity underlying Pavlovian fear conditioning occurs in the basolateral amygdala. *Neuron*, **23**, 229–32.

Fendt, M. (2001). Injections of the NMDA receptor antagonist aminophosphono-pentanoic acid into the lateral nucleus of the amygdala block the expression of fear-potentiated startle and freezing. *Journal of Neuroscience*, **21**, 4111–15.

Fendt, M. and Fanselow, M. S. (1999). The neuroanatomical and neurochemical basis of conditioned fear. *Neuroscience and Biobehavioral Reviews*, **23**, 743–60.

Frank, D. A. and Greenberg, M. E. (1994). CREB: a mediator of long-term memory from mollusks to mammals. *Cell*, **79**, 5–8.

Gean, P.-W., Chang, F.-C., Huang, C.-C., Lin, J.-H., and Way, L.-J. (1993). Long-term enhancement of EPSP and NMDA receptor-mediated synaptic transmission in the amygdala. *Brain Research Bulletin*, **31**, 7–11.

Gewirtz, J. C. and Davis, M. (1997). Second-order fear conditioning prevented by blocking NMDA receptors in amygdala. *Nature*, **388**, 471–4.

Goelet, P., Castellucci, V. F., Schacher, S., and Kandel, E. R. (1986). The long and the short of long-term memory – a molecular framework. *Nature*, **322**, 419–22.

Goosens, K. A., Hobin, J. A., and Maren, S. (2003). Auditory-evoked spike firing in the lateral amygdala and Pavlovian fear conditioning: mnemonic code or fear bias? *Neuron*, **40**, 1013–22.

Goosens, K. A. and Maren, S. (2001). Contextual and auditory fear conditioning are mediated by the lateral, basal, and central amygdaloid nuclei in rats. *Learning and Memory*, **8**, 148–55.

Grover, L. M. and Teyler, T. J. (1990). Two components of long-term potentiation induced by different patterns of afferent activation. *Nature*, **347**, 477–9.

Hall, J., Thomas, K. L., and Everitt, B. J. (2000). Rapid and selective induction of BDNF expression in the hippocampus during contextual learning. *Nature Neuroscience*, **3**, 533–5.

Hawkins, R. D., Abrams, T. W., Carew, T. J., and Kandel, E. R. (1983). A cellular mechanism of classical conditioning in Aplysia: activity- dependent amplification of presynaptic facilitation. *Science*, **219**, 400–5.

Hebb, D. O. (1949). *The Organization of Behavior*. New York: John Wiley and Sons.

Helmstetter, F. J. and Bellgowan, P. S. (1994). Effects of muscimol applied to the basolateral amygdala on acquisition and expression of contextual fear conditioning in rats. *Behavioral Neuroscience*, **108**, 1005–9.

Hollmann, M. and Heinemann, S. (1994). Cloned glutamate receptors. *Annual Review of Neuroscience*, **17**, 31–108.

Hölscher, C. (2001). *Neuronal Mechanisms of Memory Formation*. Cambridge: Cambridge University Press.

Huang, Y. Y. and Kandel, E. R. (1998). Postsynaptic induction and PKA-dependent expression of LTP in the lateral amygdala. *Neuron*, **21**, 169–78.

Huang, Y. Y., Martin, K. C., and Kandel, E. R. (2000). Both protein kinase A and mitogen-activated protein kinase are required in the amygdala for the macromolecular synthesis-dependent late phase of long-term potentiation. *Journal of Neuroscience*, **20**, 6317–25.

Huber, K. M., Mauk, M. D., and Kelly, P. T. (1995). Distinct LTP induction mechanisms: contribution of NMDA receptors and voltage-dependent calcium channels. *Journal of Neurophysiology*, **73**, 270–9.

Humeau, Y., Shaban, H., Bissiere, S., and Luthi, A. (2003). Presynaptic induction of heterosynaptic associative plasticity in the mammalian brain. *Nature*, **426**, 841–5.

Humeau, Y., Herry, C., Kemp, N., *et al.* (2005). Dendritic spine heterogeneity determines afferent-specific Hebbian plasticity in the amygdala. *Neuron*, **45**, 119–31.

Impey, S., Mark, M., Villacres, E. C., *et al.* (1996). Induction of CRE-mediated gene expression by stimuli that generate long-lasting LTP in area CA1 of the hippocampus. *Neuron*, **16**, 973–82.

Impey, S., Obrietan, K., Wong, S. T., *et al.* (1998). Cross talk between ERK and PKA is required for Ca2+ stimulation of CREB-dependent transcription and ERK nuclear translocation. *Neuron*, **21**, 869–83.

Josselyn, S. A., Shi, C., Carlezon, W. A., Jr., *et al.* (2001). Long-term memory is facilitated by cAMP response element-binding Protein over expression in the amygdala. *Journal of Neuroscience*, **21**, 2404–12.

Kandel, E. R. (1997). Genes, synapses, and long-term memory. *Journal of Cell Physiology*, **173**, 124–5.

Kandel, E. R. and Spencer, W. A. (1968). Cellular neurophysiological approaches to the study of learning. *Physiological Reviews*, **48**, 65–134.

Kapp, B. S., Frysinger, R. C., Gallagher, M., Haselton, J. R. (1979). Amygdala central nucleus lesions: effect on heart rate conditioning in the rabbit. *Physiology and Behavior*. **23**, 1109–17.

Kapp, B. S., Whalen, P. J., Supple, W. F., and Pascoe, J. P. (1992). Amygdaloid contributions to conditioned arousal and sensory information processing. In J. P. Aggleton, ed., *The Amygdala: Neurobiological Aspects of Emotion, Memory, and Mental Dysfunction*. New York: Wiley-Liss Inc., pp. 229–54.

Kelso, S. R. and Brown, T. H. (1986). Differential conditioning of associative synaptic enhancement in hippocampal brain slices. *Science*, **232**, 85–7.

Kelso, S. R., Ganong, A. H., and Brown, T. H. (1986). Hebbian synapses in hippocampus. *Proceedings of the National Academy of Sciences USA*, **83**, 5326–30.

Killcross, S., Robbins, T. W., and Everitt, B. J. (1997). Different types of fear-conditioned behavior mediated by separate nuclei within amygdala. *Nature*, **388**, 377–80.

Kim, M. and McGaugh, J. L. (1992). Effects of intra-amygdala injections of NMDA receptor antagonists on acquisition and retention of inhibitory avoidance. *Brain Research*, **585**, 35–48.

Kluver, H. and Bucy, P. C. (1939). Preliminary analysis of functions of the temporal lobe in monkeys. *Archives of Neurology and Psychiatry*, **42**, 979–97.

LeDoux, J. E., ed. (1996). *The Emotional Brain*. New York: Simon and Schuster.

LeDoux, J. E. (2000). Emotion circuits in the brain. *Annual Review of Neuroscience*, **23**, 155–84.

LeDoux, J. E., Cicchetti, P., Xagoraris, A., and Romanski, L. M. (1990). The lateral amygdaloid nucleus: sensory interface of the amygdala in fear conditioning. *Journal of Neuroscience*, **10**, 1062–9.

LeDoux, J. E. and Farb, C. R. (1991). Neurons of the acoustic thalamus that project to the amygdala contain glutamate. *Neuroscience Letters*, **134**, 145–9.

LeDoux, J. E., Iwata, J., Cicchetti, P., and Reis, D. J. (1988). Different projections of the central amygdaloid nucleus mediate autonomic and behavioral correlates of conditioned fear. *Journal of Neuroscience*, **8**, 2517–29.

Lee, H. J., Berger, S. Y., Stiedl, O., Spiess, J., and Kim, J. J. (2001a). Post-training injection of catecholaminergic drugs do not modulate fear conditioning in rats and mice. *Neuroscience Letters*, **303**, 123–6.

Lee, H. J., Choi, J. S., Brown, T. H., and Kim, J. J. (2001b). Amygdalar N-methyl-D-aspartate receptors are critical for the expression of multiple conditioned fear responses. *Journal of Neuroscience*, **21**, 4116–24.

Lee, H. J. and Kim, J. J. (1998). Amygdalar NMDA receptors are critical for new fear learning in previously fear-conditioned rats. *Journal of Neuroscience*, **18**, 8444–54.

Levy, W. B. and Steward, O. (1979). Synapses as associative memory elements in the hippocampal formation. *Brain Research*, **175**, 233–45.

Li, X. F., Phillips, R., and LeDoux, J. E. (1995). NMDA and non-NMDA receptors contribute to synaptic transmission between the medial geniculate body and the lateral nucleus of the amygdala. *Experimental Brain Research*, **105**, 87–100.

Li, X. F., Stutzmann, G. E., and LeDoux, J. L. (1996). Convergent but temporally separated inputs to lateral amygdala neurons from the auditory thalamus and auditory cortex use different postsynaptic receptors: *in vivo* intracellular and extracellular recordings in fear conditioning pathways. *Learning and Memory*, **3**, 229–42.

Liang, K. C., Hon, W., and Davis, M. (1994). Pre- and posttraining infusion of N-methyl-D-aspartate receptor antagonists into the amygdala impair memory in an inhibitory avoidance task. *Behavioral Neuroscience*, **108**, 241–53.

Lisman, J. (1994). The CaM kinase II hypothesis for the storage of synaptic memory. *Trends in Neuroscience*, **17**, 406–12.

Lynch, G. S., Dunwiddie, T., and Gribkoff, V. (1977). Heterosynaptic depression: a postsynaptic correlate of long-term potentiation. *Nature*, **266**, 737–9.

Mactutus, C. F., Riccio D. C., and Ferek, J. M. (1979). Retrograde amnesia for old (reactivated) memory: some anomalous characteristics, *Science*, **204**, 1319–20.

Magee, J. C. and Johnston, D. (1997). A synaptically controlled, associative signal for Hebbian plasticity in hippocampal neurons. *Science*, **275**, 209–13.

Malenka, R. C. (1991). The role of postsynaptic calcium in the induction of long-term potentiation. *Molecular Neurobiology*, **5**, 289–95.

Malenka, R. C. and Nicoll, R. A. (1999). Long-term potentiation – a decade of progress? *Science*, **285**, 1870–4.

Malinow, R. and Miller, J. P. (1986). Postsynaptic hyperpolarization during conditioning reversibly blocks induction of long-term potentiation. *Nature*, **320**, 529–30.

Malkani, S. and Rosen, J. B. (2000). Specific induction of early growth response gene 1 in the lateral nucleus of the amygdala following contextual fear conditioning in rats. *Neuroscience*, **97**, 693–702.

Maren, S. (1999). Long-term potentiation in the amygdala: a mechanism for emotional learning and memory. *Trends in Neurosciences*, **22**, 561–7.

Maren, S. (2000). Auditory fear conditioning increases CS-elicited spike firing in lateral amygdala neurons even after extensive overtraining. *European Journal of Neuroscience*, **12**, 4047–54.

Maren, S., Aharonov, G., Stote, D. L., and Fanselow, M. S. (1996). N-methyl-D-aspartate receptors in the basolateral amygdala are required for both acquisition and expression of conditional fear in rats. *Behavioral Neuroscience*, **10**, 1365–74.

Maren, S. and Fanselow, M. S. (1996). The amygdala and fear conditioning: has the nut been cracked? *Neuron*, **16**, 237–40.

Maren, S., Yap, S. A., and Goosens, K. A. (2001). The amygdala is essential for the development of neuronal plasticity in the medial geniculate nucleus during auditory fear conditioning in rats. *Journal of Neuroscience*, **21**, RC135.

Markram, H., Lübke, J., Frotscher, M., and Sakmann, B. (1997). Regulation of synaptic efficacy by coincidence of postsynaptic APs and EPSPs. *Science*, **275**, 213–15.

Martin, S. J., Grimwood, P. D., and Morris, R. G. M. (2000). Synaptic plasticity and memory: an evaluation of the hypothesis. *Annual Review of Neuroscience*, **23**, 649–711.

Mayford, M., Bach, M. E., Huang, Y. Y., et al. (1996). Control of memory formation through regulated expression of a CaMKII transgene. *Science*, **274**, 1678–83.

McDonald, A. J. (1984). Neuronal organization of the lateral and basolateral amygdaloid nuclei of the rat. *Journal of Comparative Neurology*, **222**, 589–606.

McDonald, A. J. (1998). Cortical pathways to the mammalian amygdala. *Progress in Neurobiology*, **55**, 257–332.

McKernan, M. G. and Shinnick-Gallagher, P. (1997). Fear conditioning induces a lasting potentiation of synaptic currents in vitro. *Nature*, **390**, 607–11.

McNaughton, B. L., Douglas, R. M., and Goddard, G. V. (1978). Synaptic enhancement in fascia dentata: cooperativity among coactive afferents. *Brain Research*, **157**, 277–93.

Misanin, J. R., Miller R. R., and Lewis, D. J. (1968). Retrograde amnesia produced by electroconvulsive shock after reactivation of a consolidated memory trace. *Science*, **160**, 554–5.

Miserendino, M. J. D., Sananes, C. B., Melia, K. R., and Davis, M. (1990). Blocking of acquisition but not expression of conditioned fear-potentiated startle by NMDA antagonists in the amygdala. *Nature*, **345**, 716–18.

Miyakawa, H., Ross, W. N., Jaffe, D., *et al.* (1992). Synaptically activated increases in Ca2+ concentration in hippocampal CA1 pyramidal cells are primarily due to voltage-gated Ca2+ channels. *Neuron*, **9**, 1163–73.

Monyer, H., Sprengel, R., Schoepfer, R., *et al.* (1992). Heteromeric NMDA receptors: molecular and functional distinction of subtypes. *Science*, **256**, 1217–21.

Muller, J., Corodimas, K. P., Fridel, Z., and LeDoux, J. E. (1997). Functional inactivation of the lateral and basal nuclei of the amygdala by muscimol infusion prevents fear conditioning to an explicit CS and to contextual stimuli. *Behavioral Neuroscience*, **111**, 683–91.

Muller, D., Joly, M., and Lynch, G. (1988). Contributions of quisqualate and NMDA receptors to the induction and expression of LTP. *Science*, **242**, 1694–7.

Nader, K., Majidishad, P., Amorapanth, P., and LeDoux, J. E. (2001). Damage to the lateral and central, but not other, amygdaloid nuclei prevents the acquisition of auditory fear conditioning. *Learning and Memory*, **8**, 156–63.

Nader, K., Schafe, G. E., and LeDoux, J. (2000a). Fear memories require protein synthesis in the amygdala for reconsolidation after retrieval. *Nature*, **406**, 722–6.

Nader, K., Schafe, G. E., and LeDoux, J. (2000b). The labile nature of consolidation theory. *Nature Reviews. Neuroscience*, **1**, 216–19.

Nakanishi, S. (1992). Molecular diversity of glutamate receptors and implications for brain function. *Science*, **258**, 597–603.

Nishiyama, M., Hong, K., Mikoshiba, K., Poo, M. M., and Kato, K. (2000). Calcium stores regulate the polarity and input specificity of synaptic modification. *Nature*, **408**, 584–8.

Pare, D., Smith, Y., and Pare, J. F. (1995). Intra-amygdaloid projections of the basolateral and basomedial nuclei in the cat: *Phaseolus vulgaris*-leucoagglutinin anterograde tracing at the light and electron microscopic level. *Neuroscience*, **69**, 567–83.

Paxinos, G. and Watson, C. (1997). *The Rat Brain in Stereotaxic Coordinates*. Sydney: Academic Press.

Pitkänen, A., Savander, V., and LeDoux, J. E. (1997). Organization of intra-amygdaloid circuitries in the rat: an emerging framework for understanding functions of the amygdala. *Trends Neuroscience*, **20**, 517–23.

Poremba, A. and Gabriel, M. (2001). Amygdalar efferents initiate auditory thalamic discriminative training-induced neuronal activity. *Journal of Neuroscience*, **21**, 270–8.

Poremba, A. and Gabriel, M. J. (1997). Amygdalar lesions block discriminative avoidance learning and cingulothalamic training-induced neuronal plasticity in rabbits. *Neuroscience*, **17**(13), 5237–44.

Quirk, G. J., Armony, J. L., and LeDoux, J. E. (1997). Fear conditioning enhances different temporal components of toned-evoked spike trains in auditory cortex and lateral amygdala. *Neuron*, **19**, 613–24.

Quirk, G. J., Repa, J. C., and LeDoux, J. E. (1995). Fear conditioning enhances short-latency auditory responses of lateral amygdala neurons: parallel recordings in the freely behaving rat. *Neuron*, **15**, 1029–39.

Rainnie, D. G., Asprodini, E. K., and Shinnick-Gallagher, P. (1993). Intracellular recordings from morphologically identified neurons of the basolateral amygdala. *Journal of Neurophysiology*, **69**, 1350–62.

Regehr, W. G. and Tank, D. W. (1990). Postsynaptic NMDA receptor-mediated calcium accumulation in hippocampal CA1 pyramidal cell dendrites. *Nature*, **345**, 807–10.

Repa, J. C., Muller, J., Apergis, J., *et al.* (2001). Two different lateral amygdala cell populations contribute to the initiation and storage of memory. *Nature Neuroscience*, **4**, 724–31.

Rodrigues, S. M., Schafe, G. E., and LeDoux, J. E. (2001). Intraamygdala blockade of the NR2B subunit of the NMDA receptor disrupts the acquisition but not the expression of fear conditioning. *Journal of Neuroscience*, **8**, 229–42.

Rogan, M., Staubli, U., and LeDoux, J. (1997). Fear conditioning induces associative long-term potentiation in the amygdala. *Nature*, **390**, 604–7.

Rogan, M. T. and LeDoux, J. E. (1995). LTP is accompanied by commensurate enhancement of auditory - evoked responses in a fear conditioning circuit. *Neuron*, **15**, 127–36.

Rogan, M. T., Weisskopf, M. G., Huang, Y.-Y., Kandel, E. R., and LeDoux, J. E. (2001). Long-term potentiation in the amygdala: implications for memory. In C. Hölscher, ed., *Neuronal Mechanisms of Memory Formation*. Cambridge: Cambridge University Press, pp. 58–76.

Romanski, L. M., LeDoux, J. E., Clugnet, M. C., and Bordi, F. (1993). Somatosensory and auditory convergence in the lateral nucleus of the amygdala. *Behavioral Neuroscience*, **107**, 444–50.

Roozendaal, B., Koolhaas, J. M., and Bohus, B. (1991). Central amygdala lesions affect behavioral and autonomic balance during stress in rats. *Physiology and Behavior*, **50**, 777–81.

Rosenblum, K., Berman, D. E., Hazvi, S., Lamprecht, R., and Dudai, Y. (1997). NMDA receptor and the tyrosine phosphorylation of its 2B subunit in taste learning in the rat insular cortex. *Journal of Neuroscience*, **17**, 5129–35.

Rosenblum, K., Dudai, Y., and Richter-Levin, G. (1996). Long-term potentiation increases tyrosine phosphorylation of the N-methyl-D-aspartate receptor subunit 2B in rat dentate gyrus in vivo. *Proceedings of the National Academy of Sciences USA*, **93**, 10457–60.

Rostas, J. A., Brent, V. A., Voss, K., *et al.* (1996). Enhanced tyrosine phosphorylation of the 2B subunit of the N-methyl-D-aspartate receptor in long-term potentiation. *Proceedings of the National Academy of Sciences USA*, **93**, 10452–6.

Sabatini, B. L. and Svoboda, K. (2000). Analysis of calcium channels in single spines using optical fluctuation analysis. *Nature*, **408**, 589–93.

Sananes, C. B. and Davis, M. (1992). N-methyl-D-aspartate lesions of the lateral and basolateral nuclei of the amygdala block fear-potentiated startle and shock sensitization of startle. *Behavioral Neuroscience*, **106**, 72–80.

Sara, S. J. (2000). Retrieval and reconsolidation: toward a neurobiology of remembering, *Learning and Memory*, Vol. **7**, pp. 73–84.

Schafe, G. E., Atkins, C. M., Swank, M. W., *et al.* (2000). Activation of ERK/MAP kinase in the amygdala is required for memory consolidation of pavlovian fear conditioning. *Journal of Neuroscience*, **20**, 8177–87.

Schafe, G. E. and LeDoux, J. (2000). Memory consolidation of auditory Pavlovian fear conditioning requires protein synthesis and protein kinase A in the amygdala. *Journal of Neuroscience*, **20**, RC96.

Schafe, G. E., Nader, K., Blair, H. T., and LeDoux, J. E. (2001). Memory consolidation of Pavlovian fear conditioning: a cellular and molecular perpective. *Trends in Neurosciences*, **24**, 540–6.

Schafe, G. E., Nadel, N. V., Sullivan, G. M., Harris, A., and LeDoux, J. E. (1999). Memory consolidation for contextual and auditory fear conditioning is dependent on protein synthesis, PKA, and MAP kinase. *Learning and Memory*, **6**, 97–110.

Schoepfer, R., Monyer, H., Sommer, B., *et al.* (1994). Molecular biology of glutamate receptors. *Progress in Neurobiology*, **42**, 353–7.

Smith, O. A., Astley, C. A., DeVito, J. L., Stein, J. M., and Walsh, R. E. (1980). Functional analysis of hypothalamic control of the cardiovascular responses accompanying emotional behavior. *Federation Proceedings*, **29**, 2487–94.

Stevens, C. F. (1998). A million dollar question: does LTP = memory? *Neuron*, **20**, 1–2.

Sweatt, J. D. (1999). Toward a molecular explanation for long-term potentiation. *Learning and Memory*, **6**, 399–416.

Sweatt, J. D. (2000). The neuronal MAP kinase cascade: a biochemical signal integration system subserving synaptic plasticity and memory. *Journal of Neurochemistry*, **76**, 1–10.

Tang, Y. P., Shimizu, E., Dube, G. R., *et al.* (1999). Genetic enhancement of learning and memory in mice. *Nature*, **401**, 63–9.

Tsien, J. Z., Huerta, P. T., and Tonegawa, S. (1996). The essential role of hippocampal CA1 NMDA receptor-dependent synaptic plasticity in spatial memory. *Cell*, **87**, 1327–38.

Walker, D. L. and Davis, M. (1997). Double dissociation between the involvement of the bed nucleus of the stria terminalis and the central nucleus of the amygdala in startle increases produced by conditioned versus unconditioned fear. *Journal of Neuroscience*, **17**(23), 9375–83.

Walker, D. L. and Davis, M. (2000). Involvement of NMDA receptors within the amygdala in short- versus long-term memory for fear conditioning as assessed with fear-potentiated startle. *Behavioral Neuroscience*, **114**, 1019–33.

Wallace, K. J. and Rosen, J. B. (2001). Neurotoxic lesions of the lateral nucleus of the amygdala decrease conditioned fear but not unconditioned fear of a predator odor: comparison with electrolytic lesions. *Journal of Neuroscience*, **21**, 3619–27.

Washburn, M. S. and Moises, H. C. (1992). Electrophysiological and morphological properties of rat basolateral amygdaloid neurons in vitro. *Journal of Neuroscience*, **12**, 4066–79.

Watkins, J. C. and Olverman, H. J. (1987). Agonist and antagonists for excitatory amino acid receptors. *Trends in Neuroscience*, **10**, 265–72.

Weinberger, N. M. (1995). Retuning the brain by fear conditioning. In M. S. Gazzaniga, ed., *The Cognitive Neurosciences*. Cambridge: MIT Press, pp. 1071–89.

Weisskopf, M. G., Bauer, E. P., and LeDoux, J. E. (1999). L-Type voltage-gated calcium channels mediate NMDA-independent associative long-term potentiation at thalamic input synapses to the amygdala. *Journal of Neuroscience*, **19**, 10512–19.

Weisskopf, M. G. and LeDoux, J. E. (1999). Distinct populations of NMDA receptors at subcortical and cortical inputs to principal cells of the lateral amygdala. *Journal of Neurophysiology*, **81**, 930–4.

Wigström, H. and Gustafsson, B. (1986). Postsynaptic control of hippocampal long-term potentiation. *Journal of Physiology*, **81**, 228–36.

Wilensky, A. E., Schafe, G. E., and LeDoux, J. E. (1999). Functional inactivation of the amygdala before but not after auditory fear conditioning prevents memory formation. *Journal of Neuroscience*, **19**, RC48.

Wilensky, A. E., Schafe, G. E., and LeDoux, J. E. (2000). The amygdala modulates memory consolidation of fear-motivated inhibitory avoidance learning but not classical fear conditioning. *Journal of Neuroscience*, **20**, 7059–66.

12

On crucial roles of hippocampal NMDA receptors in acquisition and recall of associative memory

KAZU NAKAZAWA, MATTHEW A. WILSON, AND SUSUMU TONEGAWA

12.1 Introduction

A full understanding of the mammalian brain mechanisms underlying a higher cognitive phenomenon like learning and memory requires identification of relevant events or processes occurring at multiple levels of complexity; from molecular, synaptic, and cellular levels to neuronal ensemble and brain systems levels. This is an enormous challenge for brain researchers because cognitive phenomena can be monitored only at the level of a live animal's behavior, while many of the analytical methods for the underlying mechanisms are carried out using in vitro preparations and effective in vivo methods are limited. How can we be sure that the events or processes identified by in vitro methods or by even some in vivo studies are causally related to the animals' behavioral phenotype? For simpler invertebrate systems, molecular genetics has been effective for this purpose. Organisms harboring a mutation in a specific gene can be subjected to a variety of in vitro and in vivo analyses including behavioral tests, and deficits or impairments detected at different levels of complexity can potentially be bound together using the mutation as a connecting thread.

12.2 Background

12.2.1 Experimental strategy

For the analysis of more complex mammalian systems, however, additional tricks are necessary. One significant trick would be to restrict the mutation spatially and temporally. For instance, if one can restrict deletion (i.e., null mutation) of a specific gene to a particular type of neuron present in a particular

Topics in Integrative Neuroscience: From Cells to Cognition, ed. James R. Pomerantz. Published by Cambridge University Press. © Cambridge University Press 2008.

area of the brain and only to a late phase of the animal's life, one can expect that the resulting deficits or impairments would be much more specific. Accordingly, the relationship among abnormal phenotypes at different levels of complexity could be better assessed. This is the rationale for the use of genetically and conditionally engineered mice for the study of mechanisms underlying cognitive phenomena.

12.2.2   Hippocampal network

An extensive body of evidence from cognitive, neurophysiological, and neurobiological studies has established that in both humans and animals, the hippocampus plays a crucial role in certain forms of learning and memory. The hippocampus consists of several major areas including the dentate gyrus (DG), CA3 and CA1, each of which contains several types of cells wired together in a distinct pattern (Amaral & Witter, 1989) (Figure 12.1). The hippocampus receives input from virtually all associative areas of the neocortex via the entorhinal cortex (EC). EC transmits the cortical input to DG granule cells via the perforant

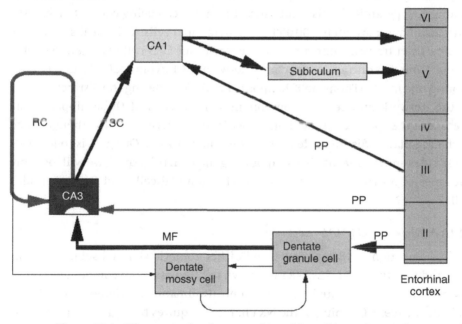

Figure 12.1   Hippocampal excitatory pathway. Most of the excitatory glutamatergic projections are depicted. Synaptic plasticity at perforant path (PP)-CA3 synapses, recurrent collateral (RC also known as commissural/associational)-CA3 synapses, and Shaffer collateral-CA1 synapses are known to be NMDA receptor dependent, while mossy fiber (MF)-CA3 synaptic plasticity occurs in an NMDA receptor-independent manner (for color image please see www.cambridge.org/9780521143400).

path (PP), which originates in its layer II stellate cells. The DG granule cells in turn send mossy fibers (MF) to CA3 where the majority of the axons synapse onto CA3 pyramidal cells that project via Schaffer collaterals to CA1 pyramidal cells. CA1 is the major exit site of the hippocampus; the information processed in the hippocampus is transmitted back to the EC either directly via CA1 pyramidal cell axons or indirectly through the subiculum. The major excitatory hippocampal loop containing DG granule cells, CA3 pyramidal cells, and CA1 pyramidal cells has received much attention and has been referred to as 'the trisynaptic pathway.' There are also other known excitatory pathways in the hippocampus. For instance, both CA3 and CA1 pyramidal cells receive direct input from the superficial layers of EC. In addition, the CA3 network is unique among those in the hippocampus in that the pyramidal cells receive robust recurrent collateral (RC; also known as commissural or associational (C/A)) input in addition to PP and MF input. Among the three types of excitatory input that CA3 pyramidal cells receive, the recurrent collateral input is the most numerous at about 12 000 per pyramidal cell in rat. The PP and MF contribute about 4000 and 50 inputs, respectively (Amaral *et al.*, 1990). Due to the recurrent synapses, the connectivity among CA3 pyramidal cells is robust, with a given cell being connected directly with 2% of approximately 600 000 other pyramidal cells. This means that each CA3 cell can transmit information to every other CA3 cell via a few synaptic connections. In contrast, connectivity between CA1 pyramidal cells is very low, around one in 130 (Thomson & Radpour, 1991). Considering the distinct feature of the network and cellular components within each of these hippocampal areas and the specific interactions between these networks, it is thought that each area plays a distinct role in the mnemonic process. Our goal is to identify these roles and the mechanisms supporting them. In this paper, we will focus on the roles of NMDA receptors (NR) in CA1 pyramidal cells and CA3 pyramidal cells.

12.2.3   *Hippocampal NMDA receptors*

Functional NRs are composed of heteromeric channel subunits using NR1 and four types of NR2s. NR1 is known to be an essential component of this voltage- and ligand-gated ion channel (Hollmann & Heinemann, 1994; Nakanishi, 1992). Opening of the NR channels requires both glutamate binding and depolarization of the postsynaptic membrane, the latter of which is primarily mediated in the hippocampus by activation of α-amino-3-hydroxy-5-methyl-4-isoxazol propionate (AMPA)/kainate receptor channels, and leads to the removal of Mg^{2+} ions from the NR channel pores. Once activated, NRs permit a transient entry of Ca^{2+} into the postsynaptic terminals, which leads to a series of changes in the postsynaptic density (PSD) and induction of long-term modifications in synaptic strength such as long-term potentiation (LTP) and long-term depression (LTD) (Bliss & Collingridge, 1993). Thus, NRs provide a molecular device for Hebbian synapses such that coincident activities in pre- and postsynaptic cells can modify the ability of one neuron to fire another. It has been demonstrated that the induction of plasticity at SC-CA1 and C/A-CA3 synapses as well as at PP-CA3 synapses is NR-dependent while that at MF-CA3 is not (Berger & Yeckel, 1991; Berzhanskaya et al., 1998; Harris & Cotman, 1986; Williams & Johnston, 1988; Zalutsky & Nicoll, 1990).

12.2.4   Role of CA1 NR in acquisition of spatial memory

Armed by Hebb's original idea (Hebb, 1949), the mechanism underlying LTP has been studied extensively as a candidate synaptic device for learning and memory. However, evidence that implicates LTP in memory has been limited to a few pharmacological studies and the claims have been contested by other studies. In addition, these pharmacological studies could not address the memory role of synaptic plasticity in a distinct area of the hippocampus because the blockade could not be reliably restricted to a specific hippocampal area.

In the middle of the 1990s, we undertook a project in which conditional gene knockout techniques were applied to NRs in CA1. We chose CA1 as the target area because SC-CA1 synapses are the most extensively studied synapses in the mammalian CNS. Further, as a major output site of the hippocampal network, its function might be expected to be most relevant for hippocampus-dependent learning and memory. Using the phage P1-derived Cre-loxP system, we were able to produce a mutant mouse line in which the NR1 gene is deleted (or knocked out) robustly only in CA1 pyramidal cells of adult mice which are one to two months of age (CA1-NR1 KO mice). These mutant mice were analyzed in comparison to control littermates using a variety of methods designed to detect deficits at different levels of complexity (Tsien et al., 1996). At the molecular level, in situ hybridization and immunohistochemical studies demonstrated that NR1 mRNA and NR protein are indeed missing in the mutants older than one month of age. Although subsequent detailed studies revealed that loss of NR1 mRNA and NR protein spread to some forebrain areas other than CA1 as the animals age, these studies confirmed that, with young adult mice, the primary site of NR1 gene deletion was CA1 pyramidal cells (Fukaya et al., 2003). In accordance with these findings at the molecular level, LTP and LTD were deficient at SC-CA1 synapses, while both LTP and LTD were normal at other types of synapses such as PP-DG synapses. Reflecting a relatively minor level of contribution of hippocampal NR channels to the basal level of synaptic transmission, the total evoked current at SC-CA1 synapses was unaffected by the NR1 gene deletion. We then subjected the CA1-NR1 KO mice to the hidden platform as well as the visible platform version of the Morris water maze and found that the mutants were specifically impaired in spatial learning.

In an effort to identify a deficit at intermediate levels between the molecular or synaptic level and the behavioral level, we examined the firing properties of individual CA1 place cells or populations of CA1 place cells by the in vivo multielectrode recording technique (McHugh *et al.*, 1996). This study revealed that the sizes of the individual place fields were on average 30% larger than those of the control littermates. Further, at the neuronal ensemble level, the ability of pairs of CA1 place cells that shared a common place field to cofire (within 200 ms) was severely impaired. Consequently, a large discrepancy existed between the actual movements of mutant mice through space and the movements predicted from place-related firing of their CA1 pyramidal cells. This observation was in contrast to the high levels of overlap between the actual and reconstructed movements of the control mice.

These studies on CA1-NR1 KO mice demonstrated that the NR-mediated function in CA1 is essential for acquisition and/or recall of long-term spatial memory. The correlative LTP and LTD deficits at SC-CA1 synapses suggest that synaptic plasticity at these synapses is an essential component of the mechanisms underlying memory. Our data also indicate that NR function and probably NR-mediated synaptic plasticity play a crucial role for the proper representation of space in the form of place cells. The finding that the formation of place cells is impaired suggests strongly that the behavioral deficit is at the acquisition rather than the recall phase of memory.

12.2.5   *Theories on the role of the CA3 recurrent network in associative memory*

Marr (1971) developed a pioneering neural network theory of the role of the hippocampus in memory storage and recall. In his theory, he considered the contribution to memory storage of modifiable connections between neurons, and the retrieval of complete memories when only fragments of the original are presented. In particular, he proposed that a recurrent network could act as an autoassociative memory system if the efficacy of the excitatory synapses were modifiable, and if the membrane potentials of primary neurons were regulated by inhibitory input that reflected total network activity. According to his theory, strengthening of recurrent excitatory connections between neurons that are activated by the original memory pattern allows storage of that pattern. When a part of the stored memory pattern is subsequently presented, recall of the whole pattern is accomplished through a process of single or multiple step iteration known as pattern completion. Marr pointed out that in the multiple-step process, primary neurons initially excited by the presentation of a fragment of the stored pattern would then activate other neurons that were a part of the original pattern, through previously strengthened recurrent connections. This process should continue until a steady firing pattern in the network is reached. The one-step recall process was called simple recall (Gardner-Medwin, 1976), while the multiple-step process was referred to as the collateral effect (Marr, 1971). Based on the observation of massive recurrent connectivity with highly modifiable synapses, area CA3 became an attractive candidate for the biological implementation of such a pattern completion network involved in the storage and retrieval of associative memory (Hasselmo et al., 1995; McNaughton & Morris, 1987; Rolls et al., 1989; Willshaw & Buckingham, 1990).

One way to interfere with the postulated memory storage and retrieval capacity of the CA3 recurrent collateral network without directly affecting plasticity of mossy fiber CA3 synapses is to target the knockout of the NR1 gene to CA3 pyramidal cells. It is expected that such mutant mice (CA3-NR1 KO mice) will be a valuable tool for addressing Marr's hypothesis directly.

12.3   Generation and characterization of CA3 NMDA receptor knockout mice

To generate CA3 pyramidal cell-specific NR1 knockout mice (CA3-NR1 KO mice), we employed the bacteriophage P1-derived Cre/loxP recombination system, which previously enabled us to produce CA1-NR1 KO mice (Tsien et al., 1996). Because earlier in situ hybridization studies had indicated that the CA3 pyramidal cell layer is a robust site of expression of KA-1, one of the kainate receptor subunits (Bahn et al., 1994; Wisden & Seeburg, 1993), we created transgenic mice in which the transcriptional regulatory region of the KA-1 gene was used to drive the expression of the Cre transgene. In one transgenic line (G32-4), the level of Cre-immunoreactivity (IR) was robust in the CA3 pyramidal cell layer in mice older than 4 weeks of age (Figure 12.2A). The spatial and temporal pattern of Cre/loxP recombination in the G32-4 Cre transgenic mouse line was examined by crossing it with a lacZ reporter mouse (Rosa26) (Soriano, 1999) and staining brain sections derived from the progeny with X-gal (Figure 12.2B–D). Cre/loxP recombination was first detectable at P14 in area CA3 of the hippocampus (data not shown). At 8 weeks of age, recombination had occurred in nearly 100% of pyramidal cells in area CA3. Recombination also occurred in a few other brain areas, but at distinctly lower frequencies: in about 10% of dentate gyrus and cerebellar granule cells, and in about 50% of cells in the facial nerve nuclei of the brain stem. These frequencies of recombination did not change in older mice (data not shown). No recombination was detected in the cerebral cortex or in the hippocampal CA1 and subicular regions. We further determined the type of the recombination-positive cells in the hippocampus by

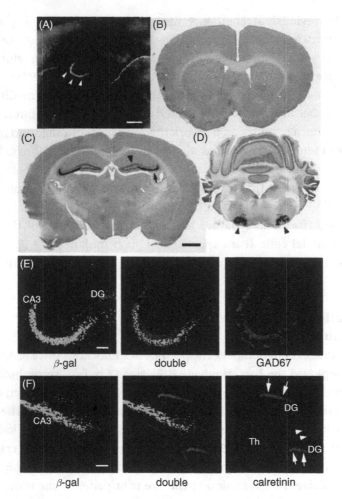

Figure 12.2 Distribution of Cre-immunoreactivity (IR) in G32-4 brain and distribution of Cre/loxP recombination mediated by G32-4 mice. (A), A sagittal Vibratome section prepared from the brain of a 4-week-old male G32-4 mouse was stained with a rabbit anti-Cre antibody, and the Cre-IR was visualized with FITC under a confocal laser microscope. The prominently stained, arc-shaped area indicated by arrowheads corresponds to the CA3 pyramidal cell layer. Scale bar: 50 μm. (B–D), Coronal Vibratome sections prepared from the brain of an 8-week-old male G32-4/ Rosa26 double transgenic mouse were stained with X-gal and counterstained with Nuclear Fast Red. No X-gal staining was observed in sections derived from the forebrain (B) while in the hippocampus the CA3 pyramidal cell layer (arrow) was the major site of X-gal staining. The dentate gyrus granule cell layer (arrowhead) was also stained by X-gal, albeit to a lesser extent (C). In the hindbrain, the facial nerve nuclei (arrowheads) were stained with X-gal (D). The scale bar shown in (C) is equivalent to 100 μm and is valid for (B–D). (E–F), Parasagittal hippocampal sections derived from the brain of an 8-week-old G32–4/Rosa26 double transgenic mouse were subjected to double

carrying out double immunofluorescence staining using a set of antibodies specific for β-galactosidase (a marker for the Cre/loxP recombination), glutamic acid decarboxylase (GAD)-67 (a marker for a subset of interneurons), and calretinin (a marker for dentate gyrus mossy cells in the mouse hippocampus) (Liu et al., 1996). Minimal overlapping staining was observed with anti-β-galactosidase and anti-GAD67 antibodies (Figure 12.2E), and with anti-β-galactosidase and anti-calretinin antibodies (Figure 12.1F). These results indicate that in area CA3 and the dentate gyrus, the Cre/loxP recombination is restricted to the pyramidal cells and the granule cells, respectively.

We crossed the G32-4 mice with floxed-NR1 (fNR1) mice (Tsien et al., 1996) in order to restrict the NR1 knockout to those cell types targeted by the G32-4 Cre transgene. Homozygous floxed, Cre-positive progeny (CA3-NR1 KO) were viable and fertile, and exhibited no gross developmental abnormalities. In situ hybridization data suggested that in the CA3 pyramidal cell layer of these mice, the NR1 gene is intact until about 5 weeks of age, starts being deleted thereafter, and is nearly completely deleted by 18 weeks of age (Figure 12.3A–D). There was no indication of deletion of the NR1 gene elsewhere in the brain throughout the animal's life. Specifically, the NR1 gene seemed to be intact in granule cells of the dentate gyrus (Figure 12.3F) and the cerebellum (Figure 12.3B,D) as well as in the facial nerve nuclei (Figure 12.3H). This is in contrast to the Cre/loxP recombination-dependent expression of the lacZ gene (see Figure 12.2C,D).

NR1-immunocytochemistry carried out using an antibody against the C-terminus of mouse NR1 in collaboration with Masahiko Watanabe (Hokkaido University, Japan) (Watanabe et al., 1998) confirmed, at the protein level, the selective and late-onset deletion of the NR1 gene in the CA3 region of the mutant mice. The distribution of the immunoreactivity (IR) was normal during the first 7 weeks after birth (data not shown). By the 18th postnatal week, however, NR1-IR had disappeared entirely from both the apical and basal dendritic areas in the CA3 region (Figure 12.3J). In contrast, normal levels of NR1-IR were maintained

---

Caption for Figure 12.2   (cont.)

immunofluorescence staining with anti-β-galactosidase (visualized by Alexa488) and anti-GAD67 (visualized by Cy3) (E), or with anti-β-galactosidase and anti-calretinin (visualized by Cy3) (F). β-galactosidase-IR (green), which appeared robustly in CA3 and to a lesser extent in the dentate gyrus, did not colocalize with GAD67-IR (red in E) or calretinin-IR (red in F), indicating that the Cre/loxP recombination in the G32-4/Rosa26 double transgenic mice is confined to pyramidal cells in CA3 and granule cells in the dentate gyrus. DG: dentate gyrus, Th: thalamus. The white arrows and arrowheads in (F) indicate somata and axon terminals of mossy cells, respectively, which are not stained by the anti-β-galactosidase. Scale bars: 10 μm (E, F) (for color image please see www.cambridge.org/9780521143400).

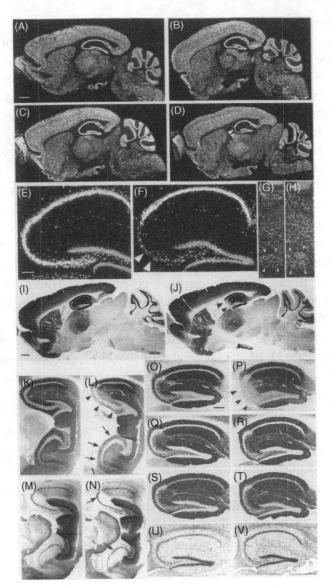

Figure 12.3 Distributions of NR1 mRNA and NR1 and other proteins in the brain of CA3-NR1 KO mice. (A–H), Dark field images of the signals of *in situ* hybridization carried out on parasagittal brain sections using a ^{33}P-labeled NR1 cRNA probe. The sources of the brains were: (A), A 5-week-old male floxed NR1 mouse (fNR1; control); (B), A 5-week-old male CA3-NR1 KO mouse (a littermate of the (A) mouse); (C, E, and G), An 18-week-old male floxed NR1 mouse; (D, F, and H), An 18-week-old male CA3-NR1 KO mouse (a littermate of the (C, E, G) mouse). Scale bar: 100 μm (A). In (E) and (F), the hippocampal regions of (C) and (D) respectively, are enlarged. In (G) and (H), the areas of the facial nerve nuclei are enlarged. In the CA3 pyramidal cell layer of the CA3-NR1 KO mice, the level of NR1 mRNA was normal until 5 weeks of age, started to decline

in the CA1 region and the dentate gyrus of the 18-week-old mutant mice. The reduction of NR1-IR in the CA3 region was observed in both dorsal and ventral hippocampus (Figure 12.3L), suggesting that the NR1 gene is deleted uniformly along the longitudinal axis of the hippocampus.

We carried out a set of cytochemical and immunocytochemical experiments to investigate the integrity of the cytoarchitecture of the mutant hippocampus (Figure 12.3O–T). Nissl staining did not reveal any obvious abnormalities (Figure 12.3U,V). Furthermore, no significant differences could be detected in the patterns of postsynaptic density-95 (PSD-95) (Valtschanoff *et al.*, 1999) (Figure 12.3Q,R) or GluR1 (AMPA-type glutamate receptor subunit 1) expression (Figure 12.3S,T). Also normal was the IR distribution of calbindin$_{D28k}$, a Ca^{2+}-binding protein known to be expressed at high levels in dentate gyrus granule cells but not in cells in the CA3 region (Watanabe *et al.*, 1998) (Figure 12.3M,N), suggesting that mossy fibers from dentate gyrus granule cells project normally to the target in their CA3 region, that is, stratum lucidum.

Caption for Figure 12.3 (cont.)

thereafter, and reached the lowest and stable level by 18 weeks of age (arrowheads in (D)). There was no indication of a reduced NR1 mRNA level in the mutant mice relative to the control littermates in any other brain area and throughout the postnatal development. In particular, the levels of NR1 mRNA in the mutants' dentate gyrus (F), cerebellum (B and D), and the facial nerve nuclei (H) are indistinguishable from those of the control littermates (E, A, C, and G). The arrowheads in (F) indicate scattered hybridization signals that are most probably derived from CA3 interneurons. The arrowheads in (G) and (H) surround the facial nerve nuclei. The scale bar in (E) is equivalent to 25 µm and is valid for (E–H). (I–T), Immunoperoxidase staining of paraffin sections of brains derived from 18-week-old male mice visualized with 3, 3'-diaminobenzidine. The primary antibodies used are: (I) to (L), anti-NR1; (M and N) anti-calbindin$_{D28k}$; (O and P) anti-NR2A; (Q and R) anti-PSD-95; (S and T) anti-GluR1. The genotypes of the mice are: (I, K, M, O, Q, and S) fNR1 (control) and (J, L, N, P, R, and T) CA3-NR1 KO (mutant). Medial parasagittal sections were used for experiments other than those in (K) to (N) for which lateral parasagittal sections were employed. In the mutants, NR1-IR was selectively deficient in the dorsal (arrowheads in (J) and (L)) as well as ventral (arrows in (L)) area CA3. This mutation did not affect the distribution of PSD-95 (R) or GluR1 (T) in the hippocampus nor in mossy fiber projections to CA3 as visualized by calbindin$_{D28k}$-IR (arrows in (N)). However, NR2A-IR was deficient in CA3 (arrowheads in (P)), presumably because the NR1 subunit needed for the release of the NR2 subunits from intra-ER retention is missing (M. Fukaya *et al.*, 2003). (U and V) Nissl staining of hippocampal sections derived from an 18-week-old male fNR1 mouse (U) and a male CA3-NR1 KO littermate (V). The mutant exhibited no gross morphological alteration. The scale bar in (I) represents 100 µm. The scale bar in (O) is equivalent to 50 µm and is valid for (K–V).

Overall, these data indicate that in the mutant mice, the NR1 gene is selectively deleted in the CA3 pyramidal cells of the hippocampus. This deletion occurs only in adult mice (older than 5 weeks of age) and does not affect the hippocampal cytoarchitecture. In the G32-4/Rosa26 mice, Cre/loxP recombination seems to be less confined to the CA3 pyramidal cells and occurs earlier in development than in the NR1 mutant mice. This is probably due in part to differences in the sensitivity of detection and in part to differences in the susceptibility of the loxP substrates to the recombinase (our unpublished observations).

To evaluate whether functional NRs are present in CA3 pyramidal cells in CA3-NR1 KO mice, Raymond Chitwood and Mark Yeckel in Daniel Johnston's laboratory (Baylor College of Medicine) conducted whole-cell patch clamp recordings on CA3 and CA1 pyramidal cells in acute hippocampal slices from adult male CA3-NR1 KO mice and their fNR1 control littermates. They compared the basic intrinsic properties and synaptically-evoked responses of CA3 and CA1 pyramidal cells. In all but two experiments, the experimenters were blind to whether the animals were control or mutant mice. There did not appear to be any differences with respect to the basic intrinsic properties of CA3 pyramidal cells in control ($n = 14$) or mutant mice ($n = 23$) (resting membrane potential (RMP): control, -67.0 ± 2.0 mV; mutant, -67.8 ± 1.6 mV; input resistance (R_N): control, 200.8 ± 17.9 MΩ; mutant, 183 ± 12.6 MΩ). Similarly, RMP and R_N did not differ for CA1 pyramidal cells in control and mutant mice (RMP: control, $n = 7$, -62.3 ± 1.4 mV; mutant, $n = 12$, -62.3 ± 0.7 mV; R_N: control, 189.8 ± 30.0 MΩ; mutant, 171.1 ± 10.8 MΩ).

In the first series of experiments, synaptically-evoked NMDA currents were pharmacologically isolated by blocking AMPA/kainate receptors (DNQX, 40 μM); in most experiments, an antagonist to GABA$_B$ receptors (CGP 35348, 50–100 μM) was also included. To fully activate NMDA currents, membrane potential-dependent blockade of NMDA channels by Mg^{2+} was reduced by omitting the Mg^{2+} ion in the bathing solution. Synaptic responses were evoked in either CA3 or CA1 with single stimulation or brief bursts of stimulation (5 pulses at 50–100 Hz) delivered to one of three afferent pathways: recurrent C/A, mossy fiber input to CA3, or Schaffer collateral input to CA1. Consistent with the immunohistochemical characterization of CA3-NR1 KO mice that showed an absence of NR1 in CA3 (Figure 12.3J), a C/A-evoked APV-sensitive NMDA current was never detected in mutant mice ($n = 10$, % block of total current, in DNQX, $96.2 \pm 1.3\%$; in DNQX/APV, $97.0 \pm 1.4\%$). In contrast, in the control mice C/A stimulation activated a slowly rising, slowly decaying current in the presence of DNQX that was blocked by APV, consistent with NR-activation ($n = 5$, % block of total current in DNQX, $72.5 \pm 3.2\%$; in DNQX/APV, $98.1 \pm 0.9\%$) (Figure 12.4A).

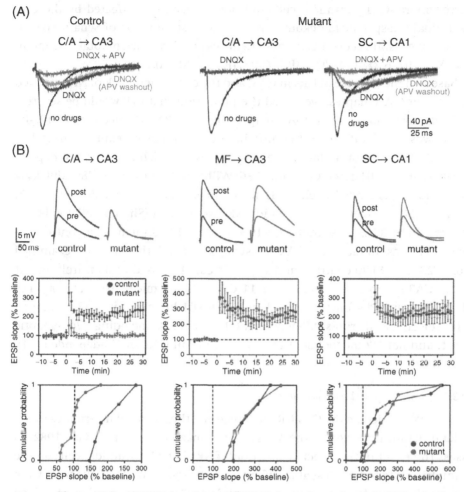

Figure 12.4   NMDAR function and NMDAR-dependent induction of LTP were absent in CA3 pyramidal cells of CA3-NR1 KO mice. Functional characterization of NMDAR-activation was performed in hippocampal slices from adult control and mutant animals (18–28 week old); experimenters were blind to the genotype of the mice. (A) Synaptic responses were evoked and NMDA currents pharmacologically isolated. *Left panel*, representative data from a control CA3 pyramidal cell showing a commissural/associational (C/A)-evoked NMDA current (isolated with 40 μM DNQX and blocked by 50 μM d, l APV; CGP 35348 was not present). *Right panel*, CA3 and CA1 EPSCs recorded from a CA3-NR1 KO mouse. As shown in this example, C/A-evoked NMDA currents were never detected in CA3 pyramidal cells of mutant animals (i.e., DNQX totally blocked fast synaptic transmission). In contrast, in a CA1 pyramidal cell from the same animal, Schaffer collateral (SC) stimulation elicited an NR-mediated EPSC. (B) Quantification of LTP induced for C/A and mossy fiber (MF) input to CA3 and SC input to CA1. *Top panel*: Representative waveforms (averages of five consecutive responses recorded at 0.05 Hz) show that C/A-CA3 LTP was selectively prevented in mutant

Furthermore, CA1 pyramidal cells did not appear to be affected by the CA3 pyramidal cell-specific knockout of NR1 because stimulation of Schaffer collaterals evoked NMDA currents in these neurons ($n = 8$, % block of total current, in DNQX, $72.9 \pm 6.2\%$; in DNQX/APV, 100%) (Figure 12.4A).

Based on the absence of NRs in CA3, and the consequent lack of NR-activated currents at C/A synapses, we tested the prediction that LTP would be severely and selectively impaired at C/A synapses in CA3-NR1 KO mice (Figure 12.4B). There was no significant difference in the induction or expression of LTP induced in control or mutant mice at synapses in which LTP does not depend on NR-activation (Harris & Cotman, 1986; Williams & Johnston, 1988; Zalutsky & Nicoll, 1990; Berger & Yeckel, 1991) (mossy fiber-CA3: control, $265 \pm 39\%$, $n = 5$; mutant, $259 \pm 45\%$, $n = 6$), or in which NRs were intact (Shaffer collateral-CA1: control, $232 \pm 37\%$, $n = 9$; mutant, $219 \pm 53\%$, $n = 10$). Similarly, in control animals LTP was induced at C/A-CA3 synapses in all the animals examined ($202 \pm 28\%$, $n = 5$). In contrast, and as predicted, LTP was almost entirely absent at C/A-CA3 synapses in nine out of 11 CA3-NR1 KO mice ($101 \pm 11\%$, $n = 11$). These data provide functional evidence that NR1 knockout in CA3 pyramidal cells selectively disrupts NR-dependent LTP in CA3, including C/A synaptic input, and not NR-independent mossy fiber LTP in CA3, or NR-dependent LTP in area CA1.

12.3.1   *Normal spatial reference memory*

We subjected the CA3-NR1 KO mice and their control littermates to the hidden platform version of the Morris water maze task (Morris *et al.*, 1982) to assess the effect of the selective ablation of NRs in CA3 pyramidal cells on the animals' ability to form a spatial reference memory. In this task, the mice were repeatedly trained over a span of several days to learn the location of a fixed platform hidden beneath polypropylene bead-covered water using multiple extramaze cues. We used 18–24-week-old male mice, and the training was carried out for 12 days, 4 trials per day. Wild-type and fNR1 mice were used as controls. No significant differences were observed in the escape latency and the

---

Caption for Figure 12.4 (cont.)

animals. *Middle panel*: Summary graphs showing the time course of potentiation after delivering 3 long trains of stimulation (100 pulses at 100 Hz concomitant with a 1 second depolarizing pulse 1 train every 20 seconds). *Bottom panel*: To better represent the results of the individual experiments, cumulative probability plots are used to graphically summarize the data; each point represents the magnitude of change relative to baseline for a given experiment 20–25 minutes (average) after high frequency stimulation (for color image please see plate section).

total distance traveled between the control and mutant mice (Figure 12.5A,B). Also indistinguishable among genotypes were the average swimming velocity (Figure 12.5C) and the proportion of the time spent in the periphery of the pool (Figure 12.5D, 'wall hugging time). The latter measure represents the degree of the animal's thigmotaxic behavior (Simon et al., 1994).

To confirm that the mice used a spatial strategy, we subjected the mutant and fNR1 control littermates to a probe trial on day 13 and assessed spatial memory by monitoring the relative radial-quadrant occupancy (Figure 12.5E). We found that both mouse strains spent significantly more time in the target radial-quadrant compared to any of the nontarget quadrants. The preferential search for the target area by both types of mice was also shown by the criterion of absolute platform occupancy (Figure 12.5F).

Subsets of the mutant and control mice that had gone through the training and testing sessions were subjected to a reversal learning task for an additional 5 days, from day 16 to day 20 (Figure 12.5A–D). In this task, the location of the hidden platform was rotated by 90 degrees, and the latency and other performance parameters were recorded. Both the mutant and control mice rapidly learned the new platform location and there was no genotype-associated difference in any of the performance parameters examined ($p > 0.05$ for all four measures). These data show that the mutant mice did not exhibit abnormal perseveration (Whishaw & Tomie, 1997).

Overall, these results indicate that the selective ablation of NRs in adult hippocampal CA3 pyramidal cells has no detectable effect on the animal's ability to form and retrieve spatial memory as determined by the standard hidden platform version of the Morris water maze task. Further, these results show that the CA3-NR1 KO mice are not impaired in motivation, motor coordination, or sensory functions required to carry out this spatial memory task.

12.3.2   Diminished recall upon partial cue removal

In order to assess the role of CA3 NRs in pattern completion at the behavioral level, we examined the dependence of spatial memory recall on the integrity of distal cues in the CA3-NR1 KO mice and their fNR1 control littermates. We first subjected subsets of the mice that had gone through the training and the probe trial sessions to one more block (4 trials) of training, one hour after the probe trial (i.e., on day 13). The purpose of this extra training was to avoid potential extinction that may have resulted from the probe trial. On day 14, we subjected these animals to a second probe trial in the same water maze except that three out of the four extramaze cues had been removed from the surrounding wall. In Figure 12.6A,B, the results of the second probe trial carried out in the partial-cue environment are compared with those of the first probe

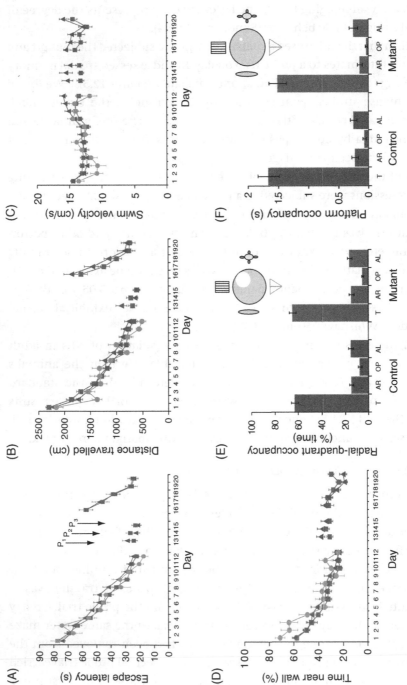

Figure 12.5 CA3-NR1 KO mice are normal in the spatial reference memory version of the Morris water maze task. Eighteen- to twenty-four-week-old male CA3-NR1 KO mice (mutant, red squares, n = 44), floxed-NR1 (fNR1; control, blue triangles, n = 37), and their wild-type littermates (control, green circles, n = 11) were subjected to training trials for 12 days, four trials per day, in a pool surrounded by four extramaze cues

trial carried out in the full-cue environment a day before with the same set of mice. In the partial-cue trial, the control mice focused their search on the phantom platform location relative to corresponding locations in the other three quadrants as much as they did in the full-cue probe trial. In contrast, the mutant mice search preference for the phantom platform location was significantly reduced by the partial cue removal.

We also monitored the effect of the partial cue removal by the criterion of relative radial-quadrant occupancy. The target radial-quadrant occupancy of the control and mutant mice were $65.9 \pm 4\%$ and $66.4 \pm 4\%$ under the full cue conditions, respectively, and $58.8 \pm 5\%$ and $44.6 \pm 5\%$ under the partial cue conditions, respectively. The effect of the partial cue removal was significant for mutants but not for controls ($F_{(3,82)} = 5.625$, $p < 0.015$; Newman-Kuels post hoc comparison for cue-removal effect on mutant mice, $p < 0.05$).

For each individual mouse, we also determined the occupancy time at the phantom platform location in the partial-cue probe trial and compared that with the phantom platform occupancy time in the earlier full-cue probe trial, yielding a 'relative recall index (RRI)' measure. As shown in Figure 12.6C, there was no effect of partial cue removal on the control mice, whereas the effect was highly significant for the mutant mice.

Caption for Figure 12.5 (cont.)

(full-cue conditions). The three types of mice did not differ significantly in escape latency (genotype effect, $F_{(2,89)} = 0.58$, $p = 0.562$) (A), distance traveled (genotype effect, $F_{(2,89)} = 1.00$, $p = 0.371$) (B), swimming velocity (genotype effect, $F_{(2,89)} = 0.61$, $p = 0.547$) (C), or time spent near the pool wall (genotype effect, $F_{(2,89)} = 0.81$, $p = 0.450$) (D). The mutant ($n = 44$) and fNR1 control ($n = 37$) mice were then subjected to a probe trial (P1) on day 13 under the full-cue conditions. The data show that mutant and control mice focused their search equally well on the target area as determined by the relative occupancy of each radial-quadrant, which is defined as the largest circle inscribed in a quadrant ($p < 0.01$ for both genotypes) (E) or absolute platform occupancy ($p < 0.01$ for both genotypes) (F). On day 14 and day 15, subsets of mice ($n = 20$ for fNR1 controls and $n = 23$ for mutants) were subjected to probe trials under partial-cue (P2) and no-cue (P3) conditions, respectively (the data are shown in Figure 12.6). One hour after each of these probe trials as well as on the day 13 probe trial, the mice were subjected to one block (4 trials) of training under the original environment (that is with the platform and the four cues all at the original locations), and the maintenance of the original memory was confirmed by the standard criteria (A–D). From day 16 to day 20, subsets of the fNR1 ($n = 14$) and mutant ($n = 16$) mice were subjected to a reversal learning task in which the location of the platform was rotated by 90 degrees. The learning was assessed by the standard criteria (A–D). T, target quadrant; AR, adjacent right quadrant; OP, opposite quadrant; AL, adjacent left quadrant (for color image please see plate section).

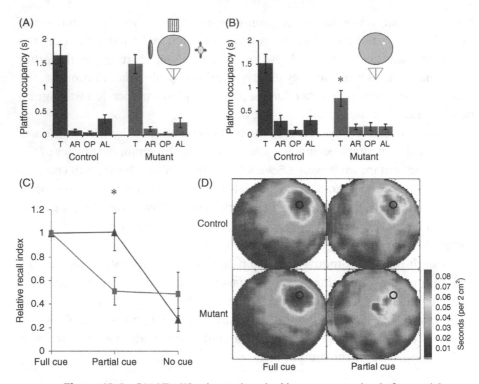

Figure 12.6   CA3-NR1 KO mice are impaired in memory retrieval after partial cue removal. The results of the probe trials carried out on day 13 under full-cue conditions (A) and on day 14 under partial-cue conditions (B) are shown using the criterion of absolute platform occupancy. The mice used are fNR1 (control; blue, $n = 20$) and CA3-NR1-KO (mutant; red, $n = 23$). The designations of the quadrants (i.e., T, AR, OP, and AL) are as described in the legend to Figure 12.5. The control mice exhibited the same level of recall under partial-cue conditions as they did under full-cue conditions, while the recall by the mutant mice was severely impaired by the partial cue removal (ANOVA for target platform occupancy, $F_{(3,82)} = 4.329$, $p < 0.007$; Newman-Keuls *post hoc* comparison for cue-removal effect on mutant mice, *$p < 0.05$). (C) The intact recall capability of control mice ($n = 18$) and its robust impairment in mutant mice ($n = 22$) under partial-cue conditions are also shown by relative recall index (RRI). RRI was defined as the ratio of the target platform occupancy on the second (P2) or third (P3) probe trial to that of the first (P1) probe trial for each animal. (C) also includes RRI of control and mutant mice under no-cue conditions. The RRI difference between the control and the mutant mice under the partial-cue conditions was highly significant (*$p < 0.009$, Mann–Whitney U-test), while that under no-cue conditions was not ($p = 0.9$, Mann–Whitney U-test). Blue triangles and red squares represent control and mutant mice, respectively. (D) The results of the full-cue and partial-cue probe trials are also shown as animals' spatial histograms during the trials. In the full-cue probe trial, both control ($n = 20$) and mutant ($n = 23$) mice focused their search at or near the phantom platform. In the partial-cue probe trial, control mice did the same, but the mutant mice spent the majority of the time at or near the center of the pool, which is the release site, and spent less time near the target site (for color image please see plate section).

This differential effect of partial cue removal on search behaviors of control and mutant mice was also indicated by a difference in how animals distributed their movements during the probe trials (Figure 12.6D). In the probe trial conducted in the full-cue environment, both mutant and control mice focused their search at or near the location of the phantom platform. A similar distribution of the animals' locations was observed for the control mice searching for the platform in the partial-cue environment. By contrast, the mutant mice spent the majority of the time at or near the release site at the center of the pool, and correspondingly spent significantly less time at or near the location of the phantom platform on the probe trial that was conducted in the partial-cue environment.

It is possible that the mutant mice performed poorly in the partial-cue probe trial compared with the fNR1 control animals because they had lost the spatial memory faster than the control mice. To test this possibility, we restored the full-cue training environment by returning the three missing cues and the platform, and subjected the same set of animals that had gone through the training and probe trials to one more block (4 trials) of training on day 14, one hour after the partial-cue probe trial. Both the mutant and control animals found the platform as fast as they did on day 12 and day 13, and there was no significant difference between the latencies of the mutant and control animals ($p = 0.32$) (Figure 12.5A). There were also no significant differences between mutant and control mice in the total path length traveled and in their thigmotaxic tendency ($p > 0.1$ for both measures) (Figure 12.5B and 12.4D), though the mutant animals swam slightly slower than control mice ($p < 0.04$) (Figure 12.5C).

To test whether the recall exhibited in the partial-cue environment depended on the remaining extramaze cue, we carried out a third probe trial (no-cue probe trial) on day 15 after removal of the entire set of the four extramaze cues. We calculated the average relative recall index (RRI) and found robust recall deficits in both control and mutant mice under these conditions (Figure 12.6C). Both the control and mutant mice retained the memory of the platform location during this no-cue probe trial, because they reached the platform efficiently in yet another block of training in the full-cue environment that was conducted one hour after the no-cue probe trial (Figure 12.5A–D, at day 15) ($p > 0.15$ for any of four measures).

In summary, under the full-cue conditions both mutant and control mice exhibited robust memory recall. When three out of the four major extramaze cues were removed, control mice still exhibited the same level of recall, while the mutants' recall capability was severely impaired.

12.3.3   CA1 place cells show preserved spatial coding

While these behavioral results demonstrate that mutant animals have an impaired ability to retrieve spatial memories when tested with a fraction of the original stimulus cues, behavioral testing alone reveals little about the precise neural mechanisms underlying this phenotype. To understand the neurophysiological consequences of CA3-NR1 disruption, CA1 place cell activity was analyzed using in vivo tetrode recording techniques. Although genetic deletion was confined to CA3 pyramidal cells, place cell recordings were made from CA1 for two reasons. First, CA1 is the final output region of the hippocampus proper and, as a consequence, CA1 activity is more likely to reflect behavioral performance than CA3 activity. Second, because most previous relevant electrophysiological tetrode recording studies have been performed on CA1 (Best *et al.*, 2001; Muller, 1996), CA1 recordings are more suitable for comparison with previously published findings of place cell activity in other genetically altered mice (McHugh *et al.*, 1996).

In total, we recorded from 188 complex spiking (pyramidal) cells and 9 putative interneurons from 5 CA3-NR1 KO mice (24 sessions) and from 155 pyramidal cells and 8 interneurons from 3 fNR1 (control) mice (19 sessions) during behavioral open field foraging (Muller & Kubie, 1987). While an analysis of the basic cellular properties of CA1 pyramidal cells revealed no difference in mean firing rate, spike width, or amplitude attenuation within bursts (Quirk *et al.*, 2001), pyramidal cells from mutant animals showed a significant decrease in complex spike bursting properties (Table 12.1). Given that a reduction in CA1 bursting may reflect a decrease in excitatory input from CA3 (Schwartzkroin & Prince, 1978; Wong & Traub, 1983) where NR1 is ablated, one might expect that reduced CA3 drive would also have an impact on the coding properties of CA1 place cells in mutant animals. However, when we examined the spatial tuning of CA1 pyramidal cells under full-cue conditions, we found no significant differences between control and mutant animals with respect to either place field size (no. of pixels above a 1 Hz threshold), or average firing rate within a cell's place field (integrated firing) (Table 12.1). Furthermore, the ability of cells with overlapping place fields to fire in a coordinated manner did not differ between control and mutant animals (Table 12.1: covariance coefficient), a result that is in sharp contrast with data from CA1-NR1 KO mice in which there was a complete lack of coordinated firing (McHugh *et al.*, 1996). These results demonstrate that spatial information within CA1 is relatively preserved despite the loss of CA3 NRs and provide a physiological correlate of the intact spatial performance of CA3-NR1 KO mice in the Morris water maze under full-cue conditions.

12.3.4   *Reduced inhibitory firing contributes to preserved spatial coding within CA1*

In addition to excitatory input from entorhinal cortex and CA3, CA1 pyramidal cells receive inhibitory input from local interneurons. Thus, CA1 output reflects a balance between excitatory and inhibitory inputs (Paulsen &

Table 12.1. *Electrophysiological properties of CA1 hippocampal neurons in familiar open field*

	Pyramidal cells		Interneurons	
	Floxed (n = 155, D = 19, N = 3)	Mutant (n = 188, D = 24, N = 5)	Floxed (n = 8, D = 19, N = 3)	Mutant (n = 9, D = 24, N = 5)
Mean firing rate (Hz)	1.175 ± 0.097	1.179 ± 0.082 (p < 0.97)	**30.96 ± 5.27**	**12.62 ± 1.73** (p < 0.003)
Spike width (μs)	328.5 ± 4.31	326.8 ± 3.70 (p < 0.76)	186.6 ± 9.7	167.2 ± 4.8 (p < 0.08)
Spike attenuation (%)	90.44 ± 0.56	90.45 ± 0.40 (p < 0.98)	N/A	N/A
Complex spike index	24.26 ± 1.21	**16.84 ± 0.83** (p < 10^{-4})	1.66 ± 0.52	1.67 ± 0.39 (p < 0.98)
Burst spike frequency (%)	**52.93 ± 1.17**	42.18 ± 1.28 (p < 10^{-4})	N/A	N/A
Integrated firing rate [$\sum$(Hz/pixel)]	549.5 ± 48.2	544.7 ± 40.0 (p < 0.94)	N/A	N/A
Place field size (no. of pixel)	125.6 ± 8.28	133.1 ± 7.27 (p < 0.50)	N/A	N/A
Covariance coefficient	0.0359 ± 0.007	0.0410 ± 0.005 (p < 0.56)	N/A	N/A

Note: The table details the properties of CA1 pyramidal cells and interneurons in both mutant and control animals during exploratory behavior. There were no statistically significant differences detected in overall firing rates, integrated firing rates, spike width, field sizes over 1 Hz, spike attenuation, and covariance coefficient between CA3-KO and control pyramidal cells (student's *t*-test). Complex spike index scores showed a 31% decrease in the mutant animals. Burst spike frequency also showed a significant reduction in the mutant cells. Interneuron firing rates also showed a 52% decrease in the mutants, suggesting reduction of CA3 to CA1 drive in the mutant mice.

Moser, 1998). In addition to a decrease in pyramidal cell bursting, we found a dramatic decrease in the firing rate of putative CA1 interneurons within CA3-NR1 KO mice (Table 12.1). This reduction in interneuron firing rate could be due to either a decrease in direct feed-forward input from CA3 onto inhibitory interneurons (Buzsaki, 1984; Mizumori *et al.*, 1989a) as a consequence of the CA3-NR1 knockout, or to a decrease in local feedback drive from CA1 pyramidal cells onto interneurons (Csicsvari *et al.*, 1998). Based on our observations, we believe that this reduction in inhibition in mutant mice compensates for the reduction of excitatory drive from CA3 thereby allowing CA1 pyramidal cells to maintain robust spatial coding. This hypothesis is consistent with previous theoretical (Marr, 1971) and experimental (Mizumori *et al.*, 1989b) studies.

12.3.5   *Partial cue removal reduces the output of CA1 place cells in CA3-NR1 KO mice*

Having established the ability of CA1 pyramidal cells from mutant animals to maintain robust spatial firing in full-cue environments, we were interested in determining whether CA1 output would be maintained following partial cue removal (Hetherington & Shapiro, 1997; O'Keefe & Conway, 1978). Animals were first allowed to explore an area for 20–30 minutes in the presence of four distal visual cues and then removed to their home cage for up to two hours. Following this two-hour delay, animals were returned to the open field with either the same four cues present (4 to 4 condition), or with three of the four cues removed (4 to 1 condition). Using three fNR1 control mice, we identified 28 and 26 complex spike cells during five "4 to 4" sessions and five "4 to 1" sessions, respectively. From five mutant mice we were able to isolate 43 and 47 complex spike cells during six "4 to 4" and six "4 to 1" recording sessions, respectively. Figure 12.7A,B shows representative examples of place fields from both mutant and control animals in the presence and partial absence of distal visual cues.

To quantify relative changes in place field properties for cells recorded across experimental conditions, we calculated, for each cell, a relative change index (RCI). Using this index, we measured three properties of CA1 output: (1) burst frequency, (2) place field size and (3) integrated firing rate (Figure 12.7C–E). Despite individual cell variation, on average in control animals there was no change in burst frequency, field size, or firing rate of cells from the cue removal conditions relative to those from the no-cue removal conditions. Thus, at the population level, the net output from CA1 was maintained for control animals under cue removal conditions. In contrast, mutant cells showed significant reductions in burst frequency, place field size, and firing rate following cue removal. Importantly, mutant place cells showed no significant changes when animals were returned to the recording environment in the presence of all four

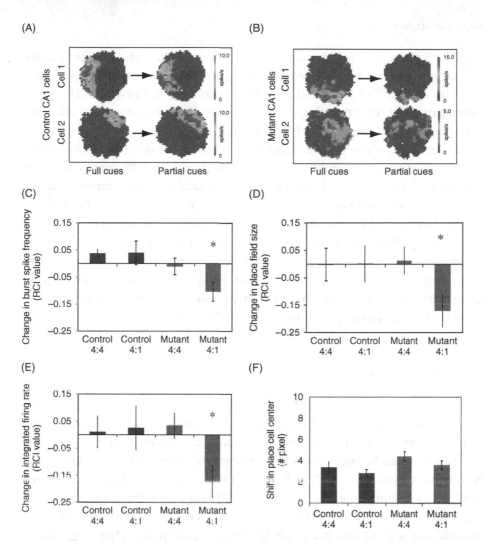

Figure 12.7 CA1 place cell activity was degraded in CA3-NR1 KO mice following partial cue removal. (A and B) Examples of the place fields before and after partial cue removal from fNR1 (control, (A)) and CA3-NR1 KO (mutant, (B)) mice. (C–E) Relative change in the place field properties for each cell recorded across two conditions was quantified using a relative change index (RCI), which is defined as the difference between the conditions divided by the sum of the conditions. Among the cells that were identified as the same cells throughout the two recording sessions, the average burst spike frequency [(C); $F_{(3,140)} = 4.16$, $p < 0.007$; Fisher's *post hoc* comparison (mutant 4:1 vs. all the other three paradigms), *$p < 0.05$], place field size over 1 Hz [(D); $F_{(3,140)} = 2.68$, $p < 0.049$; Fisher's *post hoc* comparison (mutant 4:1 vs. all the other three paradigms), *$p < 0.05$], and the integrated firing rate [(E); $F_{(3,140)} = 3.20$, $p < 0.025$; Fisher's *post hoc* comparison (mutant 4:1 vs. all the other three paradigms), *$p < 0.05$] were significantly reduced in the mutant animals (red bars) only after partial cue removal (4:1). In contrast, partial cue removal did not affect the CA1 place cell activity in the control mice (blue bars). Note that an RCI value of −0.17 is equivalent to a 30% reduction. Location of the CA1 place field center between the two recording sessions was not significantly shifted regardless of genotype and cue manipulation ((F); $F_{(3,140)} = 2.15$, $p = 0.097$) (for color image please see plate section).

distal cues. Thus, the average output from CA1 pyramidal cells was significantly reduced only for mutant cue removal experiments. Behavioral changes in the mutants might affect place cell properties such as peak firing rate. However, average running velocity in the open field across all conditions was not different in both genotypes (Kruskal-Walls test, $p = 0.70$).

Interestingly, when we examined whether the location of individual place fields shifted across conditions, we found no significant differences between mutant and control animals for either cue removal or no-cue removal conditions, suggesting that some reflection of past experience is maintained in the firing of mutant CA1 place cells even under conditions of partial cue removal (Figure 12.7F). Based on these results, we suggest that reductions in CA1 output as a consequence of reduced CA3 drive resulting from cue removal may make it more difficult for mutant animals to retrieve spatial memories. This impairment may underlie the inability of mutant animals to solve spatial memory tasks such as the water maze when only partial cues are available.

12.4   Discussion

12.4.1   CA1 is a critical site for memory storage

The formation of hippocampus-dependent memories of events and contexts involves incorporating complex configurations of stimuli into a memory trace that can be later recalled or recognized (Eichenbaum, 1997; O'Keefe & Nadel, 1978; Squire, 1992). The different sub-regions of the hippocampus are likely to serve complementary but computationally distinct roles in this process (Amaral & Witter, 1989). Previous work using CA1-NR1 KO mice demonstrated the critical role of NRs in area CA1 in the formation of spatial reference memory under conditions of fully cued memory retrieval (Tsien *et al.*, 1996). Correspondingly, these mutant mice exhibited general disruption of CA1 place cell activity (McHugh *et al.*, 1996). In contrast, we have now shown that CA3-NR1 KO mice exhibit intact spatial reference memory under conditions of fully cued memory retrieval with normal behavior and normal CA1 place cell activity. Comparison of behavioral and neuronal phenotypes between these two NR1 KO mice therefore suggests that area CA1 is a major site involved in the storage of spatial reference memory and that this memory can be formed without CA3 NRs.

12.4.2   CA3 contributes to memory recall

The previous studies of memory formation and recall with the CA1-NR1 KO mice were carried out under fully cued conditions (Tsien *et al.*, 1996). While this provided basic insights into the mechanisms of memory formation, in day-to-day life memory recall almost always occurs under the practical constraints of limited cues because of continuously changing real life contexts. This important feature of associative memory has been referred to as pattern completion (Gardner-Medwin, 1976; Hasselmo *et al.*, 1995; Hopfield, 1982; Marr, 1971; McNaughton & Morris, 1987; Willshaw & Buckingham, 1990). In the past, a substantial body of computational work has pointed out that a recurrent network with modifiable synaptic strength such as that in hippocampal area CA3 could provide this pattern completion ability. The impairment exhibited by CA3-NR1 KO mice in recalling the spatial memory following partial cue removal provides the first direct demonstration of a role of CA3 and CA3 NRs in pattern completion at the behavioral level. At the neuronal network level, pattern completion appeared as the expression of intact CA1 place cell activity under cue removal conditions in control mice, demonstrating the ability of intact CA3-CA1 networks to carry out this function. By contrast, under the same partial cue conditions, CA1 place field size in mutant mice was reduced, demonstrating incomplete memory pattern retrieval.

The residual search preference for the phantom platform location exhibited by mutant mice following partial cue removal (Figure 12.6B,D) can be interpreted as reflecting the degradation rather than the complete loss of spatial memory retrieval. This is consistent with the complementary observation of reduced place cell response with preserved place field location (Figure 12.7F), indicating decrease rather than complete disruption of reactivation of the memory trace. The partial loss of memory recall ability exhibited by mutant mice may also reflect additional recall mechanisms independent of CA3 NR function. The nature of these mechanisms remains to be examined.

It is known that while plasticity at mossy fiber-CA3 synapses is NR-independent (Berger & Yeckel, 1991; Harris & Cotman, 1986; Williams & Johnston, 1988; Zalutsky & Nicoll, 1990), plasticity at perforant path-CA3 synapses is NR-dependent (Berger & Yeckel, 1991; Berzhanskaya *et al.*, 1998). Therefore, we cannot exclude the possibility that the feed-forward input to CA3 via perforant path contributes to the observed pattern completion effects. However, the substantially greater strength of recurrent synaptic inputs relative to the contribution of the perforant path (Urban *et al.*, 2001) suggests a dominant role for the recurrent system.

12.4.3   *Model of associative memory formation and retrieval*

It has been proposed that memory can be stored in associative memory networks whose synapses are modifiable (Gardner-Medwin, 1976; Hasselmo *et al.*, 1995; Hopfield, 1982; Marr, 1971; McNaughton & Morris, 1987; Willshaw &

Buckingham, 1990). Figure 12.8 illustrates such a network that contains the basic input and output elements of the CA3 circuit. In this model inputs arriving via dentate mossy fibers and/or perforant path afferents would produce a pattern of CA3 ensemble output that reflects the pattern of inputs received. During memory acquisition under full-cue conditions in control animals, recurrent fiber synapses are modified in an NR-dependent manner to reinforce this ensemble pattern by strengthening connections between coactive neurons within the ensemble and thereby reflecting storage of the memory trace within CA3 (Figure 12.8A,B). This complete CA3 pattern, driven by full-cue input, and reinforced by recurrent connections, activates CA1 neurons and produces a pattern that serves as the output of the hippocampal circuit. The strengthening of connections between the CA3 and CA1 neurons that participated in this process reflects storage of the memory trace within CA1 (Figure 12.8A,B). Under full-cue conditions in mutant animals, the lack of NRs in the CA3 pyramidal cells prevents storage of the memory trace in the CA3 recurrent network but does not impair storage in CA1 (Figure 12.8C,D).

Under conditions of recall in control animals, presentation of all the cues activates CA3 neurons in a pattern corresponding to the original CA3 memory trace, thereby leading to reactivation of the memory trace in CA1 (Figure 12.8A). In mutant animals under full-cue conditions, although the CA3 memory trace is absent, the CA1 memory trace is reactivated directly by the incoming cues that correspond in their configuration to the pattern of the memory trace (Figure 12.8C). Reactivation of previously strengthened recurrent synapses is unnecessary for recall (Figure 12.8A–C) under full-cue conditions, as indicated in the model and confirmed by our results from recordings in CA1. Nevertheless, the reactivation may contribute to the recall process in control animals by producing a more robust input to CA1 from CA3. This possibility would be consistent with the observed reduction in CA1 inhibitory cell activity in mutant animals, suggesting that even under full-cue conditions, the strength of input from CA3 might be diminished and compensated for through homeostatic reduction of feedback or feedforward inhibitory drive. In this way a complete but weakened CA3 output pattern can provide sufficient drive to CA1 (Csicsvari *et al.*, 1998; Mizumori *et al.*, 1989). Direct measurement of CA3 output may clarify some of these issues.

Under conditions of partial cue removal, limited input activity at retrieval provides only partial activation of the CA3 output pattern in both control and mutant animals (green lines, Figure 12.8B,D). In control animals, this limited output activates previously strengthened recurrent synapses onto CA3 neurons that had participated in the original full-cue pattern (Figure 12.8B). These recurrently driven cells complete the output pattern of CA3 (red lines, Figure 12.7B),

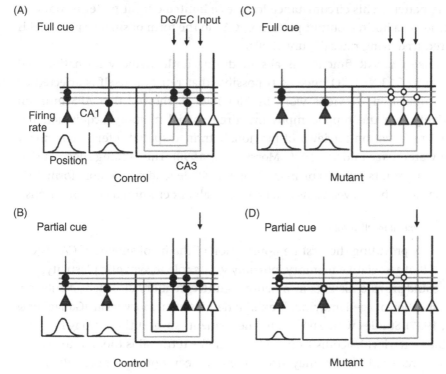

Figure 12.8   Model for a distinct role of area CA3 and CA1 in memory storage and recall. In (A) (control) and (C) (mutant), full-cue input (shown as three arrows) is provided via mossy fibers from dentate gyrus (DG) or perforant path from EC (entorhinal cortex). In (B) (control) and (D) (mutant), a fraction of the original input (partial cue shown as one arrow) is provided to activate the memory trace during recall. For detailed explanation, see Section 12.4. Red filled circles represent CA3 recurrent collateral synapses or Schaffer collateral-CA1 synapses participating in memory trace formation and its reactivation during recall. Red open circles on Schaffer collateral-CA1 synapses show the portion of the memory trace that is not activated by CA3 output. Black open circles show CA3 recurrent collateral synapses activated during recall with no memory trace. Red triangles and lines show CA3 pyramidal cell activity resulting from pattern completion through recurrent collateral firing. Green triangles and lines show CA3 pyramidal cell response to external cue information. Open triangles and black lines are silent CA3 pyramidal cells and inactive outputs. Blue triangles show CA1 pyramidal cells (for color image please see plate section).

which can then drive the full output pattern in CA1. In mutant animals, limited input drives a correspondingly limited CA3 output pattern (green line in Figure 12.8D). However, due to the lack of a memory trace in recurrent synapses, their activation is unable to drive neurons that had participated in the original full-cue pattern. This circumstance leads to a limited output pattern from CA3 that leads to a limited output pattern in CA1 in the form of smaller place fields with reduced firing rates (Figure 12.8D).

Because CA3 NR function is absent during both memory formation and retrieval in CA3-NR1 KO mice, it is possible that retrieval itself is affected by NR manipulation. Previous work by Morris *et al.* showed that AP5 infusion selectively into the hippocampus impaired spatial memory acquisition but showed no effect on retrieval of previously trained spatial reference memory in the water maze (Morris, 1989; Morris *et al.*, 1990). This finding suggests that the present results reflect a primary deficit in NR-dependent memory formation in CA3 that is then revealed as a deficit in recall under limited cue conditions.

12.4.4   General implications

By providing the first demonstration of the involvement of CA3 NR in the recall of associative memory, possibly via its role in synaptic plasticity, this study could provide insights into neurocognitive memory disorders. A substantial proportion of aged individuals exhibit deficits of memory recall (Gallagher & Rapp, 1997). Studies with early Alzheimer patients suggest that among memory variables – retrieval, acquisition, and retention – retrieval is the first to decline and such retrieval deficits may also serve as an early predictor of Alzheimer's disease (Backman *et al.*, 1999; Tuokko *et al.*, 1991). The effects of normal aging produce a CA3-selective pattern of neurochemical alterations (Adams *et al.*, 2001; Kadar *et al.*, 1998; Le Jeune *et al.*, 1996). Exposure to chronic stress, which can lead to memory deficits also selectively causes atrophy in the apical dendrites of CA3 pyramidal cells (McEwen, 1999). These results may suggest that the CA3 region plays a critical role in cognitive functions related to memory recall through pattern completion. Therefore, use of genetically engineered mice in which CA3 function is selectively altered, such as the CA3-NR1 KO mice in the present study, may help in understanding processes such as age- or stress-related neuronal changes and assist in their prevention.

On a technical level, this study along with our previous study with CA1-NR1 KO mice (McHugh *et al.*, 1996) dramatically illustrates the power of cell type-restricted, adult-onset gene manipulations in the study of molecular, cellular, and neuronal circuitry mechanisms underlying cognition. We have shown that the same neurotransmitter receptors (i.e., NMDA receptors) can play quite distinct roles in the mnemonic process – memory formation vs. memory recall – depending on where and in which neural circuitry in the hippocampus they are expressed. It is expected that other genetically engineered mice with precise spatial and/or temporal specificity will help dissect mechanisms for a variety of cognitive functions.

Acknowledgments

The part of the research on CA3-NR1 KO mice described here was conducted in collaboration with Akira Kato, Candice A. Carr (Tonegawa lab), Michael C. Quirk, Linus D. Sun (Wilson lab, MIT), Mark F. Yeckel, Raymond A. Chitwood, Daniel Johnston (Johnston lab, Baylor College of Medicine), and Masahiko Watanabe (Hokkaido University, Japan). Portions of the figures of this chapter were reproduced with permission from *Science*, Vol. 297, p. 211 by Nakazawa *et al.* (2002). This work was supported by an NIH grant (S.T.), HHMI (S.T.), and Human Frontier Science Program (K.N.).

References

Adams, M. M., Smith, T. D., Moga, D., *et al.* (2001). Hippocampal dependent learning ability correlates with N-Methyl-D-Aspartate (NMDA) receptor levels in CA3 neurons of young and aged rats. *The Journal of Comparative Neurology*, **432**, 230–43.

Amaral, D. G., Ishizuka, N., and Claiborne, B. (1990). Neurons, numbers and the hippocampal network. *Progress in Brain Research*, **83**, 1–11.

Amaral, D. G. and Witter, M. P. (1989). The three-dimensional organization of the hippocampal formation: a review of anatomical data. *Neuroscience*, **31**(3), 571–91.

Backman, L., Andersson, J. L., Nyberg, L., *et al.* (1999). Brain regions associated with episodic retrieval in normal aging and Alzheimer's disease. *Neurology*, **52**, 1861–70.

Bahn, S., Volk, B., and Wisden, W. (1994). Kainate receptor gene expression in the developing rat brain. *Journal of Neuroscience*, **14**, 5525–47.

Berger, T. W. and Yeckel, M. F. (1991). Long-term potentiation of entorhinal afferents to the hippocampus enhanced propagation of activity through the trisynaptic pathway. In M. Baudry and J. L. Davis, eds., *Long-Term Potentiation: A Debate of Current Issues*. Cambridge, MA: MIT Press, pp. 327–56.

Berzhanskaya, J., Urban, N. N., and Barrionuevo, G. (1998). Electrophysiological and pharmacological characterization of the direct perforant path input to hippocampal area CA3. *Journal of Neurophysiology*, **79**, 2111–18.

Best, P. J., White, A. M., and Minai, A. (2001). Spatial processing in the brain: the activity of hippocampal place cells. *Annual Review of Neuroscience*, **24**, 459–86.

Bliss, T. V. P. and Collingridge, G. L., (1993). A synaptic model of memory: long-term potentiation in the hippocampus. *Nature*, **361**, 31–9.

Buzsaki, G. (1984). Feed-forward inhibition in the hippocampal formation. *Progress in Neurobiology*, **22**(2), 131–53.

Csicsvari, J., Hirase, H., Czurko, A., and Buzsaki, G. (1998). Reliability and state dependence of pyramidal cell-interneuron synapses in the hippocampus: an ensemble approach in the behaving rat. *Neuron* **21**(1), 179–89.

Eichenbaum, H. (1997). Declarative memory: insights from cognitive neurobiology. *Annual Review of Psychology*, **48**, 547–72.

Fukaya, M., Kato, A., Lovett, C., Tonegawa, S., and Watanabe, M. (2003). Retention of NMDA receptor NR2 subunits in the lumen of endoplasmic reticulum in targeted NR1 knockout mice. *Proceedings of the Natural Academy of Sciences USA*, **100**(8), 4855–60.

Gallagher, M. and Rapp, P. R. (1997). The use of animal models to study the effects of aging on cognition. *Annual Review of Psychology*, **48**, 339–70.

Gardner-Medwin, A. R. (1976). The recall of events through the learning of associations between their parts. *Proceedings of the Royal Society of London B*, **194**, 375–402.

Harris, E. W. and Cotman, C. W. (1986). Long-term potentiation of guinea pig mossy fiber responses is not blocked by *N*-methyl D-aspartate antagonist. *Neuroscience Letters*, **70**, 132–7.

Hasselmo, M. E., Schnell, E., and Barkai, E. (1995). Dynamics of learning and recall at excitatory recurrent synapses and cholinergic modulation in rat hippocampal region CA3. *Journal of Neuroscience*, **15**(7 Pt 2), 5249–62.

Hebb, D. O. (1949). *The Organization of Behavior: A Neuropsychological Theory*. New York: Wiley.

Hetherington, P. A. and Shapiro, M. L. (1997). Hippocampal place fields are altered by the removal of single visual cues in a distance-dependent manner. *Behavioral Neuroscience*, **111**(1), 20–34.

Hollmann, M. and Heinemann, S. (1994). Cloned glutamate receptors. *Annual Review of Neuroscience*, **17**, 31–108.

Hopfield, J. J. (1982). Neural networks and physical systems with emergent collective computational abilities. *Proceedings of the National Academy of Sciences USA*, **79**, 2554–8.

Kadar, T., Dachir, S., Shukitt-Hale, B., and Levy, A. (1998). Sub-regional hippocampal vulnerability in various animal models leading to cognitive dysfunction. *Journal of Neural Transmission*, **105**, 987–1004.

Le Jeune, H., Cecyre, D., Rowe, W., Meaney M. J., and Quirion, R. (1996). Ionotropic glutamate receptor subtypes in the aged memory-impaired and unimpaired Long-Evans rat. *Neuroscience*, **74**, 349–63.

Liu, Y., Fujise, N., and Kosaka, T. (1996). Distribution of calretinin immunoreactivity in the mouse dentate gyrus. I. General description. *Experimental Brain Research*, **108**, 389–403.

Marr, D. (1971). Simple memory: a theory of archicortex. *Philosophical Transactions of the Royal Society of London*, **262**, 23–81.

McEwen, B. S. (1999). Stress and hippocampal plasticity. *Annual Review of Neuroscience* **22**, 105–22.

McHugh, T. J., Blum, K. I., Tsien, J. Z., Tonegawa, S., and Wilson, M. A. (1996). Impaired hippocampal representation of space in CA1-specific NMDAR1 knockout mice. *Cell*, **87**, 1339–49.

McNaughton, B. L. and Morris, R. G. M., (1987). Hippocampal synaptic enhancement and information storage within a distributed memory system. *Trends in Neurosciences*, **10**, 408–15.

Mizumori, S. J., McNaughton, B. L., Barnes, C. A., and Fox, K. B. (1989a). Preserved spatial coding in hippocampal CA1 pyramidal cells during reversible suppression of CA3c output: evidence for pattern completion in hippocampus. *Journal of Neuroscience*, **9**(11), 3915–28.

Mizumori, S. J. Y., Barnes, C. A., and McNaughton, B. L. (1989b). Reversible inactivation of the medial septum: selective effects on the spontaneous unit activity of different hippocampal cell types. *Brain Research*, **50**, 99–106.

Morris, R. G., Garrud, P., Rawlins, J. N., and O'Keefe, J. (1982). Place navigation impaired in rats with hippocampal lesions. *Nature*, **297**(5868), 681–3.

Morris, R. G. M. (1989). Synaptic plasticity and learning: selective impairment of learning in rats and blockade of long-term potentiation *in vivo* by the N-methyl-D-aspartate receptor antagonist AP5. *Journal of Neuroscience*, **9**, 3040–57.

Morris, R. G. M., Davis, S., and Butcher, S. P. (1990). Hippocampal synaptic plasticity and NMDA receptors: a role in information storage? *Philosophical Transactions of the Royal Society of London B*, **329**, 187–204.

Muller, R. (1996). A quarter of a century of place cells. *Neuron*, **17**(5), 813–22.

Muller, R. U. and Kubie, J. L. (1987). The effects of changes in the environment on the spatial firing of hippocampal complex-spike cells. *Journal of Neuroscience*, **7**(7), 1951–68.

Nakanishi, S. (1992). Molecular diversity of glutamate receptors and implications for brain function. *Science*, **258**, 597–603.

O'Keefe, J. and Conway, D. H. (1978). Hippocampal place units in the freely moving rat: why they fire where they fire. *Experimental Brain Research*, **31**(4), 573–90.

O'Keefe, J. and Nadel, L. (1978). *The Hippocampus as a Cognitive Map*. Oxford: Clarendon Press.

Paulsen, O. and Moser, E. I. (1998). A model of hippocampal memory encoding and retrieval: GABAergic control of synaptic plasticity. *Trends in Neurosciences*, **21**, 273–8.

Quirk, M. C., Blum, K. I., and Wilson, M. A. (2001). Experience-dependent changes in extracellular spike amplitude may reflect regulation of dendritic action potential back-propagation in rat hippocampal pyramidal cells. *Journal of Neuroscience*, **21**, 240–8.

Rolls, E. T., Miyashita, Y., Cahusac, P. M., *et al.* (1989). Hippocampal neurons in the monkey with activity related to the place in which a stimulus is shown. *Journal of Neuroscience*, **9**(6), 1835–45.

Schwartzkroin, P. A. and Prince, D. A. (1978). Cellular and field potential properties of epileptogenic hippocampal slices. *Brain Research*, **147**, 117–30.

Simon, P., Dupuis, R., and Costenin, J. (1994). Thigmotaxis as an index of anxiety of mice. Influence of dopaminergic transmissions. *Behavioural Brain Research*, **61**, 59–64.

Soriano, P. (1999). Generalized lacZ expression with the ROSA26Cre reporter strain. *Nature Genetics*, **21**, 70–1.

Squire, L. R. (1992). Memory and the hippocampus: a synthesis from findings with rats, monkeys, and humans. *Psychological Review*, **99**, 195–231.

Thomson, A. and Radpour, S. (1991). Excitatory connections between CA1 pyramidal cells revealed by spike triggered averaging in slices of rat hippocampus are partially NMDA receptor mediated. *European Journal of Neuroscience*, **3**, 587–601.

Tsien, J. Z., Huerta, P. T., and Tonegawa, S. (1996). The essential role of hippocampal CA1 NMDA receptor-dependent synaptic plasticity in spatial memory. *Cell*, **87**, 1327–38.

Tuokko, H., Vernon-Wilkinson, R., Weir, J., and Beattie, B. L. (1991). Cued recall and early identification of dementia. *Journal of Clinical and Experimental Neuropsychology*, **13**, 871–9.

Urban, N. N., Henze, D. A., and Barrionuevo, G. (2001). Revisiting the role of the hippocampal mossy fiber synapse. *Hippocampus*, **11**, 408–17.

Valtschanoff, J. G., Burette, A., Wenthold, R. J., and Weinberg, R. J. (1999). Expression of NR2 receptor subunit in rat somatic sensory cortex: synaptic distribution and colocalization with NR1 and PSD-95. *The Journal of Comparative Neurology*, **410**, 599–611.

Watanabe, M., Fukaya, M., Sakimura, K., *et al.* (1998). Selective scarcity of NMDA receptor channel subunits in the stratum lucidum (mossy fibre-recipient layer) of the mouse hippocampal CA3 subfield. *The European Journal of Neuroscience*, **10**, 478–87.

Whishaw, I. Q. and Tomie, J. A. (1997). Perseveration on place reversals in spatial swimming pool tasks: further evidence for place learning in hippocampal rats. *Hippocampus*, **7**(4), 361–70.

Williams, S. and Johnston, D. (1988). Muscarinic depression of long-term potentiation in CA3 hippocampal neurons. *Science*, **242**, 84–7.

Willshaw, D. J. and Buckingham, J. T. (1990). An assessment of Marr's theory of the hippocampus as a temporary memory storage. *Philosophical Transactions of the Royal Society of London B*, **329**, 205–15.

Wisden, W. and Seeburg P. H. (1993). A complex mosaic of high-affinity kainate receptors in rat brain. *Journal of Neuroscience*, **14**, 3582–98.

Wong, R. K. and Traub, R. D. (1983). Synchronized burst discharge in disinhibited hippocampal slice. I. Initiation in CA2-CA3 region. *Journal of Neurophysiology*, **49**, 442–58.

Zalutsky, R. A. and Nicoll, R. A. (1990). Comparison of two forms of long-term potentiation in single hippocampal neurons. *Science*, **248**, 1619–24.

PART IV   SENSORY PROCESSES

Overview of sensory processes

JAMES R. POMERANTZ

Understanding of sensory processes has been an ongoing concern for centuries. Consider the study of vision, for example. The early Greeks knew that seeing began in the eye and that the eye was filled with fluid – the humors. But they had no good sense of the eye's optics or of the retina's role; indeed, they thought the retina's job was to provide nutrients for the vitreous. Aristotle believed the humors were photoreceptive. The Pythagoreans believed that rays emanated outward from the eye to the external environment, leading us to wonder today as to what explanation they had in mind for why the world gets dark at night.

In 1604, one hundred years before the publication of Newton's *Optics*, the German astronomer Johannes Kepler launched a new era in vision when he noted that the eye worked as an optical instrument focusing an image sharply on the retina, observed that the retinal image is in fact oriented upside down and backwards, determined that the lens refracted light, and pinpointed the cause of myopia (before Kepler, people used spectacles to improve their vision but had no idea why curved glass sharpened their sight). There was plenty even Kepler failed to grasp however, including the actual workings of the retina. The discovery of photoreceptors – rods and cones – was over a century away, and when Treviranus officially discovered them in 1834, he misread the orientation of the retina, believing it was installed backwards in the eye (surely the light-sensitive photoreceptors could not be pointing away from the source of light and toward the dark interior of the eye socket!) This echoes the belief, apparently held by some in eras long past, that there exists a second lens in the eye that rectifies the visual image – for as everyone knows, we do not see our world upside down and backwards.

Seen against this historical backdrop, the sophistication of today's research on the neuroscience of sensation and perception comes into sharper focus. From the earliest work on the basis for sensory transduction – the conversion

Topics in Integrative Neuroscience: From Cells to Cognition, ed. James R. Pomerantz. Published by Cambridge University Press. © Cambridge University Press 2008.

at the sensory receptors of physical energy into neural signals – to today's research using tools barely imaginable not long ago, understanding how sensation works has been a challenging and rewarding area of research.

The scientific problems underlying the neuroscience of sensory processes range from the straightforward and solvable to the complex and seemingly impenetrable. Considering sensory processes in their full sweep, this part of the book could easily range the spectrum from explaining transduction at the receptors to understanding the conscious phenomenology of perception – why the world appears to us as it does. Beginning at the receptors, it might not have surprised researchers working a century ago to learn that the details of transduction would have been worked out as completely as they have today. Transduction, after all, is a straightforward problem that can be solved in detail given the benefit of instruments that allow us to peer in and observe the workings of the eyes and ears. At the level of conscious experience, however, things remain murkier, even today. How, after all, can we hope to understand how people perceive the world as they do when perception is such a private experience, inaccessible to observation or measurement? As time has shown, however, we have learned a lot, not only about transduction but about perception – about how we integrate sensory signals into a detailed and reliable perception of our environment. This part of the book is intended to illustrate our progress across this spectrum through two examples – one involving transduction in the inner ear, and the other involving the hearing and production of birdsong.

The chapter by Wooltorton, Hurley, Bao, and Eatock deals with voltage-dependent sodium currents in hair cells of the inner ear. The issue here is transduction of course, and in this case two forms of transduction. One involves sound and the auditory system, and ultimately it aims to encode the frequency and amplitude components of sound needed to represent our acoustic environment. The other involves head movement and the vestibular system, and it is targeted with encoding changes in our bodily position in space. In both cases, the transduction begins with a mechanical event – the bending of hair cells. In the former case, this bending is triggered initially by sound – the compression and rarefaction of air most typically – causing movements of membranes, bones, and ultimately of fluids in which the hair cells are bathed. In the latter case, fewer steps are involved but here too moving fluids in the inner ear cause bundles of hairs cells to deflect, in turn inducing current flow through ion channels. This current flow causes changes in membrane potential, leading in turn to changes in other ion channels further downstream. Wooltorton *et al.* differentiate among three different kinds of channels and focus on the less-well-understood hair cell Na^+ channels, ones that are controlled by sensors detecting the fluctuating voltage levels of the membrane potential rather than by detecting specific regulatory molecules binding to the channel. They explore the puzzle of those channels that are inactivated over the physiological voltage range; they look at whether multiple types of Na^+ channels inhabit the same region, serving different functions; they examine the relationship between spiking and Na^+ currents; and they ask whether Na^+ currents affect the development of immature hair cells. Wooltorton *et al.* explain much about how this works, concluding that more needs to be learned through experimentation on Na^+ channel functions, to verify the inactivation range and to determine the degree to which Na^+ currents cause spiking, noting that these experiments need to be conducted under conditions approximating natural, physiological parameters such as temperature.

The chapter by Hessler, Boettiger, and Doupe turns to songbirds, focusing on their song selectivity, singing, and synaptic plasticity. As the authors note, the neuroscience of birdsong is important for a variety of reasons, not the least of which are the many parallels birdsong has with human speech - particularly considering the element of feedback processing that is critical to successful learning early in life. Young birds learn to produce their song by listening to and forming a neural representation of the "tutor" song - with the tutors often being the birds' fathers. Later, they produce a rough copy - "plastic song" - and gradually learn to produce a closer copy of the tutor song by comparing their own vocalizations to the memory - the template - of what they have heard. We know that birds born deaf never learn to sing properly, just as humans born deaf never learn to produce speech sounds in the way their hearing siblings do. Hessler and colleagues describe clever experiments involving recording from neural sites during singing as well as during listening, testing birds of varying ages whose ability to hear and/or produce sounds has been manipulated. In this way they attempt to determine what song representations are stored, and where they are processed neurally. Specifically, neurons in the anterior forebrain pathway (AFP) form circuits tuned to compare the bird's own song with the template of the tutor song. The AFP is also particularly active during singing per se, even in deaf birds, and contains synaptic structures organized to develop temporal selectivity for song in young birds. These learning mechanisms in the AFP are not purely sensory but involve the integration of sensory and motor processes, even at the level of an individual neuron, needed for vocal imitation.

These two chapters provide fitting examples of the progress currently being made to understand sensory and perceptual processing at the neural level. One can only wonder what the next 100 years will bring. Perhaps some of our most closely held views today will turn out to be as wrong as some of the misconceptions held by such luminaries as Treviranus and Aristotle. But if the research pace today can be sustained, it seems likely that much - perhaps most - sensory processing will be understood deeply and thoroughly by the end of this century.

13

Song selectivity, singing, and synaptic plasticity in songbirds

MICHELE M. SOLIS, NEAL A. HESSLER, CHARLOTTE A. BOETTIGER, AND
ALLISON J. DOUPE

13.1 Introduction

Birdsong, like human speech, is a learned vocal behavior that requires auditory feedback. Both as juveniles, while they learn to sing, and as adults, songbirds use auditory feedback to compare their own vocalizations with an internal model of a memorized target song. Here we describe experiments that explore the properties of the songbird anterior forebrain pathway (AFP), a basal ganglia–forebrain circuit known to be critical for normal song learning and for adult modification of vocal output, but not for normal adult singing. First, neural recordings in anesthetized, juvenile birds show that single AFP neurons become specialized to process the song stimuli that are compared during sensorimotor learning. AFP neurons develop tuning to the bird's own song, and in many cases to the tutor song as well, even when these stimuli are manipulated to be very different from each other. Second, neural recordings from adult, singing birds reveal robust singing-related activity in the AFP, which is present even in deaf birds. This activity is likely to originate from premotor areas, and could represent an efference copy of motor commands for song, predicting the sensory consequences of motor commands. Finally, in vitro studies of the AFP show that recurrent synapses between neurons in the AFP outflow nucleus can undergo activity-dependent and timing-sensitive strengthening that appears to be restricted to young birds. Overall, these studies illustrate that this circuit devoted to vocal learning is not simply sensory, but rather shows highly inter-related sensory and motor processing, as is true for brain areas involved in speech. Moreover, the AFP contains synaptic mechanisms well suited to play a role in tutor song memorization and/or early refinement of song.

Topics in Integrative Neuroscience: From Cells to Cognition, ed. James R. Pomerantz. Published by
Cambridge University Press. © Cambridge University Press 2008.

Human speech and birdsong share numerous features (Doupe & Kuhl, 1999). Both are complex acoustic sequences, generated by co-ordinated actions of the vocal apparatus and the muscles of respiration. Most importantly, both speech and song are learned, and are highly dependent on hearing in early life and in adulthood: neither birds nor humans learn to vocalize normally in the absence of hearing, and as adults, both show deterioration of vocal output after hearing loss (Cowie & Douglas-Cowie, 1992; Konishi, 1965; Nordeen & Nordeen, 1992; Price, 1979; Waldstein, 1989). Songbirds thus provide a promising model system for elucidating general neural mechanisms involved in vocal learning, including how the brain may evaluate auditory feedback and use it to modify vocal output, and what synaptic mechanisms could underlie this.

Experiments to investigate the neural basis of vocal learning in songbirds are aided by a wealth of information about the behavioral time course of learning (Eales, 1985; Immelmann, 1969; Marler, 1970), and its dependence on hearing (Konishi, 1965; Price, 1979). Song learning occurs in two stages, called the sensory and sensorimotor phases (Figure 13.1A). During the sensory phase, a young bird listens to and memorizes the song of an adult tutor, often the bird's father. This memory is often called the "template." The sensorimotor phase begins later, when the young bird begins to sing; during sensorimotor learning, the juvenile uses auditory feedback to compare its own immature vocalizations ("plastic song") to its memory of the tutor song, and gradually refines and adapts its vocal output until it matches the tutor song. Thus, auditory experience of both the tutor song and the bird's own song (BOS) is required during learning. In adulthood, elimination or alteration of auditory feedback of BOS induces gradual deterioration of adult song structure (Leonardo & Konishi, 1999; Nordeen & Nordeen, 1992). These behavioral observations suggest that there must be neural circuitry involved in memorization and evaluation of song. Specifically, there must be mechanisms that compare auditory feedback from vocal output to the internal song template, and that generate signals to guide changes in vocal output.

One candidate circuit for processing and evaluating these song experiences is the anterior forebrain pathway (AFP), a basal ganglia–forebrain circuit found within a system of interconnected nuclei dedicated to song learning and production (Figure 13.1B; Nottebohm *et al.*, 1976). The AFP plays a special role during learning and song modification. Lesions of the AFP severely disrupt song learning in juveniles, whereas the same lesions do not affect song in normal adults (Bottjer *et al.*, 1984; Scharff & Nottebohm, 1991; Sohrabji *et al.*, 1990). However, lesions in adults prevent the degradation of adult song normally caused by perturbations of song production or feedback (Brainard & Doupe, 2000; Williams & Mehta, 1999). Both juvenile and adult results are

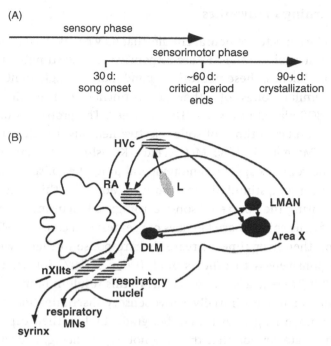

Figure 13.1 (A) Song learning occurs in two phases. For zebra finches, the sensory phase ends at ~60 days of age and the sensorimotor phase begins when birds are ~30 days old and continues until they are ≥90 days of age; thus the phases of learning overlap in this species. (B) Anatomy of the song system, which consists of two major pathways. Motor pathway nuclei are striped, and AFP pathway nuclei are in black. The motor pathway, necessary for normal song production throughout life, includes HVc, the robust nucleus of the archistriatum (RA), and the tracheosyringeal portion of the hypoglossal nucleus (nXIIts). RA also projects to nuclei involved in control of respiration. The AFP comprises Area X (X), the medial nucleus of the dorsolateral thalamus (DLM), and the lateral magnocellular nucleus of the anterior neostriatum (LMAN). The Field L complex and related areas (stippled) provide auditory input to the song system.

consistent with the idea that the AFP participates in evaluating song feedback and computing or conveying instructive signals about the quality of song, which then drive adaptive (or in case of adult deafening, nonadaptive) changes in song. The output of the AFP, the lateral magnocellular nucleus of the anterior neostriatum (LMAN), projects to the motor pathway for song, which is necessary for normal song production throughout life (Nottebohm *et al.*, 1976). Thus, the AFP is well positioned to influence activity in the motor pathway and could drive changes in vocal output. We review here experiments that implicate AFP function in the sensory and sensorimotor phases of learning, as well as in sensorimotor processing in adulthood, and describe synaptic mechanisms well suited to allow shaping of neural properties by song learning.

13.2   Song learning in juveniles

As might be expected of neural circuits that may be involved in mediating song learning, neurons in the AFP are responsive to song stimuli. In adult, anesthetized zebra finches, these neurons respond more strongly to BOS than to acoustically similar songs of other zebra finches (conspecific songs; Figure 13.2A) or BOS played in reverse (Doupe, 1997). The properties of these neurons are very similar to those of song-selective neurons first described in HVc (Figure 13.1B; Margoliash, 1983; McCasland & Konishi, 1981). Neurons that are sensitive to the complex spectral and temporal properties of song could be useful for processing song stimuli during learning. Moreover, this "song selectivity" emerges during the course of song learning: AFP neurons from birds early in the sensory learning phase (30 days of age) respond equally well to all song stimuli, and then over time increase their response to their own song while losing responsiveness to other stimuli (Doupe, 1997; Solis & Doupe, 1997; Figure 13.2B). There is a striking parallel to this result in human speech development: human infants initially show sensory discrimination of phonemes from all human languages tested, but gradually lose their capacity to accurately discriminate sounds that they are not experiencing, and improve their discrimination of the sounds of the language spoken around them (Eimas *et al.*, 1987; Kuhl, 1994; Werker & Tees, 1992). In both cases, the initial broad sensitivity endows the young organism with the capacity to learn any language or species-specific song, but this sensitivity is then narrowed and shaped by experience.

Song selectivity develops rapidly, since it is found in the AFP of zebra finches that have completed the sensory phase of learning (60 days of age: Figure 13.1A, 13.2B; Solis & Doupe, 1997). At this time zebra finches are also in the middle of the sensorimotor phase and have been producing plastic song for about a month. Thus, experience of either the bird's own or the tutor song could have shaped the selectivity of these neurons. Knowing which experience is responsible for selectivity would inform our hypotheses about AFP function during song learning. For example, neurons tuned by BOS experience could provide information about the current state of BOS, whereas those tuned by tutor song could encode the tutor song memory. When we compared the neural responses to BOS and tutor song in 60-day-old birds, we found a range of preferences for one song over the other (Figure 13.3A). Many neurons preferred BOS over tutor song, supporting a role for BOS experience in shaping selectivity. A few neurons preferred tutor over BOS, suggesting that they were tuned by tutor song experience. Finally, many neurons responded equally well to both songs. These neurons were clearly selective, because they did not respond as well to conspecific

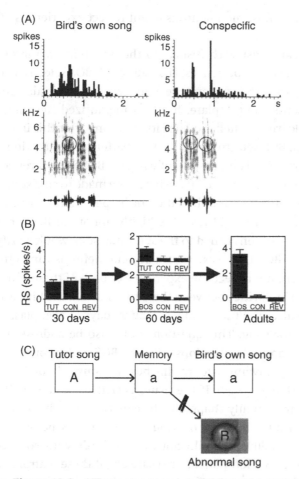

Figure 13.2 AFP neurons are song selective. (A) A song-selective neuron from an adult zebra finch. Peristimulus time histograms (PSTHs) show the greater response of a single LMAN neuron to bird's own song (BOS) than to conspecific song. Song is shown underneath each PSTH as a sonogram (plot of frequency vs. time, with the energy of each frequency band vs. time). Song-selective neurons respond to multiple acoustic features of the BOS: the circles in the sonograms identify a feature that is shared between both songs shown here and appears to elicit a response, but the figure also illustrates that many other features of BOS must contribute to the overall response of this neuron to BOS. (B) AFP neurons develop selectivity for song during development. In zebra finches of 30 days of age, LMAN neurons exhibit equivalent response strengths (RS; mean stimulus-evoked response minus background) to tutor song (TUT), conspecific song (CON), and reverse tutor song (REV). By 60 days of age, these neurons respond significantly more to TUT than to CON or to REV. In addition, BOS also elicits a much stronger response than CON and reverse BOS (REV). In adults, LMAN neurons are extremely selective for BOS. (C) When a juvenile stores a good copy of the tutor song ("A") as its template ("a"), and accurately models its own song after the template, the resulting BOS ("a") will strongly resemble the tutor song. Thus, if a

or reversed song stimuli. Thus, such neurons might reflect experiences of both BOS and tutor song.

Two important caveats exist with respect to the apparent shaping of AFP neurons by these two sensory experiences. First, although BOS selectivity might initially seem to reflect the bird's experience of its own song, it is also possible that it actually represents the template. If a bird memorized the tutor song poorly during sensory learning, then modeled its own song after this inaccurate template (Figure 13.2C), BOS selectivity would be a better representation of the template than the tutor song. The question of whether BOS indeed reflects the bird's own vocalizations could be solved if the bird were made to sing something very different from its tutor by a manipulation of its peripheral vocal system (Figure 13.2C). Since the bird would hear the highly abnormal BOS only as a result of its own singing, neurons tuned to the abnormal song would verify that it was the experience of BOS that was critical. Second, neurons tuned to both BOS and tutor song might not reflect the experience of both of these songs, but simply reflect acoustic similarities between these two stimuli: the bird is trying to model its own song after the tutor song, and by 60 days of age, plastic song often resembles the tutor song. This question could also be addressed if the acoustic similarity that normally develops between BOS and tutor song were minimized by inducing juvenile zebra finches to sing abnormal songs (Figure 13.2C; Solis & Doupe, 1999). If the neurons that respond equally well to BOS and tutor song are actually shaped by the experience of the bird's voice but respond to both stimuli because of acoustic similarities between these songs, then this kind of neuron should not exist in birds with song unlike their tutor song (Figure 13.3B, left panel). Alternatively, if these neurons reflect independent contributions of both BOS and tutor song experience to selectivity, then they should persist in birds with song unlike their tutor song, perhaps as separate neural populations (Figure 13.3B, right panel).

To induce abnormal song, we bilaterally transected the tracheosyringeal portion of the hypoglossal nerve (NXIIts) prior to song onset (~25 days of age in zebra finches; Figure 13.1A), thus denervating the muscles of the avian vocal organ (the syrinx). These juveniles therefore experienced a normal sensory phase with their tutor, but their entire experience of BOS was of the abnormal,

---

Caption for Figure 13.2 (cont.)

neuron is tuned by BOS experience only, it could also respond well to tutor song when the two songs are similar enough. This ambiguity could be resolved by making the BOS very different ("B") from the tutor song, by interfering with vocal production mechanisms; in these experiments this was done by cutting the tracheosyringeal (ts) nerves to the vocal muscles.

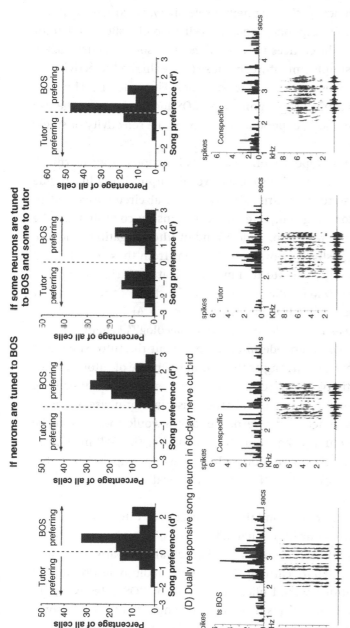

Figure 13.3 Preferences for BOS vs. tutor song by single AFP neurons. (A) Histograms show that in 60-day-old zebra finches, there is a range of preferences among LMAN neurons. The preference for each neuron is quantified with a d' value (Solis & Doupe, 1997; Theunissen & Doupe, 1998). When d' ≥ 0.5, this indicates a strong preference for BOS over tutor song; when d' ≤ −0.5, this indicates a strong preference for tutor song over BOS. Neurons with d' values in between were considered to have equivalent responses to both song stimuli. (B) Predicted results of the manipulation of BOS. *Left panel:* If neurons with equivalent responses to BOS and tutor song are shaped by BOS during development but respond to both stimuli as a result of acoustic similarities between these two songs, this type of dually responsive neuron is not expected in birds with songs unlike their tutor song, and the distribution should reveal only BOS-tuned neurons. *Right panel:* If both BOS and tutor song independently shape different neurons in the AFP, the distribution in birds with songs very different from their tutor songs is predicted to be bimodal, as shown by the histogram. (C) The observed distribution of song preferences from ts cut birds at 60 days of age. Neurons with equivalent responses to BOS and tutor song were maintained, even though these birds' songs did not resemble the tutor song. (D) Equivalent responses to tsBOS and tutor song. PSTHs show the responses of a single LMAN neuron to 13 presentations of each song. While this neuron responded equally well to tsBOS and tutor song, it did not respond well to other adult conspecific songs.

nerve cut ("ts cut") song. Song analyses demonstrated that this manipulation successfully minimized both the spectral and temporal similarity between BOS and tutor song.

Using ts cut song and tutor song as stimuli, we characterized neuronal selectivity in the AFP of ts cut birds at 60 days of age. Some neurons responded more strongly to the unique ts cut BOS ("tsBOS") than to tutor song, clearly demonstrating a role for BOS experience in shaping neural selectivity. Strikingly, a sizable proportion of neurons still responded equally well to both tsBOS and tutor song, despite the acoustic differences between these two songs (Figure 13.3C). These neurons were not simply immature, because they exhibited selectivity for tsBOS and tutor song over conspecific and reverse song (Figure 13.3D). Thus, the presence of neurons with equivalent responses to tsBOS and tutor song in these ts cut birds suggests that *both* song experiences can shape the selectivity of single neurons.

How might these different types of song selectivity function in song learning? Since BOS selectivity reflects the bird's current vocal output, it might provide information about the state of plastic song to a neural circuit involved in comparing BOS to a tutor song template stored in sensory co-ordinates. The high selectivity for BOS might also provide a kind of filter or gating function, aiding the bird in distinguishing its own vocalizations from those of others. It may also reflect in some way the pattern of motor activation during singing, as has been seen in RA (Dave & Margoliash, 2000). The function of this selectivity could be further investigated with experiments in which AFP selectivity was broadened during song learning, perhaps with pharmacological agents.

Tutor song selectivity could encode information about the tutor song, and function during sensorimotor learning as the neural reference of tutor song for birds; that is, this selectivity would result from experience of the tutor song during the sensory phase of learning. During the sensorimotor phase, the level or pattern of firing of these neurons in response to BOS would then reflect the degree to which BOS resembles the tutor song. A role for the AFP in sensory learning of the template is also supported by behavioral experiments that demonstrate a need for normal LMAN activity specifically during tutor song exposure (Basham *et al.*, 1996).

In addition, these experiments found that BOS selectivity often coexists with tutor song selectivity in the same individual AFP neurons. This "dual selectivity" may reflect a function for AFP neurons in the actual comparison of BOS and tutor song that is essential to learning. For example, auditory feedback from the bird's own vocalizations would elicit activity from BOS selective cells. If this auditory feedback of the bird's own voice also matches the tutor song, then this might elicit greater or different activity in neurons that are also tuned to the tutor song than in neurons tuned to BOS or tutor song alone. Thus, the extent to which BOS resembles the tutor might be reflected in activity of dually tuned neurons, which could then participate in the reinforcement of the motor pathway.

A further suggestion that song selectivity might not only be linked to evaluation of auditory feedback, but is actually sensitive to how well that feedback matches the target, came from studies of adult birds that were experimentally prevented from ever producing a good copy of their tutor template. We found that when we let birds that experienced NXIIts transections prior to song onset grow to adulthood, they had abnormally low song selectivity in the AFP (Solis & Doupe, 2000). Neurons were selective enough to discriminate BOS and tutor song from conspecific and reverse songs, but the degree of selectivity was less than that found in normal adults. This result suggests that selectivity is compromised by a chronic inability of birds to match their tutor song model. If true, then these neurons are not simply reflecting sensory experience, but are influenced by the degree of matching during sensorimotor learning.

Despite the joint representation of BOS and tutor song in many AFP neurons, it seems likely that a pure sensory representation of tutor song is present somewhere in the brain. Although this could be encoded by an unidentified subset of neurons lying within other song system nuclei or even within the AFP, it seems equally plausible that such a representation lies elsewhere in the brain, perhaps in the earlier high-level auditory areas that also process songs of conspecifics (Bolhuis et al., 2000; Mello et al., 1992).

13.3   Singing-related activity in the AFP

Since the auditory feedback most relevant to song learning and maintenance occurs when the bird actually sings, it was clearly critical to record AFP activity during singing. To characterize signals present in the AFP of normal adult birds, we recorded single- and multi-unit activity in LMAN during singing in adult zebra finches (Hessler & Doupe, 1999a,b). LMAN neurons fired vigorously throughout singing in adult birds (Figure 13.4), despite the fact that this nucleus is not required for normal song production. Moreover, excitation began prior to song output, indicating that at least some of the activity is independent of auditory feedback of the bird's own voice. On average, there was a consistent pattern of activity related to individual song elements, and peaks of activity tended to precede syllables. This activity resembles that reported in previous studies of singing-related premotor activity in the song control nucleus HVc (McCasland, 1987; Yu & Margoliash, 1996). This raises the possibility that much of the AFP activity during singing originates from the song motor circuit, and

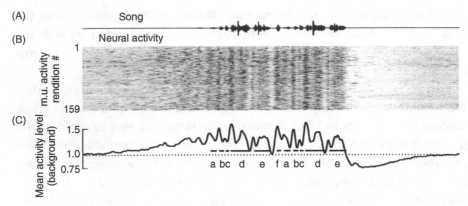

Figure 13.4 LMAN neurons exhibit strong, singing-related activity. (A) The oscillogram shows the song produced by the bird. (B) The mean level of LMAN multi-unit activity recorded in this bird before, during, and after each of 159 renditions of the song is shown below, aligned to the song. Activity level is represented by a grey scale, where black indicates high neural activity and white, low activity (Hessler & Doupe, 1999b). (C) The bottom trace shows the mean of activity during all the renditions above, illustrating the onset of AFP activity before sound, and the peaks of activity related to syllables, which are indicated by the black bars and identified with letters. The duration of the entire panel is 4.5 seconds.

may represent in part a version of the premotor signals also sent to the motor output pathway.

The properties of this singing-related activity raised the question of whether any of it is related to sensory feedback. In playback experiments, song-selective responses to auditory stimuli like those studied in anesthetized birds were apparent in LMAN of awake birds although they were variable from trial to trial and between birds (Hessler & Doupe, 1999b), and it remains to be determined whether they are present in the same neurons that show singing-related activity. Moreover, the level of activity elicited by playback of auditory stimuli was low relative to singing-related activity, making it possible that small auditory feedback signals are embedded within the robust singing-related AFP activity. As an initial step to see whether AFP activity during singing contains both sensory and motor activity, we recorded multi-unit activity from LMAN before and 1–3 days after deafening. Neural activity during singing was very similar pre- and post-deafening, indicating that much of the activity during singing is not dramatically altered by an acute loss of auditory feedback.

Although selective responses to playback of BOS had suggested that sensorimotor learning influences the AFP, the marked AFP activity during singing demonstrates very directly that this circuit is not a pure sensory pathway but, instead, a sensorimotor circuit. Its function during singing may be clarified with studies that determine whether activity in individual neurons or across a population of neurons is a mixture of motor and sensory signals, and if so, how these relate to each other. In addition, recording LMAN activity in response to altered rather than absent feedback could be an important approach to studying these neurons; this would allow multiple interleaved recordings of song-related activity with and without altered feedback, which could be useful for detecting small sensory feedback signals.

The singing-related activity in the AFP might represent an "efference copy," perhaps predicting the sensory consequences of motor commands. The properties of AFP neurons are consistent with this hypothesis. Because efference copy signals are triggered by motor commands, neurons with such signals would be expected to be active during singing, even in the absence of auditory feedback. Furthermore, if these neurons encode an internally generated prediction of the sensory outcome of a motor command to sing, then they might exhibit BOS selectivity when probed with song stimuli in playback experiments. Efference copies are often seen in sensorimotor systems (Bell, 1989; Bridgeman, 1995; von Holst & Mittelstaedt, 1950) and can be useful for providing information about intended motor activity to multiple areas of the brain, and for comparing motor instructions with the consequences of these instructions. The utility of an efference copy signal during sensorimotor learning has been explored in a computational model (Troyer & Doupe, 2000a,b). In this model, premotor activity in HVc gradually becomes associated with the resulting auditory feedback. This creates an internal prediction of the auditory feedback expected after a particular motor command is elicited. Thus, this efference copy is learned, and the role of auditory feedback is to maintain an accurate efference copy. The AFP then evaluates this sensory prediction, rather than the actual feedback. One advantage of this scheme is that it greatly shortens the normal delay between motor activity and auditory feedback, which otherwise might cause feedback evaluation signals to arrive during the motor commands for the next vocal gesture.

If a sensory prediction is learned as described above, then the considerable time it takes for altered auditory feedback to result in vocal change in adult birds (Brainard & Doupe, 2000; Leonardo & Konishi, 1999) might reflect the time necessary to revise the efference copy signal. An instructive signal for change would emerge only after consistently altered feedback changed the pattern of association of auditory feedback and motor commands in HVc. Alternatively, the time course for vocal change after deafening could reflect the time necessary for an instructive signal to take effect within the motor pathway. In this scheme, altered auditory feedback would immediately result in an instructive signal; however, a change in vocal output would not occur until the instructive signal was maintained over a certain period of time. Simultaneous recordings in the AFP and the motor pathway during singing and especially during song learning should help clarify the relationship of AFP activity to motor output and sensory feedback. Presentation of incorrect feedback might again be a useful manipulation, since altered feedback should provide a more potent signal for altering the association between motor commands and feedback in the putative efference copy than the complete absence of sound. In humans, delayed or altered auditory feedback changes vocal output much more rapidly than deafness (Cowie & Douglas-Cowie, 1992; Houde & Jordan, 1998; Lee, 1950).

13.4   Synaptic mechanisms that could underlie song learning

The above experiments implicate LMAN in processing sensory and sensorimotor information related to song, and demonstrate that the properties of LMAN neurons change during learning. Cellular properties of these neurons also change during learning: in particular, NMDA receptors (NMDARs) are strongly expressed in LMAN of young birds, and are significantly down-regulated by the end of the sensory critical period (Aamodt *et al.*, 1992). Moreover, blockade of NMDARs in LMAN during tutoring has been shown to prevent birds from producing a good copy of the tutor song (Basham *et al.*, 1996), consistent with LMAN contributing to tutor song memorization. These results raise the possibility that NMDAR-dependent long-term plasticity is present in LMAN during sensory learning. Such plasticity could contribute to the experience-dependent shaping of auditory responses in LMAN and to the memorization of tutor song.

We investigated the hypothesis that LMAN synapses of young birds can undergo activity-dependent plasticity with an in vitro zebra finch brain slice preparation (Figure 13.5A). Using slices from zebra finches early in sensory learning and not yet engaged in sensorimotor learning of song (20 days of age; Figure 13.1A; Eales, 1989; Immelmann, 1969), we made intracellular voltage recordings from LMAN principal neurons. There are two known excitatory glutamatergic inputs to these cells: afferents from the medial portion of the dorsolateral thalamus (DLM), and the recurrent axon collateral inputs that interconnect neurons within the nucleus (LMAN$_R$; Figure 13.5A). We focused on the LMAN$_R$ synapses, which can be activated by stimulating the LMAN outflow tract, because they have a significantly greater NMDAR-mediated component at the cell's resting potential (V$_{REST}$) at 20 days than do the DLM synapses (Boettiger & Doupe, 1998; Bottjer *et al.*, 1998; Livingston & Mooney, 1997).

Plasticity was induced by repeated (40×) delivery of single brief (100 msec) pulses of postsynaptic depolarizing current in conjunction with LMAN$_R$

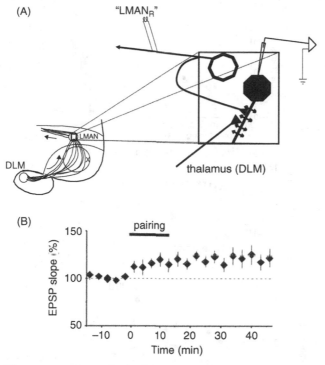

Figure 13.5 Synaptic plasticity in the LMAN slice. (A) Schematic of recording set-up. Slices were cut oblique to the parasagittal plane. The thalamic inputs to LMAN (DLM) come in from below, while the recurrent collaterals between LMAN neurons (LMAN$_R$) interconnect LMAN neurons within the nucleus. The LMAN$_R$ stimulating electrode was placed in the LMAN outflow tract, thus activating these recurrent axon collaterals. Electrode placement was adjusted such that the neuron being recorded was not antidromically activated. The recording electrode used to investigate LMAN synapses was also used to inject current and elicit bursting. (B) Summary of LMAN$_R$ data from 12 birds of approximately 20 days of age. The slope of LMAN$_R$ extracellular synaptic potentials was significantly increased 30 minutes after pairing stimulation of LMAN$_R$ inputs with postsynaptic depolarizing bursts.

stimulation. Each current injection elicited a burst of 6–10 action potentials (APs) whose duration approximated the duration of the current pulse. This pairing protocol produced a long-lasting increase of the LMAN$_R$ EPSP slope. On average, the mean LMAN$_R$ EPSP slope 30 minutes after pairing onset was increased by 21% relative to baseline (Figure 13.5B), and when stable recordings could be maintained to 60 minutes after pairing, EPSP slopes were increased by 33% relative to baseline. Consistent with many other forms of cortical and hippocampal potentiation, the induction of LMAN$_R$ LTP depended on NMDAR activation: the presence of the NMDAR blocker DL-2-amino-5-phosphonovaleric

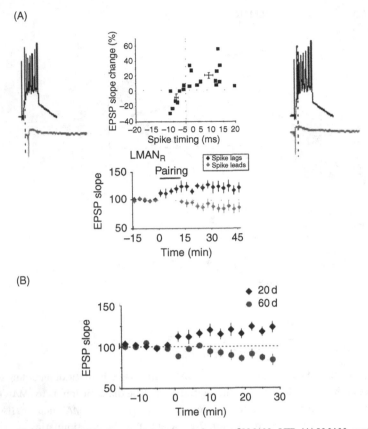

Figure 13.6 Timing- and age-dependence of LMAN$_R$ LTP. (A) LMAN$_R$ potentiation is dependent on the relative timing between the EPSP onset and the peak of the first spike elicited by the current injection; individual examples of EPSPs lagging (left inset) and leading (right inset) postsynaptic spikes are shown. The upper graph plots the percent change of LMAN$_R$ EPSP slope at 30 min vs. spike timing relative to EPSP onset. Cross-hairs denote mean $\pm$ SEM for spike lagging and spike leading data. The lower graph plots group data showing the significant difference between LMAN$_R$ EPSPs subjected to spike-lagging ($\blacklozenge$, $n = 12$) vs. spike-leading ($\blacklozenge$, $n = 8$) pairing. (B) LMAN$_R$ group data reveals the significant difference between the effects of the pairing protocol on slices from 20- to 60-days birds. At 60 days, LMAN$_R$ pairing induced no significant potentiation, instead eliciting depression.

acid (APV) during pairing blocked the increase in LMAN$_R$ responses normally observed after pairing and instead produced a small but significant depression (Boettiger & Doupe, 2001).

The changes in the LMAN$_R$ EPSP elicited by the pairing protocol also depended on the timing of the first spike elicited by the current injection relative to the onset of the EPSP (Figure 13.6A). When the first spike occurred after the LMAN$_R$ EPSP onset ("spike lags"), the LMAN$_R$ pathway was potentiated. In contrast, when the first spike in the burst preceded the EPSP onset ("spike leads"), potentiation did not occur and in some cases the LMAN$_R$ EPSP was depressed. The pairing protocol induced significantly less potentiation of LMAN$_R$ responses in spike-leading vs. spike-lagging experiments (Figure 13.6A). Thus LMAN$_R$ LTP in 20-day birds exhibits timing dependence, a computationally important feature (Roberts, 1999; Song et al., 2000) recently described in several systems (Bell et al., 1997; Bi & Poo, 1998; Debanne et al., 1998; Egger et al., 1999; Feldman, 2000; Magee & Johnston, 1997; Markram et al., 1997; Zhang et al., 1998). While the EPSP–AP burst pairing used in these experiments established this timing dependence, further experiments using a single AP will be necessary to provide a more complete description of the timing rule for LMAN$_R$ synapses. Moreover, the lack of LTP induction when the first spike of a burst preceded the EPSP, despite subsequent spikes following the EPSP, suggests that the first spike plays a critical role in determining the sign of long-term plasticity in LMAN (see also Zhang et al., 1998).

Blockade of NMDARs in LMAN during tutoring, which impairs tutor learning (Basham et al., 1996), would also have prevented the LMAN$_R$ LTP described in 20-day finches. Lack of this LTP could thus be one factor preventing the incorporation of new tutor song information in young NMDAR-blocked birds. In addition, if LMAN$_R$ LTP is critical to sensory learning, a decrease in LMAN$_R$ LTP inducibility might also occur developmentally, contributing to the normal closure of the critical period for memorization of tutor song at approximately 60 day in zebra finches (Figure 13.1A; Eales, 1985, 1987; Immelmann, 1969). To test this prediction, we paired postsynaptic bursts with LMAN$_R$ synaptic stimulation in slices from birds of 60 days of age.

The effect of the induction protocol on LMAN neurons' intrinsic synaptic inputs was strikingly different at this later age. Instead of inducing a potentiation of the LMAN$_R$ responses, a significant depression of LMAN$_R$ responses was observed at 30 minutes after spike-lagging pairing (average of -14%; Figure 13.6B). This represented a significant decrease in the ability of the pairing protocol to induce LMAN$_R$ LTP at 60 days compared to that at 20 days. While these results do not rule out the possibility that potentiation of LMAN$_R$ responses could still be induced in older birds by a less physiological protocol, they indicate that the threshold for induction of this plasticity is substantially higher by the end of sensory learning. In addition, the change in sign of the plasticity at the LMAN$_R$ synapses suggests that functionally significant changes have taken place at these connections by 60 days.

Thus, long-term synaptic plasticity of intrinsic LMAN synapses can be induced by pairing stimulation of these synapses with postsynaptic bursts of

APs, supporting the idea that excitatory feedback connections are key sites of synaptic plasticity within neural networks (Hua *et al.*, 1999). This LMAN$_R$ LTP, which depends on both NMDAR activation and the timing of the AP burst, was present at a time when sensory learning is occurring and was no longer evident by the close of the sensory critical period. This timing suggests that it may play a role in tutor song memorization, and/or in the early stages of sensorimotor evaluation and refinement of song and song-selective neurons. An advantage of the song system is that such correlations can be further tested in a straight-forward manner by manipulating learning. For instance, raising zebra finches in isolation extends the normal critical period for tutor song learning (Eales, 1987, 1989). If LMAN$_R$ LTP is critical for song memorization, it should still be present in slices from 60-day finches raised in isolation. Alternatively, if LMAN$_R$ LTP is induced by early sensorimotor matching and development of song selectivity, it might still be inducible in 60-day birds that have memorized tutor song normally but have been prevented from hearing their own voice and refining their song (for instance, by muting or otherwise preventing audible auditory feedback). Given this ability to alter the behavior very speci-fically, circuitry in LMAN, and the song system as a whole, may prove to be particularly advantageous for pursuing a causal link between experience-dependent changes in synaptic strength and the learning of a complex behavior.

Finally, such spike timing-dependent LMAN$_R$ plasticity provides a simple and plausible mechanism for storage and recognition of a temporal pattern (Abbott & Blum, 1996; Gerstner *et al.*, 1993). This plasticity could be useful for generating connectivity within LMAN that reflects the temporal pattern of DLM-afferent activity elicited by the tutor song, and thus can predict that pattern; that is, if different subsets of DLM afferents fire at different time points in response to the sound of the tutor song, LMAN$_R$ LTP would cause LMAN neurons activated by DLM at one point in time to strengthen their connections onto LMAN neurons activated by DLM at a subsequent time point (Figure 13.7). In contrast, because of the spike-timing dependence of LMAN$_R$ LTP, the reciprocal LMAN$_R$ connections would weaken or remain static. These changes in synaptic strength over the course of sensory learning would come to represent the temporal pattern of DLM-afferent activation in response to tutor song. Circuitry organized in this fashion could represent a memory of the tutor song, reminiscent of a proposed model for sequence prediction in the hippocampus (Abbott & Blum, 1996). During sensorimotor learning, such circuitry could then preferentially reinforce motor sequences produced by the bird that sound adequately similar to the tutor song (Troyer & Doupe, 2000a,b).

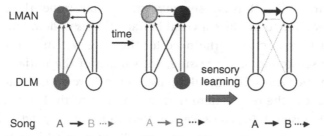

LMAN

time

sensory
learning

DLM

Song   A → B ···►   A → B ···►   A → B ···►

Figure 13.7   A simple model depicting a possible role for LMAN plasticity in song learning. During sensory learning, LMAN plasticity may establish a prediction within the recurrent circuitry of the temporal pattern of DLM afferent activation elicited by tutor song. A segment of tutor song "A" would elicit firing in a subset of DLM projection neurons (left panel, shown in medium gray), which in turn would activate a subset of LMAN neurons (also in medium gray), including their recurrent projections onto other LMAN neurons (middle panel, light gray). The LMAN neurons (shown in black, middle panel) activated by collateral inputs (light gray) and simultaneously by DLM inputs responding to the next chunk of song "B" (middle panel, shown in dark gray) would experience the conjunction required for LMAN$_R$ LTP. Over the course of sensory learning, the spike-timing dependent strengthening of LMAN$_R$ synapses would come to reflect the temporal pattern of DLM afferent activation by tutor song (right panel). During subsequent sensorimotor learning, the production of the correct A-B sequence could lead to firing of strong LMAN$_R$ inputs driven by A coincident with spikes driven by B, leading to enhanced LMAN neuronal activity; this could represent an instructive signal for guiding vocal motor output at RA.

13.5   Conclusions

The studies here used a combination of neurophysiological studies and behavioral manipulations to investigate the function of the AFP, investigating not only normal birds at different stages of development but also animals in which the usual relationship between vocal motor output and sensory input had been in some way disrupted. The results revealed that AFP neurons develop selectivity during learning for both BOS and tutor song, are strongly active during singing, even in deaf birds, and have synaptic mechanisms appropriate for developing temporal selectivity for song.

AFP neurons appear to reflect multiple sensory and motor aspects of song, suggesting that these processes are almost inextricably entangled, even at the level of single neurons. In this respect, birdsong is reminiscent of human speech (Doupe & Kuhl, 1999): electrical stimulation of a single language area can affect both production and perception of speech (Ojemann, 1991), and some cortical neurons respond differently to the same word depending on whether it was spoken by the subject, or by someone else (Creutzfeldt *et al.*, 1989). Perhaps this entanglement indicates that the primary task assigned to the song system, and to many speech areas as well, is not sensory learning, but rather the sensori-motor learning required to produce a vocal imitation. This undertaking alone may be sufficient to have created the need for the song system, and to have specialized it for sensorimotor processing, with much of the initial sensory processing and memorizing of songs taking place elsewhere in the brain.

It is also relevant to the results here that the AFP is a cortical-basal ganglia circuit (Bottjer & Johnson, 1997; Luo & Perkel, 1999). Such basal ganglia circuits are well conserved evolutionarily, and are generally implicated in motor and reinforcement learning – functions critical to sensorimotor learning of song. In primates, striatal neurons have predictive information related to movement and reward, and might participate in comparisons of motor output to internal models (Hikosaka *et al.*, 1989; Hollerman *et al.*, 1998; Tremblay *et al.*, 1998). Spike-timing-dependent plasticity similar to that observed here could be involved in generating such predictions. Like mammalian basal ganglia, AFP neurons could receive or even compute reinforcement signals, and transfer them to the motor pathway. Because the AFP is a discrete basal ganglia–forebrain circuit specialized for one well-defined behavior, it may prove a particularly tractable system for elucidating the neural signals present in these structures, both at circuit and synaptic levels, and their function in the learning and modification of sequenced motor acts.

Acknowledgments

The work described here was supported by the NIH (MH55987 and NS34835 to AJD, MH11896 to CAB, NS00913 to NAH), a National Sciences Foundation graduate fellowship (MMS), and the John Merck Fund and the EJLB Foundation (AJD). M. S. Brainard provided thoughtful comments on an earlier version of the manuscript and P. Puri provided invaluable editorial assistance.

References

Aamodt, S. M., Kozlowski, M. R., Nordeen, E. J., and Nordeen, K. W. (1992). Distribution and developmental change in [3H]MK-801 binding within zebra finch song nuclei. *Journal of Neurobiology*, **23**, 997–1005.

Abbott, L. F. and Blum, K. I. (1996). Functional significance of long-term potentiation for sequence learning and prediction. *Cerebral Cortex*, **6**, 406–16.

Basham, M. E., Nordeen, E. J., and Nordeen, K. W. (1996). Blockade of NMDA receptors in the anterior forebrain impairs sensory acquisition in the zebra finch (Poephila guttata). *Neurobiology of Learning and Memory*, **66**, 295–304.

Bell, C. (1989). Sensory coding and corollary discharge effects in mormyrid electric fish. *Journal of Experimental Biology*, **146**, 229–53.

Bell, C. C., Han, V. Z., Sugawara, Y., and Grant, K. (1997). Synaptic plasticity in a cerebellum-like structure depends on spike timing, synaptic strength and cell type. *Nature*, **387**, 278-81.

Bi, G. and Poo, M.-M. (1998). Synaptic modifications in cultured hippocampal neurons: dependence on spike timing, synaptic strength, and postsynaptic cell type. *Journal of Neuroscience*, **18**, 10464-72.

Boettiger, C. A. and Doupe, A. J. (1998). Intrinsic and thalamic excitatory inputs onto songbird LMAN neurons differ in their pharmacological and temporal properties. *Journal of Neurophysiology*, **79**, 2615-28.

Boettiger, C. A. and Doupe, A. J. (2001). Developmentally restricted synaptic plasticity in a songbird nucleus required for song learning. *Neuron*, **31**, 809-18.

Bolhuis, J. J., Zijlstra, G. G. O., den Boer-Visser, A. M., and Van der Zee, E. A. (2000). Localized neuronal activation in the zebra finch brain is related to the strength of song learning. *Proceedings of the National Academy of Sciences USA*, **97**, 2282-5.

Bottjer, S. W., Brady, J. D., and Walsh, J. P. (1998). Intrinsic and synaptic properties of neurons in the vocal-control nucleus lMAN from in vitro slice preparations of juvenile and adult zebra finches. *Journal of Neurobiology*, **37**, 642-58.

Bottjer, S. W. and Johnson, F. (1997). Circuits, hormones, and learning: vocal behavior in songbirds. *Journal of Neurobiology*, **33**, 602-18.

Bottjer, S. W., Miesner, E. A., and Arnold, A. P. (1984). Forebrain lesions disrupt development but not maintenance of song in passerine birds. *Science*, **224**, 901-3.

Brainard, M. S. and Doupe, A. J. (2000). Interruption of a basal ganglia-forebrain circuit prevents plasticity of learned vocalizations. *Nature*, **404**, 762-6.

Bridgeman, B. (1995). A review of the role of efference copy in sensory and oculomotor control systems. *Annals of Biomedical Engineering*, **23**, 409-22.

Cowie, R. and Douglas-Cowie, E. (1992). Postlingually acquired deafness: speech deterioration and the wider consequences. In W. Winter, ed., *Trends in Linguistics*. Mouton de Gruyter, Berlin: Mouton de Gruyter.

Creutzfeldt, O., Ojemann, G., and Lettich, E. (1989). Neuronal activity in the human lateral temporal lobe. II. Responses to the subjects own voice. *Experimental Brain Research*, **77**, 476-89.

Dave, A. and Margoliash, D. (2000). Song replay during sleep and computational rules for sensorimotor vocal learning. *Science*, **270**, 812-16.

Debanne, D., Gahwiler, B. H., and Thompson, S. M. (1998). Long-term synaptic plasticity between pairs of individual CA3 pyramidal cells in rat hippocampus slice cultures. *Journal of Physiology*, **507**, 237-47.

Doupe, A. J. (1997). Song- and order-selective neurons in the songbird anterior forebrain and their emergence during vocal development. *Journal of Neuroscience*, **17**, 1147-67.

Doupe, A. J. and Kuhl, P. K. (1999). Birdsong and human speech: common themes and mechanisms. *Annual Review of Neuroscience*, **22**, 567-631.

Eales, L. A., (1985). Song learning in zebra finches: some effects of song model availability on what is learnt and when. *Animal Behavior*, **33**, 1293-300.

Eales, L. A. (1987). Song learning in female-raised zebra finches: another look at the sensitive phase. *Animal Behavior*, **35**, 1356–65.

Eales, L. A. (1989). The influences of visual and vocal interaction on song learning in zebra finches. *Animal Behavior*, **37**, 507–8.

Egger, V., Feldmeyer, D., and Sakmann, B. (1999). Coincidence detection and changes of synaptic efficacy in spiny stellate neurons in rat barrel cortex. *Nature Neuroscience*, **2**, 1098–105.

Eimas, P. D., Miller, J. L., and Jusczyk, P. W. (1987). On infant speech perception and language acquisition. In S. Harnard, ed., *Categorical Perception*. New York: Cambridge University Press, pp. 161–95.

Feldman, D. E. (2000). Timing-based LTP and LTD at vertical inputs to layer II/III pyramidal cells in rat barrel cortex. *Neuron*, **27**, 45–56.

Gerstner, W., Ritz, R., and van Hemmen, J. L. (1993). Why spikes? Hebbian learning and retrieval of time-resolved excitation patterns. *Biology Cybernetics*, **69**, 503–15.

Hessler, N. A. and Doupe, A. J. (1999a). Social context modulates singing-related neural activity in the songbird forebrain. *Nature Neuroscience*, **2**, 209–11.

Hessler, N. A. and Doupe, A. J. (1999b). Singing-related neural activity in a dorsal forebrain-basal ganglia circuit of adult zebra finches. *Journal of Neuroscience*, **19**, 10461–81.

Hikosaka, O., Sakamoto, M., and Usui, S. (1989). Functional properties of monkey caudate neurons. III. Activities related to expectation of target and reward. *Journal of Neurophysiology*, **61**, 814–32.

Hollerman, J. R., Tremblay, L., and Schultz, W. (1998). Influence of reward expectation on behavior-related neuronal activity in primate striatum. *Journal of Neurophysiology*, **80**, 947–63.

Houde, J. F. and Jordan, M. I. (1998). Sensorimotor adaptation in speech production. *Science*, **36**, 1213–16.

Hua, S. E., Houk, J. C., and Mussa-Ivaldi, F. A. (1999). Emergence of symmetric, modular, and reciprocal connections in recurrent networks with Hebbian learning. *Biology Cybernetics*, **81**, 211–25.

Immelmann, K. (1969). Song development in the zebra finch and other estrildid finches. In R. A. Hinde, ed., *Bird Vocalizations*. London: Cambridge University Press, pp. 61–74.

Konishi, M. (1965). The role of auditory feedback in the control of vocalization in the white-crowned sparrow. *Zeitschrift fuer Tierpsychologie*, **22**, 770–83.

Kuhl, P. K. (1994). Learning and representation in speech and language. *Current Opinion Neurobiology*, **4**, 812–22.

Lee, B. S. (1950). Effects of delayed speech feedback. *Journal of the Acoustical Society of America*, **22**, 824–6.

Leonardo, A. and Konishi, M. (1999). Decrystallization of adult birdsong by perturbation of auditory feedback. *Nature*, **399**, 466–70.

Livingston, F. S. and Mooney, R. (1997). Development of intrinsic and synaptic properties in a forebrain nucleus essential to avian song learning. *Journal of Neuroscience*, **17**, 8997–9009.

Luo, M. and Perkel, D. J. (1999). A GABAergic, strongly inhibitory projection to a thalamic nucleus in the zebra finch song system. *Journal of Neuroscience*, **19**, 6700–11.

Magee, J. C. and Johnston, D. (1997). A synaptically controlled, associative signal for Hebbian plasticity in hippocampal neurons. *Science*, **275**, 209–13.

Margoliash, D. (1983). Acoustic parameters underlying the responses of song-specific neurons in the white-crowned sparrow. *Journal of Neuroscience*, **3**, 1039–57.

Markram, H., Lübke, J., Frotscher, M., and Sakmann, B. (1997). Regulation of synaptic efficacy by coincidence of postsynaptic APs and EPSPs. *Science*, **275**, 213–15.

Marler, P. (1970). A comparative approach to vocal learning: song development in white-crowned sparrows. *Journal of Comparative and Physiological Psychology Monographs*, **71**, 1–25.

McCasland, J. S. (1987). Neuronal control of bird song production. *Journal of Neuroscience*, **7**, 23–39.

McCasland, J. S. and Konishi, M. (1981). Interaction between auditory and motor activities in an avian song control nucleus. *Proceedings of the National Academy of Sciences USA*, **78**, 7815–19.

Mello, C. V., Vicario, D. S., and Clayton, D. F. (1992). Song presentation induces gene expression in the songbird forebrain. *Proceedings of the National Academy of Sciences USA*, **89**, 6818–22.

Nordeen, K. W. and Nordeen, E. J. (1992). Auditory feedback is necessary for the maintenance of stereotyped song in adult zebra finches. *Behavioral Neural Biology*, **57**, 58–66.

Nottebohm, F., Stokes, T. M., and Leonard, C. M. (1976). Central control of song in the canary, *Serinus canarius*. *Journal of Comparative Neurology*, **165**, 457–86.

Ojemann, G. A. (1991). Cortical organization of language. *Journal of Neuroscience*, **11**, 2281–7.

Price, P. H. (1979). Developmental determinants of structure in zebra finch song. *Journal of Comparative and Physiology Psychology*, **93**, 260–77.

Roberts, P. D. (1999). Computational consequences of temporally asymmetric learning rules: I. Differential Hebbian learning. *Journal of Computation in Neuroscience*, **7**, 235–46.

Scharff, C. and Nottebohm, F. (1991). A comparative study of the behavioral deficits following lesions of the various parts of the zebra finch song system: implications for vocal learning. *Journal of Neuroscience*, **11**, 2896–913.

Sohrabji, F., Nordeen, E. J., and Nordeen, K. W. (1990). Selective impairment of song learning following lesions of a forebrain nucleus in the juvenile zebra finch. *Behavioral Neurology Biology*, **53**, 51–63.

Solis, M. M. and Doupe, A. J. (1997). Anterior forebrain neurons develop selectivity by an intermediate stage of birdsong learning. *Journal of Neuroscience*, **17**, 6447–62.

Solis, M. M. and Doupe, A. J. (1999). Contributions of tutor and bird's own song experience to neural selectivity in the songbird anterior forebrain. *Journal of Neuroscience*, **19**, 4559–84.

Solis, M. M. and Doupe, A. J. (2000). Compromised neural selectivity for song in birds with impaired sensorimotor learning. *Neuron*, **25**, 109–21.

Song, S., Miller, K. D., and Abbott, L. F. (2000). Competitive Hebbian learning through spike-timing-dependent synaptic plasticity. *Nature Neuroscience*, **3**, 919–23.

Theunissen, F. E. and Doupe, A. J. (1998). Temporal and spectral sensitivity of complex auditory neurons in the nucleus HVc of male zebra finches. *Journal of Neuroscience*, **18**, 3786–802.

Tremblay, L., Hollerman, J. R., and Schultz, W. (1998). Modifications of reward expectation-related neuronal activity during learning in primate striatum. *Journal of Neurophysiology*, **80**, 964–77.

Troyer, T. and Doupe, A. J. (2000a). An associational model of birdsong sensorimotor learning I. Efference copy and the learning of song syllables. *Journal of Neurophysiology*, **84**(3), 1204–23.

Troyer, T. and Doupe, A. J. (2000b). An associational model of birdsong sensorimotor learning. II. Temporal hierarchies and the learning of song sequence. *Journal of Neurophysiology*, **84**, 1224–39.

von Holst, E. and Mittelstaedt, H. (1950). Das Reafferenzprinzip. Wechselwirkungen zwischen Zentralnervensystem und Peripherie. *Naturwissenschaften*, **37**, 464–76.

Waldstein, R. S. (1989). Effects of postlingual deafness on speech production: implications for the role of auditory feedback. *Journal of the Acoustical Society of America*, **88**, 2099–114.

Werker, J. F. and Tees, R. C. (1992). The organization and reorganization of human speech perception. *Annual Review of Neuroscience*, **15**, 377–402.

Williams, H. and Mehta, N. (1999). Changes in adult zebra finch song require a forebrain nucleus that is not necessary for song production. *Journal of Neurobiology*, **39**, 14–28.

Yu, A. C. and Margoliash, D. (1996). Temporal hierarchical control of singing in birds. *Science*, **273**, 1871–5.

Zhang, L. I., Tao, H. W., Holt, C. E., Harris, W. A., and Poo, M.-M. (1998). A critical window for cooperation and competition among developing retinotectal synapses. *Nature*, **395**, 37–44.

14

Voltage-dependent sodium currents in hair cells of the inner ear

JULIAN R. A. WOOLTORTON, KAREN M. HURLEY, HONG BAO,
AND RUTH ANNE EATOCK

14.1 Introduction

The hair cell is the mechanosensory cell of the auditory and vestibular organs of the inner ear. Sounds and head movements deflect the hair cells' apical bundles of specialized microvilli, inducing current flow through mechano-sensitive ion channels in the bundles. The resulting change in membrane potential – the receptor potential – in turn modulates diverse voltage-gated ion channels in the basolateral membrane. The most numerous channels are potassium (K^+)-selective and may be voltage- and/or calcium (Ca^{2+})-activated. Flow of current through K^+ channels tends to drive the hair cell towards its resting potential, providing negative feedback on the transduction current or, in some cases, amplifying the voltage response through electrical resonance. The properties of hair cell K^+ channels have been the focus of many studies, in part because of the opportunity to link diversity in the repertoire of K^+ channels to sensory signaling (Fettiplace & Fuchs, 1999). The voltage-gated Ca^{2+} channels of hair cells have been investigated because of their functional significance as activators of K^+ current (e.g., Art & Fettiplace, 1987; Hudspeth & Lewis, 1988) and/or mediators of chemical transmission (e.g., Beutner et al., 2001; Engel et al., 2002; Parsons et al., 1994).

The voltage-gated sodium (Na^+) currents of hair cells have only recently attracted significant attention. Because they have fast inactivation kinetics and frequently very negative voltage ranges of inactivation, hair cell Na^+ currents can be negligible during standard voltage protocols, so that their distribution is not fully characterized. Furthermore, the negative inactivation range of many of the channels raises questions about their availability in the physiological range of membrane potentials. In this chapter, we review

Topics in Integrative Neuroscience: From Cells to Cognition, ed. James R. Pomerantz. Published by
Cambridge University Press. © Cambridge University Press 2008.

the sometimes fragmentary literature on hair cell Na^+ channels, with the following questions in mind: What is the functional significance of those Na^+ channels, reported in a majority of cases, that are largely inactivated over the physiological voltage range? Do different kinds of Na^+ channels play different roles? How prevalent is hair cell spiking, and how much does it depend on Na^+ current? Does Na^+ current in immature hair cells play a developmental role? We begin with a brief introduction to voltage-gated Na^+ channels in general.

14.2   Overview of sodium channels

Voltage dependent Na^+ channels are central to the initiation and propagation of action potentials in excitable cells. They have rapid kinetics, with activation and inactivation time constants often under 1 ms, and are responsible for the initial upstroke (depolarization) in the action potentials of neurons and cardiac muscle cells (Hille, 2001). Loss of normal Na^+ channel function can lead to death when it occurs in the heart (as in Long-QT, Brugada and Lev-Lenegre syndromes; for review, see Napolitano *et al.*, 2003), or dysfunction when it occurs in the brain (causing epilepsy: Escayg *et al.*, 2000; Lossin *et al.*, 2003; Ohmori *et al.*, 2002). In this chapter we refer to voltage-gated Na^+ channels as Na^+ channels and neglect other kinds of Na^+ channels, such as amiloride-sensitive Na^+ channels.

Each Na^+ channel comprises an α subunit that forms the channel pore and, in many cases, auxiliary (β) subunits. In mammals, there are nine known α subunits (Table 14.1), denoted $Na_V 1.x$, where $x = 1-9$, and 4 β subunits, denoted βx, where $x = 1-4$ (for review, see Goldin *et al.*, 2000; for the recently identified $\beta 4$, see Yu *et al.*, 2003). Na^+ channels are thought to consist of one α subunit and one or two different β subunits (e.g., Hartshorne & Catterall, 1984; Maier *et al.*, 2004; Malhotra *et al.*, 2001; Roberts & Barchi, 1987). The α subunits confer many of the biophysical and pharmacological properties of the Na^+ channel and can function in the absence of β subunits; as we will see later, there is molecular evidence for multiple α subunits in hair cells. β subunits cannot form channels by themselves, but substantially modulate electrophysiological properties, such as voltage-dependent steady-state inactivation curves and inactivation kinetics (for review, see Isom, 2002). Nothing is known about the distribution of β subunits in hair cells.

The Na^+ channels were classically characterized by their biophysical and pharmacological properties, especially their voltage ranges of activation and inactivation and their sensitivity to block by tetrodotoxin (TTX) or divalent cations. *TTX-sensitive* and *TTX-insensitive* Na^+ channels (Table 14.1) are

TTX sensitivity	K_D	Type	Former names	Gene symbol	Localization	$V_{1/2,act}$, mV	$V_{1/2,inact}$, mV	τ_{act}, µs	τ_{inact}, ms	Preparation
TTX sensitive	1–25 nM[1–6,24]	Na$_V$1.1	Rat I, HNSCI, GPBI	SCN1A	CNS	−17 ± 4[1] −23.6 ± 1.2[17]	−35 ± 2[1] −64.1 = 1.1[17]	—	τ_1 0.3, τ_2 4[17]	Oocytes[1] HEK[17]
		Na$_V$1.2	Rat II, HBSCII	SCN2A	CNS	−18 ± 5[1] −22.0 ± 0.3 (7)[18]	−42 ± 4[1] −61[18]	140[26]	0.4[18] 0.6[26]	Oocytes[1,26] HEK[18]
		Na$_V$1.3	Rat III	SCN3A	CNS	−23 ± 3 (11)[3] −25.5 ± 1.6 (24)[19] −12.1 ± 1.5 (19)[20] −28.2 ± 0.3 (8)[18]	−44 ± 2 (11)[3] −65 ± 1.5 (25)[19] −47.5 ± 1.2 (18)[20] −71.6 ± 2.0 (17)[18]	—	0.7[3] 0.95[19] 0.8[20] 0.4[18]	CHO[3,20] HEK[3,19]
		Na$_V$1.4	SkM1, µ1	SCN4A	Skeletal muscle	−27.0 ± 0.8 (31)[21] −40 ± 4 (6)[22]	−72 ± 1 (31)[21]	289 ± 23 (20)[21,−30 mV]	0.51 ± 0.05 (10)[21] 0.44[22]	HEK[18,21,22]
		Na$_V$1.6	NaCh6, PN4, CerIII	SCN8A	CNS, PNS	−8.8 ± 4 (5)[24]	−55 ± 3 (5)[24]	—	1.3[24] 1[27]	Oocytes[24] Transfected DRGs[27]
		Na$_V$1.7	NaS, hNE-Na, PN1	SCN9A	PNS	−31 ± 3.8 (4)[6] −25.8 ± 0.8 (45)[21]	−78 ± 1.1 (4)[6] −78 ± 1 (45)[21]	303 ± 17 (25)[21,−30 mV]	0.77 ± 0.03 (10)[21]	Oocytes[6] HEK[21]
TTX insensitive	150 nM–2 µM[7–11]	Na$_V$1.5	SkM2, H1	SCN5A	Heart	−47.8 ± 0.5 (14)[18] −56 ± 5 (5)[22] −34.4 ± 2.5 (6)[23]	−92.1 ± 1.2 (14)[18] −81.6 ± 1.4 (6)[23]	480 ± 60 (6)[23]	0.6[18] 0.62[22]	HEK[18,22] B104 cells[23]
	31 µM–>100 µM[12–16]	Na$_V$1.8	SNS, PN3, NaNG	SCN10A	DRG	−16 ± 2.6 (38)[25]	−34 ± 6.5 (38)[25]	320 ± 30 (10)[25]	1.0 ± 0.09 (6)[23] 3.5 ± 0.52 (10)[25]	Cultured DRGs[25]
		Na$_V$1.9	NaN, SNS2, PN5, NaT	SCN11A	PNS	−47 ± 1 (17)[15] −58 ± 2.2 (38)[25]	−44 ± 1 (10)[15] −55 ± 1.3 (38)[25]	430 ± 50 (10)[25]	5.7 ± 0.57 (10)[25]	Cultured DRGs[15,25]

Notes: Where possible, data are given as means ± SEM. Where standard errors are unavailable, values have been rounded. All data obtained at room temperature. CNS and PNS: central and peripheral nervous system; DRG: dorsal root ganglia; K_D: dissociation constant for TTX; $V_{1/2}$ = potential at which half of the cell's Na$^+$ channels are activated ($V_{1/2,act}$) or inactivated ($V_{1/2,inact}$); τ: time constant for activation (act) and inactivation (inact) at 0 mV, unless otherwise stated.

[1] Smith and Goldin, 1998; [2] Noda et al., 1986; [3] Chen et al., 2000; [4] Moran et al., 2003; [5] Dietrich et al., 1998; [6] Sangameswaran et al., 1997; [7] DiFrancesco et al., 1985; [8] Frelin et al., 1986; [9] Sheets and Hanck, 1992; [10] Yamamoto et al., 1993; [11] Kuo et al., 2002; [12] Akopian et al., 1996; [13] Sangameswaran et al., 1996; [14] Rabert et al., 1998; [15] Cummins et al., 1999; [16] Rugiero et al., 2003; [17] Lossin et al., 2003; [18] O'Leary, 1998; [19] Cummins et al., 2001; [20] Meadows et al. 2002; [21] Cummins et al., 1998; [22] Sheets and Hanck, 1999; [23] Gu et al., 1997; [24] Smith et al., 1998; [25] Renganathan et al., 2002; [26] Stühmer et al., 1987; [27] Herzog et al., 2003

blocked by low nanomolar and high nanomolar to micromolar concentrations, respectively. Sometimes TTX-insensitive channels are referred to as 'TTX-resistant'. Na^+ channels are also differentially sensitive to block by divalent cations such as cadmium (Cd^{2+}). Cd^{2+} concentrations that block 50% of the Na^+ current (IC_{50} values) are between 50 and 250 μM for TTX-insensitive cardiac channels ($Na_V1.5$; e.g., DiFrancesco *et al.*, 1985; Favre *et al.*, 1995; Frelin *et al.*, 1986; Yamamoto *et al.*, 1993) and are greater than 5 mM for TTX-sensitive channels (e.g., Frelin *et al.*, 1986; Roy & Narahashi, 1992). What little information exists on the effects of Cd^{2+} on the highly TTX-insensitive $Na_V1.8$ and $Na_V1.9$ subunits suggests that they are insensitive (Rugiero *et al.*, 2003). Thus, Cd^{2+} sensitivity provides an alternative method of discriminating between voltage-gated Na^+ channels. A single residue in the pore domain of the α subunit is responsible for both the TTX sensitivity and the Cd^{2+} sensitivity. In TTX-sensitive, Cd^{2+}-insensitive subunits, the critical residue is a tyrosine or phenylalanine, whereas in the TTX-insensitive, Cd^{2+}-sensitive $Na_V1.5$ subunit it is a cysteine (e.g., Backx *et al.*, 1992; Satin *et al.*, 1992; Favre *et al.*, 1995) and in the highly TTX-insensitive $Na_V1.8$ and $Na_V1.9$ subunits it is a serine (e.g., Dib-Hajj *et al.*, 1998; Sangameswaran *et al.*, 1996; Sivilotti *et al.*, 1997).

The α subunits also differ in such biophysical parameters as the voltage range and time course of activation and inactivation. Figure 14.1A illustrates typical voltage protocols used to record Na^+ currents and to measure activation and inactivation parameters. The voltage dependence is illustrated by activation and inactivation curves (Figure 14.1B), which are typically fit by Boltzmann functions and characterized by midpoints (voltages of half-maximal activation, $V_{1/2,act}$, or inactivation, $V_{1/2,inact}$) and steepness factors ('s' values, the voltage range corresponding to an *e*-fold increase in current). Activation ranges are generally positive to resting potential, but the midpoints vary over a large range, from ~-60 mV to -10 mV (Table 14.1). Voltage ranges for steady-state inactivation (Figure 14.1B) show similar variability, with $V_{1/2,inact}$ values ranging from ~-90 mV to -30 mV (Table 14.1).

The time course and extent of activation and inactivation also vary between Na^+ channels. Activation time course is typically fit by an exponential term raised to the third power and inactivation time course by a monoexponential function (Hodgkin & Huxley, 1952). For most channels, activation and inactivation are both rapid (time constants 0.3–1 ms; Table 14.1) and complete. Channels comprising the subunits that are least sensitive to TTX ($Na_V1.8$ and $Na_V1.9$), however, have unusually long inactivation time constants (3.5–6 ms; Table 14.1) and incomplete inactivation (Baker & Bostock, 1997; Chen & Lucero, 1999; Magistretti & Alonso, 1999; Rugiero *et al.*, 2003).

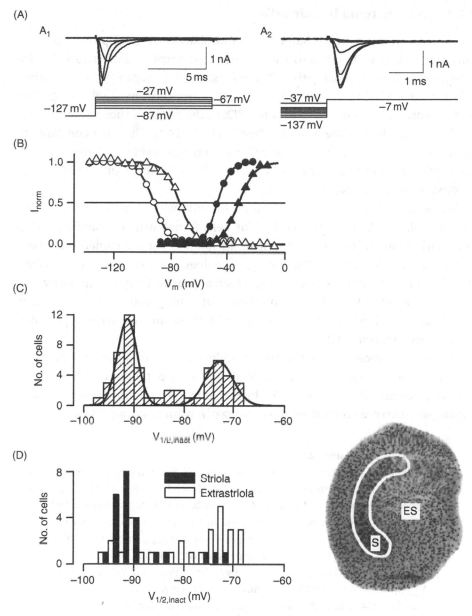

Figure 14.1 Two populations of Na$^+$ channels in hair cells of the immature rat utricular epithelium. (A) Na$^+$ currents evoked by activation (A$_1$) and inactivation (A$_2$) voltage protocols. Whole-cell currents were recorded from a hair cell in the striolar zone of the epithelium, with the ruptured patch version of the patch clamp method (see photomicrograph in D). Holding potential − 67 mV. Protocols: A$_1$, 10-ms iterated depolarizing steps followed a 20-ms prepulse to − 127 mV; A$_2$, A 10-ms depolarization to − 7 mV followed iterated 20-ms prepulses. Online leak subtraction was accomplished with a +P, −P/4 protocol (see Bao *et al.*, 2003 for details). Larger currents

14.3 Na$^+$ currents in hair cells

According to their biophysical and pharmacological properties, Na$^+$ currents in hair cells fall into three categories: negatively-inactivating, TTX-sensitive; negatively-inactivating, TTX-*insensitive*; less negatively inactivating, TTX-sensitive ("–/TTX-S," "–/TTX-I," "+/TTX-S," respectively, Table 14.2). The TTX-insensitive currents have K$_D$'s for TTX in the range of those described for cardiac channels and the Na$_V$1.5 subunits (Table 14.1). The time constants of activation and inactivation of hair cell Na$^+$ currents (Table 14.2) overlap with those of most known subunits, from Na$_V$1.1 to Na$_V$1.7, except for the highly TTX-insensitive subunits, Na$_V$1.8 and Na$_V$1.9.

While the importance of Na$^+$ channels for spiking cells such as neurons and cardiac cells is clear, their role in hair cells is not firmly established. It is generally assumed that they participate in spiking, but the evidence for Na$^+$-based spikes is weak when $V_{1/2,inact}$ values are negative to –80 mV (Section 14.3.1.1). In these hair cells, which appear to be in the majority, the Na$^+$ channels should be largely inactivated at resting potential – that is they should become significantly available for activation only following hyperpolarizing inputs (Section 14.3.1.1).

In contrast, recent experiments on rodent hair cells have revealed Na$^+$ currents that are only partly inactivated at resting potential and help shape action potentials (Section 14.3.1.2). In the immature rat utricle, a vestibular organ, such currents coexist with more negatively inactivating, TTX-insensitive

---

Caption for Figure 14.1 (cont.)

correspond to the more positive voltage steps in A$_1$ and to the more hyperpolarized prepulses in A$_2$. K$^+$ currents were blocked by 100% substitution of K$^+$ by Cs$^+$, both inside and outside the cell, and 5 mM extracellular 4-AP. (B) Activation (*filled symbols*) and inactivation (*open symbols*) curves for the cell in A (*circles*), and a second hair cell from the extrastriolar zone (*triangles*). V$_m$, membrane potential; I$_{norm}$, current normalized to maximum current. Data fit with a single Boltzmann function. Striolar cell: V$_{1/2, inact}$ –92 mV, slope (S) 5.4, V$_{1/2, act}$ –47 mV, S 4.5; Extrastriolar cell: V$_{1/2, inact}$ –74 mV, S 5.5; V$_{1/2, act}$ –32 mV, S 5.4. (C) Two populations of Na$^+$ currents. Distribution of V$_{1/2, inact}$ values ($n = 54$ cells; 2 mV bins) is bimodal. Gaussian fits yielded mean for the two populations of –91 ± 0.1 mV and –73 ± 0.3 mV. (D) The two populations of Na$^+$ currents were differentially distributed across the utricular epithelium. Photomicrograph (right, courtesy of S. Desai and A. Lysakowski, University of Illinois, Chicago) shows the crescent-shaped striolar and surrounding extrastriola zones, as revealed by labeling with calretinin antibody. Most (83%) cells in the striola (*filled bars*) had V$_{1/2, inact}$ values negative to –84 mV, compared to just 33% in the extrastriola (*open bars*). Modified from Figure 2 and Figure 6 in Wooltorton *et al.* (2007). Used with permission from The American Physiological Society.

Table 14.2. Na^+ currents in hair cells

Organ	Species	Age	$V_{1/2(act)}$, mV (no. of cells)	$V_{1/2(inact)}$, mV (no. of cells)	τ_{act}, μs (no. of cells)	τ_{inact}, ms (no. of cells)	TTX effect (block or K_D)	Classification	Papain/ semi-intact
Cochlea	Alligator	2 months[1]	−36	−100	TP $1320^{-24\,mV}$	$1.33^{-24\,mV}$	80% block (100 nM)	−/TTX-S	P
	Guinea pig	Adult[2]	−37	−100	—	—	90% block (100 nM)	−/TTX-S	P I
	Mouse	E16.5–P12[3] (IHCs)	34–37 °C: −30.5 (11)*	34–37 °C: −71.4 (6)*	$\tau\ 32^{0\,mV}$	$0.15^{0\,mV}$	K_D 5 nM	+/TTX-S	I
	Rat	P0–P18[4] (OHCs)	−40 ± 3.5 (22)	23 °C: −93 ± 1.2 (10) 36 °C: −85 ± 0.7 (10)	TP <500 (4)$^{-10\,mV}$	0.3 ± 0.04 (4)$^{-10\,mV}$	K_D 475 nM	−/TTX-I	I
Saccule	Goldfish	Mature[5]	—	Fully inact at −70 mV	—	—	100% block (300 nM)	−/TTX-S	P
Utricle	Mouse	E15–P0+[6]	−40 ± 5.3 (56)	−88 ± 6.1 (50)	—	—	Max 24% block (300–1000 nM)	−/TTX-I	I
		P1–Adult[7] (neonatal and type II)	—	−104 ± 3.7 (5)	TP $630^{-29\,mV}$	$0.7^{-29\,mV}$	K_D 350 nM	−/TTX-I	I
	Rat	P0–P4[8]	−43 ± 0.6 (29)	−91 ± 0.5 (30)	—	—	—	−/TTX-I	I
			−35 ± 0.7 (22)	−75 ± 0.9 (24)	—	—	—	+/TTX-S	
		P1–P3[8]	−45 ± 1.5 (5)	−112 ± 1.9 (5)	—	—	55% block (500 nM)	−/TTX-I	P
			−34 ± 1.6 (3)	−83 ± 2.6 (3)	—	—	75% block (50 nM)	+/TTX-S	
		P0–P2[9] (neonatal and type II)	−39 ± 1.8 (16)	−80 ± 3.6 (7)	$\tau\ 110 \pm 11\ (7)^{+5\,mV}$	0.3 ± 0.01 (10)$^{+15\,mV}$	100% block (100 nM)	+/TTX-S	I

Table 14.2. (cont.)

Organ	Species	Age	$V_{1/2(act)}$, mV (no. of cells)	$V_{1/2(inact)}$, mV (no. of cells)	Act, μs (no. of cells)	τ_{inact}, ms (no. of cells)	TTX effect (block or K_D)	Classification	Papain/ semi-intact
Canal	Chick	P14–P21[10]	—	—	—	—	100% block (100 nM)	?/TTX-S	P
		E14–adult[11]	—	Immature: −96 (5)* Adult: −89 (10)*	TP 600 (10)$^{-10\,mV}$	0.4$^{-10\,mV}$	K_D 15 nM (immature)	−/TTX-S	I
	Rat	P5–P22[8]	−43 ± 1.8 (7)	−105 ± 2.2 (6)	—	—	—	−/TTX-I[†]	P

Where possible, data are given as means ± SEM. Where standard errors are unavailable, values have been rounded. All data obtained at room temperature unless otherwise stated. * Obtained by fitting averaged data from (number of cells). Act, activation data: τ (time constant) or TP (time to peak) at given potential. τ_{inact}, time constant of inactivation.

Classification: −, $V_{1/2,inact} < -84$ mV; +, $V_{1/2,inact} > -84$ mV; TTX-S, TTX-sensitive; TTX-I, TTX-insensitive.

[†] TTX-insensitivity assumed on the basis of Cd^{2+} sensitivity. P, cells dissociated enzymatically with papain; I, cells recorded from semi-inact preparations, such as epithelial whole mounts or slices.

[1] Evans and Fuchs, 1987;   [2] Witt et al., 1994;   [3] Marcotti et al., 2003b;   [4] Oliver et al., 1997;   [5] Sugihara and Furukawa, 1989;   [6] Géléoc et al., 2004;   [7] Rüsch and Eatock, 1997;   [8] Current chapter,   [9] Chabbert et al., 2003 (for complete study, age range was E20–P8 + P21);   [10] Sokolowski et al., 1993;   [11] Masetto et al., 2003.

currents (Section 14.3.2.1). Reverse transcription polymerase chain reaction (RT-PCR) experiments on the rat utricle have suggested multiple molecular candidates for the three kinds of hair cell currents (Section 14.3.2.2).

Although mature hair cells in some inner ear epithelia express Na^+ currents, the Na^+ currents in rodent cochlear and utricular hair cells are down-regulated during development (Section 14.3.3). This has led to speculation that Na^+ currents are critical to activity-driven development within the sensory epithelia and possibly at higher stages in the auditory or vestibular pathways. This kind of argument holds special power in the cochlea, where inner hair cell Na^+ currents disappear at hearing onset and therefore have no sensory function.

14.3.1   Do hair cells make Na^+ spikes?

There are two parts to this question: Under what conditions do hair cells spike? Are the spikes created by the influx of Na^+ or Ca^{2+} or both? Hair cells have fast-activating Ca^{2+} currents to mediate vesicular release of the excitatory transmitter (e.g., Art & Fettiplace, 1987; Bao et al., 2003; Lelli et al., 2003; Lewis & Hudspeth, 1983; Roberts et al., 1991; Zidanic & Fuchs, 1995). These currents are activated by depolarization in about the same voltage range as the Na^+ currents and therefore potentially make substantial contributions to spikes.

14.3.1.1   Spiking in hair cells with negatively inactivating Na^+ current

The Na^+ currents that have been reported in mature hair cells have steady-state inactivation curves with midpoints negative to $-84\,mV$ and a fairly narrow operating range of voltage (Table 14.2; see example with open circles in Figure 14.1B). Mature hair cells with such currents are found in the low frequency zones of the alligator basilar papilla (Evans & Fuchs, 1987) and the goldfish saccule (Sugihara & Furukawa, 1989), both auditory organs, and in the chick semicircular canal (Masetto et al., 2003), which detects angular head movements. These currents are all TTX sensitive. In addition, small samples of hair cells from mature mouse utricles (Rüsch & Eatock, 1997) and 3-week-old rat semicircular canals (e.g., Figure 14.3) had negatively inactivating Na^+ currents. TTX sensitivity was not tested in mature rodent hair cells; in immature rodent hair cells, the negatively inactivating Na^+ currents are TTX insensitive (Géléoc et al., 2004; Oliver et al., 1997; Rüsch & Eatock, 1997; see Section 14.3.2.1).

In hair cells, resting membrane potentials usually fall between $-50\,mV$ and $-70\,mV$ (Dallos et al., 1982; Dallos, 1985; Kros et al., 1998; Marcotti et al., 1999; Russell & Kossl, 1991). Even at the negative end of this range, relatively few Na^+ channels are likely to be available for activation from resting potential. This arrangement casts doubt on the ability of the currents to influence the receptor potential and contribute to spikes, and indeed, the evidence supporting their contributions is not strong. In alligator cochlear hair cells, spikes were observed from resting potential (Evans & Fuchs, 1987), but their slow time course was consistent with Ca^{2+} spikes reported in other hair cells. Goldfish saccular hair cells can produce spikes with both a slow Ca^{2+} component and a fast Na^+ component (Sugihara & Furukawa, 1989), but in these experiments the resting potential was unphysiologically negative (-90 to -100 mV) because of a steep K^+ gradient. Thus, it is not clear that Na^+ would contribute to spiking from resting potential *in vivo*.

In slice preparations of the chick semicircular canal, both embryonic and mature hair cells expressed negatively inactivating Na^+ currents, although the inactivation range was more positive in mature hair cells ($V_{1/2,inact}$ -89 mV vs. -96 mV; Masetto *et al.*, 2003). For hair cells with resting potentials much more negative than the population averages (-60 to -70 mV), mixed Na^+/Ca^{2+} spikes could be evoked at the offset of hyperpolarizing prepulses or from resting potential. TTX application showed that Na^+ current modestly enhanced the speed and size of these spikes.

Thus, while Na^+ contributions to spikes have been observed in a number of hair cells with negatively inactivating Na^+ currents, there are two important caveats. First, Ca^{2+} influx is a major, if not dominant, contributor to the spikes. Second, it is not clear that Na^+ would contribute to spikes *in vivo*. We discuss two possible explanations for this rather surprising problem. One is that, *in vivo*, the inactivation range is more positive and/or the resting potential is more negative than measured experimentally. The other possibility is that under certain conditions, a negatively inactivating Na^+ current can still make an appreciable contribution to the receptor potential.

Is there more overlap between physiological potentials and inactivation range than experiments suggest?

First, the estimates of resting potential may be wrong. Resting potential may be altered by the methods used to record it, whether intracellular (sharp) microelectrodes or whole-cell patch electrodes. Most forms of damage might be expected to depolarize the cells, and the more negative true hair cell potentials are, the more impact Na^+ current will have. In olfactory neurons, where Na^+ currents have been described with a similarly negative inactivation range (Qu *et al.*, 2000), it has been argued that resting potential must be unusually negative in order to exploit the Na^+ current. But in hair cells, experimental manipulations may equally well hyperpolarize the hair cells, by damaging the sensitive transduction apparatus and removing that source of inward current. Moreover, the activation range of voltage-gated Ca^{2+} channels places constraints on the resting potential in hair cells. If hair cells are to transmit information about small and, in some cases, bi-directional stimuli, then their resting potentials must be close to or overlap the activation range of the Ca^{2+} channels, so that resting transmitter release is modulated by the receptor potential. Thus, we do not expect true resting potentials in hair cells to be significantly negative to $-60\,mV$, at which most hair cell Ca^{2+} channels begin to activate (reviewed in Bao et al., 2003; Zidanic & Fuchs, 1995).

Alternatively or additionally, the measured inactivation range may be wrong. The inactivation range of voltage-gated Na^+ channels is susceptible to modulation by intracellular ATP (Choi et al., 2003; El Sherif et al., 2001), intracellular papain (Cota & Armstrong, 1989; Gonoi & Hille, 1987), and channel glycosylation (Tyrrell et al., 2001). Two manipulations shown to affect the properties of voltage-gated currents in hair cells are temperature and extracellular papain. Most Na^+ current data have been collected at room temperature and therefore not at physiological temperature for avian and mammalian hair cells. Data from the rat cochlea show that temperature may have a significant effect on the inactivation range. At room temperature, Na^+ currents of immature rat outer hair cells had $V_{1/2,inact}$ values of $-93\,mV$, on average $30\,mV$ negative to resting potential (Oliver et al., 1997; Table 14.2). At $36\,°C$, the inactivation range shifted positively by $8\,mV$. Such shifts could significantly increase the number of available Na^+ channels at resting potential – unless temperature causes a parallel shift in resting potential, as was observed in mouse utricular hair cells (Rüsch & Eatock, 1996).

The extracellular papain treatment that has often been used to isolate hair cells can affect the voltage dependence and kinetic parameters of measured currents, as shown for Ca^{2+} currents and Ca^{2+}-activated K^+ currents in frog saccular hair cells (Armstrong & Roberts, 1998, 2001). We have evidence that extracellular papain negatively shifts the Na^+ current inactivation range without affecting the activation range (Table 14.2). The negatively inactivating current from rat utricular hair cells in the semi-intact epithelium (not exposed to papain) had a $V_{1/2,inact}$ value of $-91 \pm 0.5\,mV$ (mean $\pm$ SEM; $n = 30$ hair cells), significantly more positive than the value obtained from papain-isolated hair cells ($-112 \pm 1.9\,mV$, $n = 5$ cells; $P < 0.001$, unpaired Student's t-test; Table 14.2). Papain also negatively shifted the inactivation range of a more positively activating Na^+ current in the same preparation, although by just $8\,mV$ (Table 14.2).

In frog saccular hair cells, extracellular papain removed the inactivation of Ca^{2+}-activated K^+ channels (Armstrong & Roberts, 2001), apparently by cleaving extracellular components of an auxiliary β subunit. Papain may have an analogous effect on Na^+ channel β subunits. Each β subunit (probably one or two per channel, see Section 14.2) interacts with the pore-forming α subunit via an Ig V-like motif in the extracellular domain (McCormick et al., 1998). Ig V-like domains contain a consensus sequence that can be cleaved by papain (Chamow *et al.*, 1990): if extracellular papain cleaves the β subunits of hair cell Na$^+$ channels at this site, it might remove a modulatory influence on the inactivation range. β subunits may shift inactivation negatively ($\beta1$ with Na$_V$1.1 or Na$_V$1.8: Isom *et al.*, 1992; Smith & Goldin, 1998; Smith *et al.*, 1998), positively ($\beta3$ with Na$_V$1.5: Fahmi *et al.*, 2001) or not at all ($\beta2$ with Na$_V$1.1: Smith & Goldin, 1998; $\beta4$ with Na$_V$1.2, Na$_V$1.4 and Na$_V$1.5; Yu *et al.*, 2003).

Thus, cell preparation or recording procedures could exaggerate the distance between resting potential and the inactivation range of Na$^+$ currents. Ideally, one would like to know the parameters for hair cells not exposed to enzymes, at appropriate temperature, in physiological salines and recorded in the perforated patch mode of whole-cell recording, which preserves internal second messengers (Horn & Marty, 1988). This rather heroic combination has never been tried at one time. Is it possible that hair cells really do have Na$^+$ currents that are largely inactivated at resting potential?

In support of this argument, the very negative inactivation ranges have been recorded in diverse hair cell preparations, some at appropriate temperatures (alligator cochlea, goldfish saccule, rat cochlea), others from semi-intact epithelia (mouse and rat utricle, chick semicircular canal, rat cochlea), and still others with the perforated patch method (rat semicircular canal). Despite the negative inactivation range, a very small number of Na$^+$ channels would still be available for activation. For hair cells with high input resistances, current through just a few Na$^+$ channels may affect the receptor potential. For example, some rodent vestibular type II cells have input resistances in excess of $1\,G\Omega$ (Chen & Eatock, 2000). Given a driving force at $-70\,mV$ of $\sim150\,mV$ and a single-channel conductance of $19\,pS$ (Hille, 2001), it would take just a handful of open Na$^+$ channels (<5) to depolarize a 1-$G\Omega$ membrane by $10\,mV$.

Most mature hair cells with Na$^+$ channels are sensitive to relatively low stimulus frequencies – below $400\,Hz$ in alligator or fish auditory organs and below $30\,Hz$ in chick and rodent canals. This may reflect the inability of the membrane potential to follow stimuli at frequencies above a value determined by the membrane time constant. At higher frequencies, phase-locked voltage oscillations fall off and the membrane registers an average depolarization (e.g., Holt *et al.*, 1997; Holton & Weiss, 1983; Russell & Sellick, 1983), which would further inactivate the Na$^+$ channels. Evans and Fuchs (1987) hypothesized that spikes in hair cells facilitate time-locking of afferent activity to low frequency sounds. Spikes would presumably trigger release of large amounts of neurotransmitter, guaranteeing postsynaptic spike activity that is time-locked, with a synaptic delay, to presynaptic spikes.

In summary, the functionality of the negatively inactivating Na$^+$ channels is not yet clear because of several uncertainties. The inactivation range reported in mature hair cells may be excessively negative as a consequence of papain treatment and/or inappropriate temperatures. After accounting for such effects, however, the inactivation range may still be mostly negative to resting potential, leaving only a small fraction of the total number of channels available for activation. On the other hand, for hair cells with high input resistances, currents through small numbers of Na$^+$ channels may significantly speed up spikes or subspiking depolarizations. Moreover, the numbers of available Na$^+$ channels will increase under certain conditions: hyperpolarizations followed by depolarizations that are rapid enough to activate the channels before inactivation sets in.

14.3.1.2 *Spiking in hair cells with positively inactivating Na$^+$ currents*

Evidence for function is much more secure for the more positively inactivating Na$^+$ currents that have been recently identified in immature rodent hair cells (V$_{1/2,\text{inact}}$ values positive to -84 mV). These hair cells spike in physiological conditions, and recent data support a specific mechanism whereby such spiking facilitates synaptogenesis (Section 14.3.3.2).

Chabbert *et al.* (2003) and Marcotti *et al.* (2003b) have described more positively inactivating Na$^+$ currents in immature rat and mouse hair cells (Table 14.2). In inner hair cells in a semi-intact preparation of the mouse cochlea at mammalian temperature, Marcotti *et al.* (2003b) showed that both Na$^+$ and Ca^{2+} currents contribute to spiking from resting potential. While Ca^{2+} currents were both necessary and sufficient to produce spikes, the addition of Na$^+$ current reduced the time for the membrane to reach spike threshold and the rate of rise of spikes, and the increased spike rate (e.g., from $\sim$10 to 15 spikes/s in an example in which spiking was evoked by injecting a small depolarizing current).

The inactivation range reported by Chabbert *et al.* (2003) for the immature rat utricle is significantly positive of that reported by Rüsch and Eatock (1997) for the immature mouse utricle. In the next section, we describe data from rodent vestibular epithelia in more detail, and include new results that may explain the apparent discrepancy between reported inactivation ranges.

14.3.2 *Multiple Na$^+$ channel types in rodent vestibular hair epithelia*

14.3.2.1 *Whole-cell Na$^+$ currents*

The peripheral vestibular system of mammals comprises five organs per ear: three semicircular canals, which detect angular head movements, and two otolith organs (the saccule and utricle), which detect linear head movements and head tilt. The vestibular epithelia of mammals, birds and reptiles have hair cells of two morphological classes: type I and type II. In rodents, electrophysiological differences between the two hair cell types emerge in the first postnatal week, when type I hair cells acquire a very negatively activating and large K^+ conductance, $g_{K,L}$ (Eatock & Hurley, 2003; Géléoc *et al.*, 2004; Hurley *et al.*, 2006; Rüsch *et al.*, 1998). Recordings from hair cells in rodent canal and utricular epithelia in the first postnatal month reveal that many express voltage-gated Na^+ currents. But the measured properties vary with species (rat vs. mouse), developmental stage, epithelium type (canal vs. utricle), and hair cell type.

Rüsch and Eatock (1997) reported that ~40% of immature or type II hair cells in the semi-intact mouse utricle (postnatal day [P] 1–adult) expressed a Na^+ current that was both negatively inactivating and TTX insensitive (Table 14.2). These currents therefore resembled those reported in rat outer hair cells by Oliver *et al.* (1997). Na^+ currents were almost never seen in hair cells that had acquired the type I-specific K^+ conductance, $g_{K,L}$.

In more recent reports, Na^+ currents from semi-intact preparations of the young rodent utricle have more positive inactivation ranges and high TTX sensitivity (Chabbert *et al.*, 2003; Lennan *et al.*, 1999). The $V_{1/2,inact}$ values obtained by Chabbert *et al.* (2003) in the early postnatal rat utricle are ~25 mV positive to that previously reported by Rüsch and Eatock (1997) and Géléoc *et al.* (2004). This Na^+ current disappears with development (Section 14.3.3.1), unlike the negatively inactivating current reported by Rüsch and Eatock (1997) and Géléoc *et al.* (2004). These apparently contradictory observations can be reconciled if rodent utricles express two Na^+ currents, one positively inactivating current that disappears with maturation, and one negatively activating current that may persist in some mature cells. As we illustrate here, our recent data provide some support for this hypothesis by showing concurrent expression of the two Na^+ currents in the first postnatal week (Wooltorton *et al.*, 2007).

Figure 14.1A shows whole-cell currents recorded from hair cells in the semi-intact rat utricular epithelium (P0–P4) under conditions that isolate voltage-gated Na^+ and Ca^{2+} currents. Different voltage protocols are used to determine the voltage ranges of activation (A_1) (Figure 14.1A) and inactivation (A_2) (Figure 14.1A), which are plotted as activation and inactivation curves in Figure 14.1B. Figure 14.1B shows data from the cell in Figure 14.1A and from a cell with a more positive voltage dependence. The Na^+ currents of these two cells are representative of two populations expressed by the immature rat utricular epithelium. The distribution of $V_{1/2, inact}$ values (Figure 14.1C) has two modes: fitting with two Gaussians yields mean values of -91 ± 0.5 mV ($n = 30$) and -75 ± 0.9 mV ($n = 24$). The activation ranges of the two Na current types also differed significantly ($V_{1/2, \text{act}} = -43 \pm 0.6$ mV, $n = 29$ and -35 ± 0.7 mV, $n = 22$; $P < 0.001$). Thus, two Na^+ current populations are co-expressed in one epithelium at one developmental stage.

Why did one group only report the negatively inactivating current and the other group only report a more positively inactivating current? Our recent data suggest a combination of two factors: selective sampling of different epithelial zones and pooling of the data from the two populations. Mammalian vestibular epithelia have distinct anatomical regions (Goldberg, 1991; Lindeman, 1973). The utricular epithelium has a curved swath, the striola, surrounded by a peripheral zone called the extrastriola. These regions are associated with distinctive morphologies and vestibular afferent response properties (Baird et al., 1988; Goldberg et al., 1990; Lindeman, 1973) and can be visualized with calretinin immunostaining (Desai et al., 2005b; Leonard & Kevetter, 2002; photomicrograph in Figure 14.1D). Figure 14.1D shows that the distribution of Na^+ channels differs with zone in the immature rat utricular epithelium: 83% (21/24) of striolar hair cells had negatively inactivating Na^+ currents vs. just 33% (10/30) of extrastriolar hair cells. The significance of these regional differences in the developing rat utricle is not clear. The striola develops slightly in advance of the extrastriola (Rüsch et al., 1998; Sans & Chat, 1982); thus, one possibility is that regional variation in the first postnatal week arises because the less negatively inactivating Na^+ current is an immature form and more prevalent in the less mature extrastriola.

Based on our results, we suggest that a very negative inactivation range was reported in the immature mouse utricle (Géléoc et al., 2004; Rüsch & Eatock, 1997) because the analyzed data were predominately from the striola, while the results of Chabbert et al. (2003) are consistent with pooling of data from small samples of two Na^+ current populations. Their values for $V_{1/2,\text{inact}}$ (-80 ± 3.6 mV, $n = 7$) and $V_{1/2, \text{act}}$ (-39 ± 1.8 mV, $n = 16$) are intermediate between the values for our two populations and not significantly different from the values for our pooled results: $V_{1/2,\text{inact}} = -84 \pm 1.2$ mV ($n = 54$) and $V_{1/2,\text{act}} = -39 \pm 0.7$ mV ($n = 51$).

In experiments on enzymatically dissociated rat utricular hair cells, we found that the two Na^+ current populations were differentially sensitive to TTX (Figure 14.2). The voltage dependencies of the Na^+ currents of dissociated cells fell into two categories, as observed in the semi-intact preparation. (They were shifted negatively relative to data from the semi-intact epithelium, which we attribute to papain; see Section 14.3.1.1.) 50 nM TTX blocked the less negatively inactivating currents by $76 \pm 8.1\%$ ($n = 3$; Figure 14.2A), consistent with the reported K_D's of TTX-sensitive subunits (1–20 nM). In contrast, 500 nM TTX blocked more negatively inactivating Na^+ currents by $55 \pm 4.8\%$ ($n = 5$;

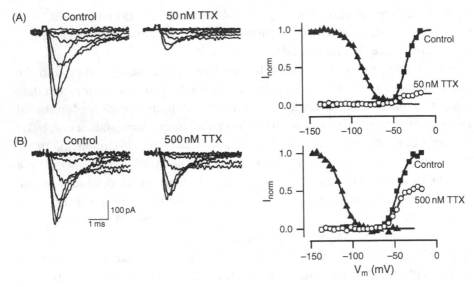

Figure 14.2 Pharmacological evidence for two Na^+ currents in immature rat utricular hair cells. Cells were isolated from rat utricles following enzymatic treatment, which shifted the Na^+ currents' inactivation ranges negatively relative to values in the semi-intact preparation (see text). *Left panels*: Currents elicited by the activation protocol (Figure 14.1A_1) in control external solution or with TTX added. The sustained current observed after Na^+ current inactivation is through L-type Ca^{2+} channels (Bao *et al.*, 2003). *Right panels*: Activation curves (*filled squares*) and inactivation curves (*filled triangles*) in control conditions plus activation curves in TTX (*open circles*). Curves are normalized to the peak value in control conditions. (A) Data from a hair cell with the less negative $V_{1/2, \text{inact}}$ ($-88\,mV$; $S = 8.6\,mV$). 50 nM TTX reduced the maximum current by 86%, consistent with a TTX sensitive Na^+ channel. (B) Data from a hair cell with the more negative $V_{1/2, \text{inact}}$ ($-114\,mV$, $S = 7.2\,mV$). 500 nM TTX reduced the maximum current by 45%, consistent with a TTX-insensitive channel. Modified from Figure 5 in Wooltorton *et al.* (2007). Used with permission from The American Physiological Society.

Figure 14.2B), consistent with the K_D's for negatively inactivating Na^+ currents in the mouse utricle ($\sim$350 nM; Rüsch & Eatock, 1997) and the rat cochlea ($\sim$475 nM; Oliver *et al.*, 1997), and for cardiac TTX-insensitive currents (150 nM–2 µM: e.g., Arreola *et al.*, 1993; Brown *et al.*, 1981; Krafte *et al.*, 1991; White *et al.*, 1993; Yoshida, 1994).

In a study of hair cells dissociated from the rat anterior semicircular canal (P4–P22), all 34 cells, including 15 type I cells, expressed a Na^+ current (Figure 14.3A). The current was negatively inactivating, with voltage dependence similar to that recorded from dissociated rat utricular hair cells (Table 14.2), and Cd^{2+}-sensitive (Figure 14.3B). The Cd^{2+} sensitivity suggests that the negatively

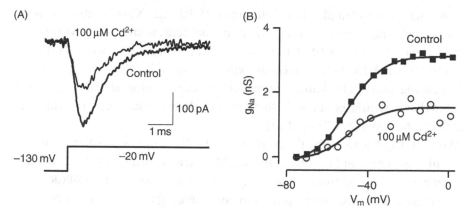

Figure 14.3 Negatively inactivating Na^+ currents are Cd^{2+} sensitive. Data from a hair cell isolated from the rat anterior semicircular canal (P22) following enzymatic treatment (see Bao et al., 2003 for Methods). (A) Currents evoked by steps from $-130\,mV$ to $-20\,mV$ in control external medium and in external medium with $100\,\mu M\,Cd^{2+}$. $V_{1/2,\,inact}$ $-110\,mV$. (B) Conductance–voltage activation curves in control external solution (filled squares) and in Cd^{2+} (open circles). $100\,\mu M\,Cd^{2+}$ blocked the maximum conductance by 47% and in another cell (not shown) by 42%. In two other cells, $200\,\mu M\,Cd^{2+}$ blocked the conductance by 45% and 67%. These values are consistent with the potency of Cd^{2+} block on cardiac TTX-insensitive Na^+ channels (see text).

inactivating current in rat canal hair cells is TTX insensitive (see Section 14.2), similar to the negatively inactivating current in mouse and rat utricular hair cells.

14.3.2.2 Na^+ channel subunit expression in the rat utricular epithelium

Based on the inactivation range, TTX insensitivity and Cd^{2+} sensitivity, we hypothesize that $Na_V1.5$ channels carry the negatively inactivating current in rat vestibular hair cells and possibly in immature rat outer hair cells as well (Oliver et al., 1997). As shown in Table 14.1, the voltage ranges of activation and inactivation of heterologously expressed $Na_V1.5$ channels match well with those of the negative Na^+ current population recorded in semi-intact preparations of hair cells. RT-PCR experiments show that $Na_V1.5$ and a number of TTX-sensitive α subunits are expressed by the rat utricular epithelium (Wooltorton et al., 2007; see below).

A pharmacological and biophysical approach cannot determine the molecular identities of the TTX-sensitive currents in hair cells because there are six TTX-sensitive α subunits with overlapping biophysical properties (Table 14.1). In rat utricle, RT-PCR has been used to identify candidates from expression of messenger RNA (mRNA) by either single cells (Chabbert et al., 2003; Mechaly et al., 2005) or the entire epithelium (Wooltorton et al., 2007). Chabbert and colleagues investigated the expression of neuronal TTX-sensitive α subunits ($Na_V1.1$, 1.2,

1.3, .6, and 1.7) in utricular hair cells from P1–P3 rats. Nine combinations of these five subunits were detected in 13 individual cells, with the following order of prevalence: $Na_V1.6$ (in 10 of 13 cells), $Na_V1.2$ (7/13), $Na_V1.7$ (4/13), $Na_V1.3$ (3/13), and $Na_V1.1$ (1/13). Individual cells expressed up to four isoforms, a remarkable heterogeneity. The known properties of these isoforms are sufficiently similar that it would be difficult to recognize their separate contributions in whole-cell Na^+ currents (Table 14.1).

We used RT-PCR to probe for all nine known Na^+ channel α subunits in rat vestibular epithelia and ganglia at P1 and P21. Utricular and semicircular canal epithelia were peeled from underlying tissue; the material for RT-PCR comprised cells from nonsensory epithelium surrounding the sensory epithelium, plus the hair cells, supporting cells and possibly nerve terminals of the sensory epithelium. At P1, all five neuronal TTX-sensitive subunits ($Na_V1.1$, 1.2, 1.3, 1.6, and 1.7) were expressed in the epithelia, as expected from the single-cell results of Chabbert and colleagues (Chabbert *et al.*, 2003; Mechaly *et al.*, 2005). We also detected the TTX-sensitive skeletal muscle subunit ($Na_V1.4$) and the TTX-insensitive cardiac muscle subunit ($Na_V1.5$), which Chabbert and colleagues (2003) did not probe for. At P21, we again detected $Na_V1.1$, 1.2, 1.3, 1.5, and 1.6, but no longer saw $Na_V1.4$ and $Na_V1.7$ message in the epithelia.

The ganglia expressed all of the subunits found in the epithelia plus $Na_V1.7$ at P21 and the two subunits that are highly insensitive to TTX, $Na_V1.8$ and $Na_V1.9$. We had not expected to see $Na_V1.8$ and $Na_V1.9$ expression in the epithelia because their biophysical properties do not match those of hair cell Na^+ currents (Section 14.2). It is interesting to find them in the vestibular ganglia as they are expressed in other sensory ganglia (dorsal root and trigeminal ganglia; Akopian *et al.*, 1996; Dib-Hajj *et al.*, 1998; Sangameswaran *et al.*, 1996).

14.3.3   The role of Na^+ currents in inner ear development

14.3.3.1 Na^+ currents in rodent hair cells decrease after birth

Kros, Marcotti and colleagues have shown that in mouse inner hair cells, developmental changes in Na^+, Ca^{2+}, and K^+ currents have clear effects on spike generation (Kros *et al.*, 1998; Marcotti *et al.*, 2003a,b). Early postnatal hair cells generate larger and faster spikes than embryonic hair cells, reflecting growth in Na^+ and Ca^{2+} currents from embryonic day (E) 16.5 to P8. From P12 on, Na^+ currents are eliminated, Ca^{2+} currents are reduced to approximately one-third their peak value, and a number of K^+ currents appear; probably as a result of all of these changes, the inner hair cells cease to spike. Beutner and Moser (2001) also reported the developmental changes in mouse inner hair cell Ca^{2+} currents, and Oliver *et al.* (1997) described a similar trend in Na^+ current amplitude in rat outer hair cells. P12 has special significance in the rodent cochlea because it marks the maturation of a number of key features such as outer hair cell electromotility and the onset of hearing (reviewed in Eatock & Hurley, 2003).

Chabbert *et al.* (2003) found that in rat utricular hair cells, as in rodent cochlear hair cells (Marcotti *et al.*, 2003b; Oliver *et al.*, 1997), Na^+ currents declined with maturation. (As discussed in Section 14.3.2.1, these Na^+ currents had more positive inactivation ranges than those reported in mature hair cells of the mouse utricle and rat canal.) The percentage of hair cells expressing Na^+ current peaked at >90% at P1, then fell off gradually to 5% at P21. The average peak Na^+ current (for those hair cells that expressed Na^+ current) also peaked at P1. These changes resemble those described for rodent cochlear hair cells, both inner and outer (Marcotti *et al.*, 2003b; Oliver *et al.*, 1997), except shifted earlier by a few days to one week.

In rodent vestibular epithelia, over 90% of hair cells are born by P1 (Ruben, 1967) and 50–60% become type I hair cells (Desai & Lysakowski, 2005a,b); thus, the high incidence of Na^+ current at P1 shows that immature hair cells of both types (I and II) express Na^+ currents. Neither Chabbert *et al.* (2003) nor Rüsch and Eatock (1997) detected Na^+ currents in differentiated type I hair cells. In contrast, type I hair cells from semicircular canals do not appear to lose Na^+ currents upon differentiation, either in chick (Masetto *et al.*, 2003) or in rat, as we have found (Section 14.3.2.1).

Expression of Na^+ channel α subunits was similar in the whole epithelia at P1 and P21, except for the apparent absence of $Na_V1.4$ and $Na_V1.7$ at P21 (Section 14.3.2.2). The loss of these subunits could underlie the reduction in Na^+ current with age (Chabbert *et al.*, 2003). RT-PCR only provides candidates for the possible components of Na^+ channel proteins, however. For example, our RT-PCR on epithelia showed $Na_V1.2$ mRNA expression at both P1 and P21, but antibody staining for $Na_V1.2$ suggests that the cellular sources of $Na_V1.2$ mRNA shift during this period (Chabbert *et al.*, 2003). At P0–P3, the $Na_V1.2$ antibody labeled hair cells strongly, but by P20 staining was more prevalent in supporting cells. As a result, $Na_V1.2$ is another candidate for the TTX-sensitive, less negatively inactivating Na^+ channel that disappears with age.

14.3.3.2 Possible roles of Na^+ current in development

In mouse inner hair cells, changes in the amplitude of Na^+ currents have a similar time course to changes in Ca^{2+} current levels (Marcotti *et al.*, 2003b). Changes in Ca^{2+} currents will affect neurotransmitter release. Indeed, Beutner and Moser (2001) noted that developmental changes in Ca^{2+} current levels correlate in time with changes in the amount of exocytosis (fusion of synaptic vesicles with the presynaptic membrane, measured as increases in membrane capacitance) and in the number of presynaptic ribbons and postsynaptic bouton terminals (Sobkowicz *et al.*, 1982, 1986). These correlations are consistent with the hypothesis that most voltage-gated Ca^{2+} channels in hair cells are located at active zones (Roberts *et al.*, 1990); thus, the more postsynaptic nerve terminals that a hair cell contacts, the more active zones and Ca^{2+} channels it has and, consequently, the more vesicle fusion occurs. That all of these changes occur hand in hand with changes in Na^+ channel expression raises the possibility that mixed Na^+/Ca^{2+} spikes play an important role in the dynamic synaptogenesis that characterizes the early postnatal cochlea.

By boosting spikes and transmitter release, Na^+ channels could affect afferent synapse formation through Hebbian mechanisms. This could have both pre- and post-synaptic effects, for example through Ca^{2+}-mediated changes on gene expression (Beutner & Moser, 2001). There is evidence that before hearing onset, spontaneous spiking in mammalian and avian cochlear nerve fibers drives spike activity at higher levels of the auditory system, and that this input is crucial to normal development of the pathway (reviewed in Rübsamen & Lippe, 1998). This spiking could originate in either the cochlear fibers or the hair cells.

Recent experiments by Chabbert *et al.* (2003) address the alternative hypothesis that Na^+ channel activity in hair cells affects synapse formation by modulating the release of neurotrophic factors. Growth of eighth-nerve afferents into the inner ear requires both neurotrophin secretion from inner ear epithelia and the neurotrophin receptors on the afferents (see reviews by Pirvola & Ylikoski, 2003; Rubel & Fritzsch, 2002). In the rodent vestibular periphery, the formation of hair cell-afferent synapses is particularly vigorous during the first two postnatal weeks (e.g., Desmadryl & Sans, 1990), and innervation of the epithelia depends on the neurotrophin brain derived growth factor (BDNF) and its receptor (TrkB) (Don *et al.*, 1997; Ernfors *et al.*, 1994). Chabbert *et al.* (2003) showed that both hair cells and supporting cells in neonatal (P0–P3) rat utricular epithelia are labeled by BDNF antibody. They further showed that electrical stimulation of the epithelia elicits BDNF release, and that this release is inhibited by TTX, implicating Na^+ channel activity. By P20, BDNF antibody mostly labels supporting cells and BDNF release no longer has a TTX-dependent or electrically driven component, although there is a baseline (constitutive) release. Chabbert *et al.* (2003) speculate that the activity-dependent BDNF release is critical to formation and survival of synapses during development while the constitutive pathway is important for maintaining innervation.

Na^+ channels may also play a role in the *post*synaptic effect of BDNF: In hippocampal neurons and human neuroblastoma cells, TTX-insensitive $Na_V1.9$ channels can be activated by BDNF without changes in voltage, probably via activation of TrkB receptors (Blum *et al.*, 2002). Such a mechanism might also occur in vestibular afferents, given that $Na_V1.9$ mRNA is present in vestibular ganglia (Section 14.3.3.1).

14.4   Concluding remarks

A survey of the hair cell literature on Na^+ currents yields three basic types (Table 14.2): negatively inactivating, TTX-sensitive channels; negatively inactivating, TTX-insensitive channels; and more positively inactivating, TTX-sensitive channels. Published reports have all assumed a uniform channel type in a given preparation, but recent data from the rat utricle show that TTX-insensitive, negatively inactivating channels and TTX-sensitive, less negatively inactivating channels may be expressed simultaneously within an epithelium. Such heterogeneity may have been missed in other inner ear epithelia. Indeed, even in the rat utricle, TTX sensitivity has not been tested on enough cells to rule out the presence of the third class of Na^+ current, the TTX-sensitive, negatively inactivating current. Identification of the molecular substrates of these three currents should facilitate screening of other inner ear epithelia for the possible presence of multiple Na^+ channel types. It might turn out that only certain channels are down-regulated with maturation, and that other channels persist to contribute to sensory signaling. We hypothesize that the positively inactivating, TTX-sensitive class is an immature form and the more negatively inactivating currents are more mature forms. Na^+ currents are rare in mature hair cells of the mammalian cochlea and possibly the utricle, but appear to be more widely expressed at maturity in avian and possibly mammalian semicircular canals as well as in the low frequency zones of certain auditory organs.

Further understanding of Na^+ channel functions in hair cells requires better documentation of their properties and influence in physiological conditions. Hair cell spikes have a strong Ca^{2+} component, and, in some cases, Na^+ current contributions become clear only after background hyperpolarizations relieve Na^+ channel inactivation. Two experimental priorities are to confirm, under physiological conditions, the inactivation range and the extent to which Na^+ currents contribute to spiking or subthreshold voltage changes. In vivo conditions may be approximated in vitro by recording at body temperature with the perforated-patch method from hair cells in a semi-intact epithelial preparation, thereby avoiding undesirable effects of inappropriate temperature, loss of second messengers, and enzymes on voltage-dependent channels and resting potentials. It is presumably no accident that the most convincing data on hair cell spiking were obtained in a semi-intact preparation at mammalian temperature (Marcotti et al., 2003b), and that in these conditions Na^+ currents had a clear impact on spike time course and the approach to spike threshold.

Acknowledgments

The work in our laboratory is supported by NIH grant DC02290 and by Karim Al-Fayed Neurobiology of Hearing funds. We thank Jasmine Garcia for technical help and comments on the manuscript.

References

Akopian, A. N., Sivilotti, L., and Wood, J. N. (1996). A tetrodotoxin-resistant voltage-gated sodium channel expressed by sensory neurons. *Nature*, **379**, 257–62.

Armstrong, C. E. and Roberts, W. M. (1998). Electrical properties of frog saccular hair cells: distortion by enzymatic dissociation. *Journal of Neuroscience*, **18**, 2962–73.

Armstrong, C. E. and Roberts, W. M. (2001). Rapidly inactivating and non-inactivating calcium-activated potassium currents in frog saccular hair cells. *Journal of Physiology*, **536**, 49–65.

Arreola, J., Spires, S., and Begenisich, T. (1993). Na$^+$ channels in cardiac and neuronal cells derived from a mouse embryonal carcinoma cell line. *Journal of Physiology*, **472**, 289–303.

Art, J. J. and Fettiplace, R. (1987). Variation of membrane properties in hair cells isolated from the turtle cochlea. *Journal of Physiology*, **385**, 207–42.

Backx, P. H., Yue, D. T., Lawrence, J. H., Marbán, E., and Tomaselli, G. F. (1992). Molecular localization of an ion-binding site within the pore of mammalian sodium channels. *Science*, **257**, 248–51.

Baird, R. A., Desmadryl, G., Fernández, C., and Goldberg, J. M. (1988). The vestibular nerve of the chinchilla. II. Relation between afferent response properties and peripheral innervation patterns in the semicircular canals. *Journal of Neurophysiology*, **60**, 182–203.

Baker, M. D. and Bostock, H. (1997). Low-threshold, persistent sodium current in rat large dorsal root ganglion neurons in culture. *Journal of Neurophysiology*, **77**, 1503–13.

Bao, H., Wong, W. H., Goldberg, J. M., and Eatock, R. A. (2003). Voltage-gated calcium channel currents in type I and type II hair cells isolated from the rat crista. *Journal of Neurophysiology*, **90**, 155–64.

Beutner, D. and Moser, T. (2001). The presynaptic function of mouse cochlear inner hair cells during development of hearing. *Journal of Neuroscience*, **21**, 4593–9.

Beutner, D., Voets, T., Neher, E., and Moser, T. (2001). Calcium dependence of exocytosis and endocytosis at the cochlear inner hair cell afferent synapse. *Neuron*, **29**, 681–90.

Blum, R., Kafitz, K. W., and Konnerth, A. (2002). Neurotrophin-evoked depolarization requires the sodium channel Na$_V$1.9. *Nature*, **419**, 687–93.

Brown, A. M., Lee, K. S., and Powell, T. (1981). Sodium current in single rat heart muscle cells. *Journal of Physiology*, **318**, 479–500.

Chabbert, C., Mechaly, I., Sieso, V., *et al.* (2003). Voltage-gated Na$^+$ channel activation induces both action potentials in utricular hair cells and brain-derived neurotrophic factor release in the rat utricle during a restricted period of development. *Journal of Physiology*, **553**, 113–23.

Chamow, S. M., Peers, D. H., Byrn, R. A., *et al.* (1990). Enzymatic cleavage of a CD4 immunoadhesin generates crystallizable, biologically active Fd-like fragments. *Biochemistry*, **29**, 9885–91.

Chen J. W. Y. and Eatock, R. A. (2000). Major potassium conductance in type I hair cells from rat semicircular canals: characterization and modulation by nitric oxide. *Journal of Neurophysiology*, **84**, 139–51.

Chen, N. and Lucero, M. T. (1999). Transient and persistent tetrodotoxin-sensitive sodium currents in squid olfactory receptor neurons. *Journal of Comparative Physiology A: Neuroethology, Sensory, Neural, and Behavioral Physiology*, **184**, 63–72.

Chen, Y. H., Dale, T. J., Romanos, M. A., *et al.* (2000). Cloning, distribution and functional analysis of the type III sodium channel from human brain. *European Journal of Neuroscience*, **12**, 4281–9.

Choi, E. J., Hong, M. P., Kyoo, S. Y., *et al.* (2003). ATP modulation of sodium currents in rat dorsal root ganglion neurons. *Brain Research*, **968**, 15–25.

Cota, G. and Armstrong, C. M. (1989). Sodium channel gating in clonal pituitary cells. The inactivation step is not voltage dependent. *Journal of General Physiology*, **94**, 213–32.

Cummins, T. R., Aglieco, F., Renganathan, M., *et al.* (2001). $Na_V1.3$ sodium channels: rapid repriming and slow closed-state inactivation display quantitative differences after expression in a mammalian cell line and in spinal sensory neurons. *Journal of Neuroscience*, **21**, 5952–61.

Cummins, T. R., Dib-Hajj, S. D., Black, J. A., *et al.* (1999). A novel persistent tetrodotoxin-resistant sodium current in SNS-null and wild-type small primary sensory neurons. *Journal of Neuroscience*, **19**, RC43.

Cummins, T. R., Howe, J. R., and Waxman, S. G. (1998). Slow closed-state inactivation: a novel mechanism underlying ramp currents in cells expressing the hNE/PN1 sodium channel. *Journal of Neuroscience*, **18**, 9607–19.

Dallos, P. (1985). Membrane potential and response changes in mammalian cochlear hair cells during intracellular recording. *Journal of Neuroscience*, **5**, 1609–15.

Dallos, P., Santos-Sacchi, J., and Flock, A. (1982). Intracellular recordings from cochlear outer hair cells. *Science*, **218**, 582–4.

Desai, S. S., Ali, H., and Lysakowski, A. (2005a). Comparative morphology of rodent vestibular periphery. II. Cristae ampullares. *Journal of Neurophysiology*, **93**, 267–80.

Desai, S. S. and Lysakowski, A. (2005b). Comparative morphology of rodent vestibular periphery. I. Saccular and utricular maculae. *Journal of Neurophysiology*, **93**, 251–66.

Desmadryl, G. and Sans, A. (1990). Afferent innervation patterns in crista ampullaris of the mouse during ontogenesis. *Brain Research., Developmental Brain Research*, **52**, 183–9.

Dib-Hajj, S. D., Tyrrell, L., Black, J. A., and Waxman, S. G. (1998). NaN, a novel voltage-gated Na channel, is expressed preferentially in peripheral sensory neurons and down-regulated after axotomy. *Proceedings of the National Academy of Sciences USA*, **95**, 8963–8.

Dietrich, P. S., McGivern, J. G., Delgado, S. G., *et al.* (1998). Functional analysis of a voltage-gated sodium channel and its splice variant from rat dorsal root ganglia. *Journal of Neurochemistry*, **70**, 2262–72.

DiFrancesco, D., Ferroni, A., Visentin, S., and Zaza, A. (1985). Cadmium-induced blockade of the cardiac fast Na channels in calf Purkinje fibres. *Proceedings of the Royal Society of London B: Biological Sciences*, **223**, 475–84.

Don, D. M., Newman, A. N., Micevych, P. E., and Popper, P. (1997). Expression of brain-derived neurotrophic factor and its receptor mRNA in the vestibuloauditory system of the bullfrog. *Hearing Research*, **114**, 10–20.

Eatock, R. A. and Hurley, K. M. (2003). Functional development of hair cells. In. R. Romand and I. Varela-Nieto, eds., *Development of the Auditory and Vestibular Systems 3: Molecular Development of the Inner Ear*. San Diego: Academic Press, pp. 389–448.

El Sherif, Y., Wieraszko, A., Banerjee, P., and Penington, N. J. (2001). ATP modulates Na$^+$ channel gating and induces a non-selective cation current in a neuronal hippocampal cell line. *Brain Research*, **904**, 307–17.

Engel, J., Michna, M., Platzer, J., and Striessnig, J. (2002). Calcium channels in mouse hair cells: function, properties and pharmacology. *Advances in Otorhinolaryngology*, **59**, 35–41.

Ernfors, P., Lee, K. F., and Jaenisch, R. (1994). Mice lacking brain-derived neurotrophic factor develop with sensory deficits. *Nature*, **368**, 147–50.

Escayg, A., MacDonald, B. T., Meisler, M. H., *et al.* (2000). Mutations of SCN1 A, encoding a neuronal sodium channel, in two families with GEFS + 2. *Nature Genetics*, **24**, 343–5.

Evans, M. G. and Fuchs, P. A. (1987). Tetrodotoxin-sensitive, voltage-dependent sodium currents in hair cells for the alligator cochlea. *Biophysical Journal*, **52**, 649–52.

Fahmi, A. I., Patel, M., Stevens, E. B., *et al.* (2001). The sodium channel β-subunit SCN3b modulates the kinetics of SCN5a and is expressed heterogeneously in sheep heart. *Journal of Physiology*, **537**, 693–700.

Favre, I., Moczydlowski, E., and Schild, L. (1995). Specificity for block by saxitoxin and divalent cations at a residue which determines sensitivity of sodium channel subtypes to guanidinium toxins. *Journal of General Physiology*, **106**, 203–29.

Fettiplace, R. and Fuchs, P. A. (1999). Mechanisms of hair cell tuning. *Annual Review of Physiology*, **61**, 809–34.

Frelin, C., Cognard, C., Vigne, P., and Lazdunski, M. (1986). Tetrodotoxin-sensitive and tetrodotoxin-resistant Na$^+$ channels differ in their sensitivity to Cd^{2+} and Zn^{2+}. *European Journal of Pharmacology*, **122**, 245–50.

Géléoc, G. S. G., Risner, J. R., and Holt, J. R. (2004). Developmental acquisition of voltage-dependent conductances and sensory signalling in hair cells of the embryonic mouse inner ear. *Journal of Neuroscience*, **24**, 11148–59.

Goldberg, J. M. (1991). The vestibular end organs: morphological and physiological diversity of afferents. *Current Opinion in Neurobiology*, **1**, 229–35.

Goldberg, J. M., Desmadryl, G., Baird, R. A., and Fernández, C. (1990). The vestibular nerve of the chinchilla. V. Relation between afferent discharge properties and peripheral innervation patterns in the utricular macula. *Journal of Neurophysiology*, **63**, 791–804.

Goldin, A. L., Barchi, R. L., Caldwell, J. H., *et al.* (2000). Nomenclature of voltage-gated sodium channels. *Neuron*, **28**, 365–8.

Gonoi, T. and Hille, B. (1987). Gating of Na channels. Inactivation modifiers discriminate among models. *Journal of General Physiology*, **89**, 253–74.

Gu, X. Q., Dib-Hajj, S., Rizzo, M. A., and Waxman, S. G. (1997). TTX-sensitive and – resistant Na$^+$ currents, and mRNA for the TTX-resistant rH1 channel, are expressed in B104 neuroblastoma cells. *Journal of Neurophysiology*, **77**, 236–46.

Hartshorne, R. P. and Catterall, W. A. (1984). The sodium channel from rat brain. Purification and subunit composition. *Journal of Biological Chemistry*, **259**, 1667–75.

Herzog, R. I., Liu, C., Waxman, S. G., and Cummins, T. R. (2003). Calmodulin binds to the C terminus of sodium channels Na$_V$1.4 and Na$_V$1.6 and differentially modulates their functional properties. *Journal of Neuroscience*, **23**, 8261–70.

Hille, B. (2001). *Ion Channels of Excitable Membranes*. Sunderland: Sinauer Associates, Inc.

Hodgkin, A. L. and Huxley, A. F. (1952). The components of membrane conductance in the giant axon of Loligo. *Journal of Physiology*, **116**, 473–96.

Holt, J. R., Corey, D. P., and Eatock, R. A. (1997). Mechanoelectrical transduction and adaptation in hair cells of the mouse utricle, a low-frequency vestibular organ. *Journal of Neuroscience*, **17**, 8739–48.

Holton, T. and Weiss, T. F. (1983). Receptor potentials of lizard cochlear hair cells with free-standing stereocilia in response to tones. *Journal of Physiology*, **345**, 205–40.

Horn, R. and Marty, A. (1988). Muscarinic activation of ionic currents measured by a new whole-cell recording method. *Journal of General Physiology*, **92**, 145–59.

Hudspeth, A. J. and Lewis, R. S. (1988). Kinetic analysis of voltage- and ion-dependent conductances in saccular hair cells of the bull-frog, *Rana catesbeiana*. *Journal of Physiology*, **400**, 237–74.

Hurley, K. M., Gaboyard, S., Zhong, M., *et al.* (2006). M-like K$^+$ currents in type I hair cells and calyx afferent endings of the developing rat utricle. *Journal of Neuroscience*, **26**, 10253–69.

Isom, L. L. (2002). β subunits: players in neuronal hyperexcitability? *Novartis Foundation Symposium*, **241**, 124–38.

Isom, L. L., De Jongh, K. S., Patton, D. E., *et al.* (1992). Primary structure and functional expression of the β1 subunit of the rat brain sodium channel. *Science*, **256**, 839–42.

Krafte, D. S., Volberg, W. A., Dillon, K., and Ezrin, A. M. (1991). Expression of cardiac Na channels with appropriate physiological and pharmacological properties in Xenopus oocytes. *Proceedings of the National Academy of Sciences USA*, **88**, 4071–4.

Kros, C. J., Ruppersberg, J. P., and Rüsch, A. (1998). Expression of a potassium current in inner hair cells during development of hearing in mice. *Nature*, **394**, 281–4.

Kuo, C. C., Lin, T. J., and Hsieh, C. P. (2002). Effect of Na$^+$ flow on Cd^{2+} block of tetrodotoxin-resistant Na$^+$ channels. *Journal of General Physiology*, **120**, 159–72.

Lelli, A., Perin, P., Martini, M., *et al.* (2003). Presynaptic calcium stores modulate afferent release in vestibular hair cells. *Journal of Neuroscience*, **23**, 6894–903.

Lennan, G. W. T., Steinacker, A., and Lehouelleur, J. (1999). Ionic currents and current-clamp depolarisations of type I and type II hair cells from the developing rat utricle. *Pflügers Archiv*, **438**, 40–6.

Leonard, R. B. and Kevetter, G. A. (2002). Molecular probes of the vestibular nerve. I. Peripheral termination patterns of calretinin, calbindin and peripherin containing fibers. *Brain Research*, **928**, 8–17.

Lewis, R. S. and Hudspeth, A. J. (1983). Voltage- and ion-dependent conductances in solitary vertebrate hair cells. *Nature*, **304**, 538–41.

Lindeman, H. H. (1973). Anatomy of the otolith organs. *Advances in Otorhinolaryngology*, **20**, 405–33.

Lossin, C., Rhodes, T. H., Desai, R. R., *et al.* (2003). Epilepsy-associated dysfunction in the voltage-gated neuronal sodium channel SCN1 A. *Journal of Neuroscience*, **23**, 11289–95.

Magistretti, J. and Alonso, A. (1999). Biophysical properties and slow voltage-dependent inactivation of a sustained sodium current in entorhinal cortex layer-II principal neurons: a whole-cell and single-channel study. *Journal of General Physiology*, **114**, 491–509.

Maier, S. K. G., Westenbroek, R. E., McCormick, K. A., *et al.* (2004). Distinct subcellular localization of different sodium channel α and β subunits in single ventricular myocytes from mouse heart. *Circulation*, **109**, 1421–7.

Malhotra, J. D., Chen, C., Rivolta, I., *et al.* (2001). Characterization of sodium channel α- and β-subunits in rat and mouse cardiac myocytes. *Circulation*, **103**, 1303–10.

Marcotti, W., Géléoc, G. S. G., Lennan, G. W. T., and Kros, C. J. (1999). Transient expression of an inwardly rectifying potassium conductance in developing inner and outer hair cells along the mouse cochlea. *Pflügers Archiv*, **439**, 113–22.

Marcotti, W., Johnson, S. L., Holley, M. C., and Kros, C. J. (2003a). Developmental changes in the expression of potassium currents of embryonic, neonatal and mature mouse inner hair cells. *Journal of Physiology*, **548**, 383–400.

Marcotti, W., Johnson, S. L., Rüsch, A., and Kros, C. J. (2003b). Sodium and calcium currents shape action potentials in immature mouse inner hair cells. *Journal of Physiology*, **552**, 743–61.

Masetto, S., Bosica, M., Correia, M. J., *et al.* (2003). Na^{+} currents in vestibular type I and type II hair cells of the embryo and adult chicken. *Journal of Neurophysiology*, **90**, 1266–78.

McCormick, K. A., Isom, L. L., Ragsdale, D., *et al.* (1998). Molecular determinants of Na^{+} channel function in the extracellular domain of the β1 subunit. *Journal of Biological Chemistry*, **273**, 3954–62.

Meadows, L. S., Chen, Y. H., Powell, A. J., Clare, J. J., and Ragsdale, D. S. (2002). Functional modulation of human brain Na$_V$1.3 sodium channels, expressed in mammalian cells, by auxiliary β1, β2 and β3 subunits. *Neuroscience*, **114**, 745–53.

Mechaly, I., Scamps, F., Chabbert, C., Sans, A., and Valmier, J. (2005). Molecular diversity of voltage-gated sodium channel alpha subunits expressed in neuronal and non-neuronal excitable cells. *Neuroscience*, **130**, 389–96.

Moran, O., Picollo, A., and Conti, F. (2003). Tonic and phasic guanidinium toxin-block of skeletal muscle Na channels expressed in mammalian cells. *Biophysical Journal*, **84**, 2999–3006.

Napolitano, C., Rivolta, I., and Priori, S. G. (2003). Cardiac sodium channel diseases. *Clinical Chemistry and Laboratory Medicine*, **41**, 439–44.

Noda, M., Ikeda, T., Suzuki, H., *et al.* (1986). Expression of functional sodium channels from cloned cDNA. *Nature*, **322**, 826–8.

Ohmori, I., Ouchida, M., Ohtsuka, Y., Oka, E., and Shimizu, K. (2002). Significant correlation of the SCN1A mutations and severe myoclonic epilepsy in infancy. *Biochemical and Biophysical Research Communications*, **295**, 17–23.

O'Leary, M. E. (1998). Characterization of the isoform-specific differences in the gating of neuronal and muscle sodium channels. *Canadian Journal of Physiology and Pharmacology*, **76**, 1041–50.

Oliver, D., Plinkert, P., Zenner, H. P., and Ruppersberg, J. P. (1997). Sodium current expression during postnatal development of rat outer hair cells. *Pflügers Archiv: European Journal of Physiology*, **434**, 772–8.

Parsons, T. D., Lenzi, D., Almers, W., and Roberts, W. M. (1994). Calcium-triggered exocytosis and endocytosis in an isolated presynaptic cell: capacitance measurements in saccular hair cells. *Neuron*, **13**, 875–83.

Pirvola, U. and Ylikoski, J. (2003). Neurotrophic factors during inner ear development. *Current Topics in Developmental Biology*, **57**, 207–23.

Qu, W., Moorhouse, A. J., Rajendra, S., and Barry, P. H. (2000). Very negative potential for half-inactivation of, and effects of anions on, voltage-dependent sodium currents in acutely isolated rat olfactory receptor neurons. *Journal of Membrane Biology*, **175**, 123–38.

Rabert, D. K., Koch, B. D., Ilnicka, M., *et al.* (1998). A tetrodotoxin-resistant voltage-gated sodium channel from human dorsal root ganglia, hPN3/SCN10A. *Pain*, **78**, 107–14.

Renganathan, M., Dib-Hajj, S., and Waxman, S. G. (2002). $Na_V 1.5$ underlies the 'third TTX-R sodium current' in rat small DRG neurons. *Brain Research. Molecular Brain Research*, **106**, 70–82.

Roberts, R. H. and Barchi, R. L. (1987). The voltage-sensitive sodium channel from rabbit skeletal muscle. Chemical characterization of subunits. *Journal of Biological Chemistry*, **262**, 2298–303.

Roberts, W. M., Jacobs, R. A., and Hudspeth, A. J. (1990). Colocalization of ion channels involved in frequency selectivity and synaptic transmission at presynaptic active zones of hair cells. *Journal of Neuroscience*, **10**, 3664–84.

Roberts, W. M., Jacobs, R. A., and Hudspeth, A. J. (1991). The hair cell as a presynaptic terminal. *Annals of the New York Academy of Sciences*, **635**, 221–33.

Roy, M. L. and Narahashi, T. (1992). Differential properties of tetrodotoxin-sensitive and tetrodotoxin-resistant sodium channels in rat dorsal root ganglion neurons. *Journal of Neuroscience*, **12**, 2104–111.

Rubel, E. W. and Fritzsch, B. (2002). Auditory system development: primary auditory neurons and their targets. *Annual Review of Neuroscience*, **25**, 51–101.

Ruben, R. J. (1967). Development of the inner ear of the mouse: a radioautographic study of terminal mitoses. *Acta Otolaryngologica. Supplementum*, **220**, 1–31.

Rübsamen, R. and Lippe, W. R. (1998). The development of cochlear function. In E. W. Rubel, A. N. Popper, and R. R. Fay, eds., *Development of the Auditory System*. New York: Springer-Verlag, pp. 193–270.

Rugiero, F., Mistry, M., Sage, D., *et al.* (2003). Selective expression of a persistent tetrodotoxin-resistant Na^+ current and $Na_V1.9$ subunit in myenteric sensory neurons. *Journal of Neuroscience*, **23**, 2715–25.

Rüsch, A. and Eatock, R. A. (1996). A delayed rectifier conductance in type I hair cells of the mouse utricle. *Journal of Neurophysiology*, **76**, 995–1004.

Rüsch, A. and Eatock, R. A. (1997). Sodium currents in hair cells of the mouse utricle. In E. R. Lewis, G. R. Long, R. F. Lyon, C. R. Steele, P. M. Narins, and E. Hecht-Poinar, eds., *Diversity in Auditory Mechanics*. Singapore: World Scientific Press, pp. 549–55.

Rüsch, A., Lysakowski, A., and Eatock, R. A. (1998). Postnatal development of type I and type II hair cells in the mouse utricle: acquisition of voltage-gated conductances and differentiated morphology. *Journal of Neuroscience*, **18**, 7487–501.

Russell, I. J. and Kossl, M. (1991). The voltage responses of hair cells in the basal turn of the guinea-pig cochlea. *Journal of Physiology*, **435**, 493–511.

Russell, I. J. and Sellick, P. M. (1983). Low-frequency characteristics of intracellularly recorded receptor potentials in guinea-pig cochlear hair cells. *Journal of Physiology*, **338**, 179–206.

Sangameswaran, L., Delgado, S. G., Fish, L. M., *et al.* (1996). Structure and function of a novel voltage-gated, tetrodotoxin-resistant sodium channel specific to sensory neurons. *Journal of Biological Chemistry*, **271**, 5953–6.

Sangameswaran, L., Fish, L. M., Koch, B. D., *et al.* (1997). A novel tetrodotoxin-sensitive, voltage-gated sodium channel expressed in rat and human dorsal root ganglia. *Journal of Biological Chemistry*, **272**, 14805–9.

Sans, A. and Chat, M. (1982). Analysis of temporal and spatial patterns of rat vestibular hair cell differentiation by tritiated thymidine radioautography. *Journal of Comparative Neurology*, **206**, 1–8.

Satin, J., Kyle, J. W., Chen, M., *et al.* (1992). A mutant of TTX-resistant cardiac sodium channels with TTX-sensitive properties. *Science*, **256**, 1202–5.

Sheets, M. F. and Hanck, D. A. (1992). Mechanisms of extracellular divalent and trivalent cation block of the sodium current in canine cardiac Purkinje cells. *Journal of Physiology*, **454**, 299–320.

Sheets, M. F. and Hanck, D. A. (1999). Gating of skeletal and cardiac muscle sodium channels in mammalian cells. *Journal of Physiology*, **514**, 425–36.

Sivilotti, L., Okuse, K., Akopian, A. N., Moss, S., and Wood, J. N. (1997). A single serine residue confers tetrodotoxin insensitivity on the rat sensory-neuron-specific sodium channel SNS. *FEBS Letters*, **409**, 49–52.

Smith, M. R., Smith, R. D., Plummer, N. W., Meisler, M. H., and Goldin, A. L. (1998). Functional analysis of the mouse Scn8a sodium channel. *Journal of Neuroscience*, **18**, 6093–102.

Smith, R. D. and Goldin, A. L. (1998). Functional analysis of the rat I sodium channel in xenopus oocytes. *Journal of Neuroscience*, **18**, 811–20.

Sobkowicz, H. M., Rose, J. E., Scott, G. E., and Slapnick, S. M. (1982). Ribbon synapses in the developing intact and cultured organ of Corti in the mouse. *Journal of Neuroscience*, **2**, 942–57.

Sobkowicz, H. M., Rose, J. E., Scott, G. L., and Levenick, C. V. (1986). Distribution of synaptic ribbons in the developing organ of Corti. *Journal of Neurocytology*, **15**, 693–714.

Sokolowski, B. H., Stahl, L. M., and Fuchs, P. A. (1993). Morphological and physiological development of vestibular hair cells in the organ-cultured otocyst of the chick. *Developmental Biology*, **155**, 134–46.

Stühmer, W., Methfessel, C., Sakmann, B., Noda, M., and Numa, S. (1987). Patch clamp characterization of sodium channels expressed from rat brain cDNA. *European Biophysics Journal*, **14**, 131–8.

Sugihara, I. and Furukawa, T. (1989). Morphological and functional aspects of two different types of hair cells in the goldfish sacculus. *Journal of Neurophysiology*, **62**(6), 1330–43.

Tyrrell, L., Renganathan, M., Dib-Hajj, S. D., and Waxman, S. G. (2001). Glycosylation alters steady-state inactivation of sodium channel $Na_V1.9/NaN$ in dorsal root ganglion neurons and is developmentally regulated. *Journal of Neuroscience*, **21**, 9629–37.

White, J. A., Alonso, A., and Kay, A. R. (1993). A heart-like Na^+ current in the medial entorhinal cortex. *Neuron*, **11**, 1037–47.

Witt, C. M., Hu, H.-Y., Brownell, W. E., and Bertrand, D. (1994). Physiologically silent sodium channels in mammalian outer hair cells. *Journal of Neurophysiology*, **72**, 1037–40.

Wooltorton, J. R. A., Gaboyard, S., Hurley, K. M., *et al.* (2007). Developmental changes in two voltage-dependent sodium currents in utricular hair cells. *Journal of Neurophysiology*, **97**, 1684–1704.

Yamamoto, Y., Fukuta, H., and Suzuki, H. (1993). Blockade of sodium channels by divalent cations in rat gastric smooth muscle. *Japanese Journal of Physiology*, **43**, 785–96.

Yoshida, S. (1994). Tetrodotoxin-resistant sodium channels. *Cellular and Molecular Neurobiology*, **14**, 227–44.

Yu, F. H., Westenbroek, R. E., Silos-Santiago, I., *et al.* (2003). Sodium channel $\beta4$, a new disulfide-linked auxiliary subunit with similarity to $\beta2$. *Journal of Neuroscience*, **23**, 7577–85.

Zidanic, M. and Fuchs, P. A. (1995). Kinetic analysis of barium currents in chick cochlear hair cells. *Biophysical Journal*, **68**, 1323–36.

Index